Quality in Nuclear Medicine

Andor W.J.M. Glaudemans
Jitze Medema • Annie K. van Zanten
Rudi A.J.O. Dierckx
Editors

C.T.B. (Kees) Ahaus
Guest Editor

Quality in Nuclear Medicine

Springer

Editors
Andor W.J.M. Glaudemans
Department of Nuclear Medicine and Molecular Imaging
University Medical Center Groningen
University of Groningen
Groningen
The Netherlands

Annie K. van Zanten
Department of Nuclear Medicine and Molecular Imaging
University Medical Center Groningen
University of Groningen
Groningen
The Netherlands

Jitze Medema
Department of Nuclear Medicine and Molecular Imaging
University Medical Center Groningen
University of Groningen
Groningen
The Netherlands

Rudi A.J.O. Dierckx
Department of Nuclear Medicine and Molecular Imaging
University Medical Center Groningen
University of Groningen
Groningen
The Netherlands

Guest Editor
C.T.B. (Kees) Ahaus
Dutch Institute for Healthcare Improvement
Utrecht
The Netherlands

ISBN 978-3-319-81537-4 ISBN 978-3-319-33531-5 (eBook)
DOI 10.1007/978-3-319-33531-5

Softcover reprint of the hardcover 1st edition 2016

This Springer imprint is published by Springer Nature
The registered company is Springer International Publishing AG Switzerland

Foreword

Historically, nuclear medicine emerged at the end of the nineteenth century. Henri Becquerel and Marie Curie discovered the mysterious rays of uranium and named them radioactivity. From the middle of the last century, the production and application of pharmaceuticals and diagnostic tests developed seriously. During the last decades, imaging by the new developed camera systems such as the single photon emission computed tomography (SPECT) camera and the positron emission tomography (PET) camera, both in the last years often combined with computed tomography (CT) and/or magnetic resonance imaging (MRI), opened new perspectives in the contribution of nuclear medicine towards health care.

With the introduction of high-tech equipment, robotics and process technology new challenges appeared. Application of radioactivity in research (preclinical, in volunteers and in patients) and in a clinical setting require that safety risks and strict rules have to be taken into account. Nuclear disasters in the past have shown us the health damage of radiation and the long-term effects it can have on people and environment. In contrast to the nuclear industry, health-care organizations are not used to applying prospective risk assessment techniques other than as part of their medical assessments. More specifically, medical doctors and research staff may not always be aware of the risks. They perceive regulations as curtailing their opportunities.

The editors of this book have identified this issue. Therefore, the focus of this book covers more than only the scientific successes. The aim of this book is to provide professionals with an integrated approach to quality and quality management aspects concerning nuclear medicine. Nuclear medicine as a mainstream in research and in clinical diagnostics and treatment of metabolic and organ disorders requires the involvement of an interdisciplinary team of experts. Experts in the field of nuclear medicine, physics, radiation safety, good clinical practice (GCP) and good manufacturing practice (GMP), mechanical engineering, quality control, and ICT are needed. All of those themes are covered in this textbook. The contributions are from professionals with many years of experience in the field of nuclear medicine.

Special acknowledgment concerns Prof. Rudi Dierckx, Head of the Department of Nuclear Medicine and Molecular Imaging of the University Medical Center Groningen, as the initiator of this textbook. No one better than Prof. Dierckx knows that, to achieve excellent quality as well as an excellent institute in nuclear medicine, a long and thrilling journey must be taken. Therefore, one could see the chapters in this book as the keystone to this success.

Groningen, The Netherlands
April 2016

Alexander van der Star

Preface

The Department of Nuclear Medicine and the PET center at the University Hospital Groningen obtained their first ISO-9001 certification in the year 2000, actually also a first for the hospital. Using the European Foundation for Quality Management (EFQM) model, in 2015, the newly established department of Nuclear Medicine and Molecular Imaging switched its focus from management domains towards results for different stakeholders. In 2011, the department obtained the Institute for Dutch Quality price 3 stars (INK, Instituut voor Nederlandse Kwaliteit). The formal trajectory towards excellence ended in 2015 with the EFQM recognition 4 stars being awarded. Similar to Japanese arrow shooting the movement, that is, the road towards excellence, was more important than the target. This multi-author textbook wants to share this enthusiasm and expertise from the Groningen network.

Nuclear medicine is a specialty characterized by the use of open sources of radioactivity for diagnosis and therapy. Hence, quality assurance in such an environment may not be considered a luxury. Moreover, from the beginning of the specialty production of radiopharmaceuticals on site and sensitivity of crystal detectors to fluctuations also prompted the need for structured quality controls. In nuclear medicine in Europe, it was Utrecht in the Netherlands under the guidance of Prof. Peter van Rijk being the first to recognize the importance of an umbrella for quality assurance encompassing all processes and to obtain ISO-certification in 1998. Other centers in Belgium such as Gent and later on Leuven, and Groningen in the Netherlands thus in 2000 quickly followed building on this expertise.

Meanwhile the domain changed rapidly, for example, with the breakthrough of informatics, hybrid imaging, and molecular medicine. In the Netherlands and Belgium, the weight of the juridical framework became primarily European, with, the European medical device directory, Euratom directives or, for example, European legislation on good manufacturing practice (GMP), on good clinical practice (GCP), on privacy of patient data, etc. A trend towards harmonization globally further builds upon this layer, as may be seen, for example, in research guidelines (International Commission on Harmonization) or through the efforts of international organizations such as the International Atomic Energy Agency (IAEA).

Also stakeholders in health care have become more demanding and more explicit in their expectations. In the Netherlands or Belgium, now certification or accreditation of the whole hospital is required, no longer as a differentiator, but now as a qualifier only, for example, in order to obtain contracts form health insurance companies. ISO (health) certification, Joint Commission International (JCI), and NIAZ-Qmentum, just to name the top three in the Low Countries, are labels requiring involvement, not only from all clinical departments, but also from all facilitating departments. In a university hospital or university medical center, research, training, and teaching may be included within the scope of quality assurance. In these settings, nuclear medicine may be evaluated no longer only as a department, but rather, for example, in the chain of a care trajectory through "tracing audits" or in the setting of an audit of multidisciplinary investigator-driven research.

Finally, quality may have many faces, but it is clear their number increased and furthermore diversified in a growing demand for clinical governance. Keywords may include transparency, ownership, responsibility, documentation, involvement of stakeholders, cost control, efficiency, and efficacy. Quality instruments nowadays encompass, for example, lean six sigma, Deming circle (PDCA, Plan Do Check Act), prospective risk inventarisation, Prisma analysis, safe incident reporting, evidence base medicine, and clinical guidelines or recommendations, but also retrospective analysis of clinical files of deceased patients, supply chain management, or hostmanship. Personalized medicine not only implies precision medicine, but also, for example, experience-based co-design, attention for the level of understanding of different groups of customers, or medical decision support. Balance scorecards, quality parameters, and other key performance indicators are instruments to keep hold on the growing information on quality, as in the end all is quality related.

Can we deliver quality without the aforementioned tools? Yes, we can. But similar to the aviation industry we have learned that when lives are at stake, safety needs to be assured. Moreover, stakeholders expect more in return for the given societal and individual responsibility and investments. On the other hand, it should be clear that the tools are not the goal, but only the means on the quest for quality and excellence.

This multi-author textbook was written by experts in the field to provide a global view and hopefully at the same time a practical view on quality in nuclear medicine. Moreover, it hopes to provide not only tools, but also an understanding and foster enthusiasm to do better. Ours is a beautiful specialty, but it is in permanent transition as is the outer world. We hope this book would be of help to some in the field at this point in time.

Ars longa, vita brevis.

Groningen, The Netherlands
Andor W.J.M. Glaudemans
Jitze Medema
Annie K. van Zanten
Rudi A.J.O. Dierckx
Utrecht, The Netherlands
C.T.B. (Kees) Ahaus

Contents

Part I

Laws, Standards and Guidelines

The Road to Excellence: A Case Study of the Application of GMP, ISO 9001 and the EFQM Excellence Model in a Nuclear Medicine Department

1

Lidia S. van Huizen and C.T.B. (Kees) Ahaus

Abstract

Definitions are introduced to give insight in the field of work of quality management in relation to responsibilities in NMMI. A relational model visualises the relationships when working on the road to quality excellence. The standards such as GMP, GCP, ISO 9001 and EFQM with examples can help put these models to practise. The road of NMMI in the University Hospital in Groningen presented in boxes gives lessons learned. Additionally the A3 model to prioritise issues on the road to quality excellence is explained.

1.1 Introduction to Quality and Excellence

University hospitals are organisations in which knowledge and innovation regarding cure and care come together in an academic setting. Medical–technical development and high-tech equipment are used in complex multidisciplinary care pathways in centres in which diverse healthcare professionals work together.

This entails responsibility for the ethics, sustainability, reliability and validity of diagnoses and patient treatment, in research and in educating the next generation of healthcare professionals. The field of nuclear medicine assumed this responsibility

L.S. van Huizen (✉)
Senior Consultant Quality and Patient Safety, Department UMC-staff Quality, University of Groningen, University Medical Center Groningen, Groningen, The Netherlands

Kerteza, Worldwide Consultancy and Training Institute for Health Care Organizations, Kasterlee, Belgium
e-mail: l.s.van.huizen@umcg.nl

C.T.B. (Kees) Ahaus
Organisational Unit, Faculty of Economics and Business, Centre of Expertise Healthwise, Groningen, The Netherlands

A.W.J.M. Glaudemans et al. (eds.), *Quality in Nuclear Medicine*,
DOI 10.1007/978-3-319-33531-5_1

and designed a quality management system (QMS) to ensure the sustainability of its (diagnostic) procedures. European and national societies developed guidelines for most of the diagnostic procedures to guarantee reliable and valid diagnoses. For the most part, this began with establishing procedures related to the risks of using equipment, the safe production of radiopharmaceuticals and the careful evaluation of the imaging process, thereby resulting in a QMS and periodic audits to assess their compliance with the standards. In applying the QMS, the field of nuclear medicine evolved towards excellence in patient care, research and education.

How this evolution unfolded from quality to excellence in quality is explained in this chapter, which includes examples of how this evolution worked for the Department of Nuclear Medicine and Molecular Imaging at the University Medical Centre Groningen (hereafter referred to as NMMI).

1.2 Quality Definitions and Standards in Quality Management

First, it is important to define what is meant by quality in health care and, particularly, in the field of nuclear medicine. Subsequently, the quality improvement cycle and the road to excellence, which is achieved by applying standards and models, will be discussed. It is relevant to describe in a systemic way the roles and responsibilities of professionals and quality staff or supportive staff in health care. Donabedian (Donabedian 1993) argued that we need to agree on (a) the meaning of quality in health care, (b) the relevant actors or players and (c) the configuration of the stage or playing field (Donabedian 1993).

1.2.1 Quality Definitions

In quality management and certification, the ISO 9000 family of standards is widely used as a reference for QMSs. The terms and definitions related to quality and quality management are listed in ISO 9000, whilst ISO 9001 comprises the requirements of the QMS. For health care, a translation of specific terms is undertaken, and these are then added to facilitate their implementation in healthcare organisations (NEN-EN-15224, Health care services – quality management systems 2012a).

The quality of a product or service is not easily defined as various definitions can be found in the literature. Reeves and Bednar (Reeves and Bednar 1994) typify the different definitions of quality. The rather internally or manufacturing-focused definition of ISO emphasises the specified or expected characteristics of a product or service. Other definitions are more externally focused and marketing-based ("Quality is meeting and/or exceeding customers' expectations" (Reeves and Bednar 1994)) or can be considered value-based ("Quality is related to both the actual use and the price of the product" (Reeves and Bednar 1994)). Quality can even be seen as "the highest form", as we can all recognise excellent quality when we see it.

1.2.1.1 Quality

Quality refers to the degree to which a set of inherent characteristics fulfils requirements (ISO 9000) (ISO 9000:2005).

The term "quality" can be used with adjectives such as poor, good or excellent, which makes it a relative and not an absolute concept. In the second definition, "inherent" can be seen as opposed to "assigned", which means that quality exists in something, especially as a permanent characteristic.

These definitions do not consider the different perspectives of stakeholders in the field in which an organisation is working. Within the nuclear medicine field, stakeholders—for example, the patient, the referring healthcare professional, the organisation or the government—may have expectations of different qualities.

1.2.1.2 Quality in Health Care

In our work, we use quality defined as the "degree to which a set of inherent characteristics fulfils requirements" (ISO 9000:2005). To make quality in health care measurable and controllable, the quality characteristics of clinical processes must be identified and described. In the healthcare-specific NEN-EN 15224 (ISO 9001 for Healthcare) standard, the patients' or customers' requirements for healthcare services must be specified according to effectiveness, safety, availability, timeliness/accessibility, continuity of care, respect for patient values and preferences, and appropriateness, aspects of efficiency, fair distribution and evidence must be considered.(NEN-EN-15224, Health care services – quality management systems 2012a) These requirements or expectations are similar to the six aims for improvement mentioned by the Institute of Medicine in its well-known report titled "Crossing the Quality Chasm: Safe, Effective, Efficient, Personalized, Timely and Equitable" (Institute of Medicine 2001).

A precondition for delivering a high quality of products and services is the quality of an organisation. All activities that aim to strengthen the quality of the organisation can be considered quality management.

1.2.1.3 Quality Management

This refers to the coordinated activities that aim to direct and control an organisation with regard to quality (ISO 9000:2005).

The direction and control of an organisation with regard to quality generally include the establishment of a quality policy and quality objectives, quality planning, quality control, quality assurance and quality improvement. Based on these quality management activities, the organisation provides a "justified trust" related to the quality that is delivered, and it views the improvement of the organisation's performance as a permanent objective.

In the primary process of a nuclear medicine organisation, different types of standards need to be fulfilled on the production floor. By implementing a QMS, the learning or self-cleansing ability of the organisation becomes important. Subsequently, standards of excellence take this a step further. The relationships between quality control, quality assurance and total quality management are visualised in Fig. 1.1. In the primary process, quality control provides trust; in the QMS,

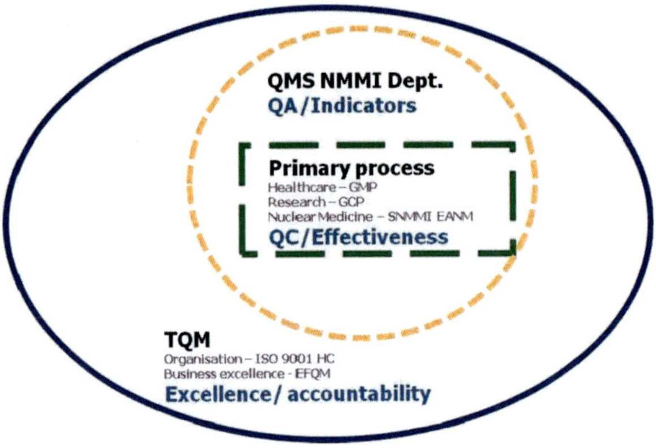

Fig. 1.1 Visualisation of the relationships between different standards and quality focus at different levels (*QMS* quality management system, *NMMI Dept.* Department of Nuclear Medicine and Molecular Imaging, *QA* quality assurance, *GMP* good manufacturing practice, *GCP* good clinical practice, *SNMMI* Society of Nuclear Medicine and Molecular Imaging, *EANM* European Association of Nuclear Medicine, *QC* quality control, *HC* health care, *EFQM* European Foundation of Quality Management)

quality assurance and quality improvement using performance indicators are embedded; and in total quality management, the expectations of all stakeholders are important. At each level, a focus on quality improvement brings the organisation to the level of excellence. This requires leadership and a strategy of striving for excellence.

In Fig. 1.1, we depict the relationships between different standards regarding quality control, assurance, improvement and excellence. The inner rectangle represents the primary process with the quality control checks and guidelines which are specific to the field of work. The middle circle is about the quality assurance of the primary and supporting processes and about quality improvement based on the Deming cycle: plan–do–check–act. Finally, in the outer circle, the business is led by total quality management with clear accountability and a focus on excellence.

1.2.2 Standards and Models

The Department of NMMI at UMCG produces its radiopharmaceuticals in close collaboration with, and under the supervision of, the hospital pharmacy, and it has not only a good manufacturing practice (GMP) licence but also ISO 9001 certification and an INK/EFQM recognition. In this section, we discuss different standards which can be used in quality control and (total) quality management: GMP, GCP, ISO 9001 (for health care) and the EFQM excellence model.

Radiopharmaceutical production can be executed according to GMP in relation to the European Pharmacopoeia. NMMI works collaboratively with the Society of

Nuclear Medicine and Molecular Imaging (SNMMI) and the European Association of Nuclear Medicine (EANM). NMMI advocates the use of standardised procedures for diagnoses and patient treatment in order to create a sustainable QMS. For the protection of the patients, personnel and environment, NMMI adheres to the Radiation Protection Act. For basic research and development of new radiopharmaceuticals and nuclear medicine procedures, compliance with good clinical practice (GCP)/the Helsinki Rules, which govern research on humans and legislation related to research on animals, is mandatory.

1.2.2.1 Good Manufacturing Practice (GMP) (De Vos et al. 2005)

Radiopharmaceuticals must be manufactured in accordance with GMP guidelines; strict adherence to these guidelines is mandatory and is monitored by agencies that control authorisation and licencing for the manufacture and sale of pharmaceutical products, for example. These guidelines provide minimum requirements that a pharmaceutical product manufacturer must meet to ensure that the products are of a high quality and do not pose any risk to the consumer or public. Table 1.1 provides examples of the GMP criteria in a nuclear medicine field.

Table 1.1 GMP criteria and examples for applying these in a nuclear medicine field

GMP	Examples
Environmental requirement	Production is in clean areas with required air characteristics
Personnel	Personnel are trained in disciplines relevant to the manufacturing of sterile and radioactive products
	High standards of personal hygiene are applied
	Authorities and responsibilities are clearly defined (e.g. the release of a batch)
	Safety rules of radiation control are respected
Premises and equipment	The design of laboratories fulfils all requirements regarding radiation protection, cleanliness and sterility
	Cross-contamination of radioactive air with nonradioactive air is prevented
	Critical equipment is listed, calibrated, tested and maintained
Production	Standard operating procedures (SOPs) are available, reviewed and kept up to date
	Quality control and (double) checks are applied in addition to release procedures
	The dispensation, packaging and transportation of radiopharmaceuticals comply with national and international regulations
Labelling	Products are identified by permanently attached labels
Production and distribution records	Records of production batches provide a complete account of the manufacturing history
Quality assurance and quality control	Quality control requires detailed instructions for testing and analysis
	Quality assurance includes the review of the production process

1.2.2.2 Good Clinical Practice (GCP)

GCP follows the International Conference on Harmonisation (ICH) of GCP guidelines. GCP is an international quality standard that is provided by the ICH, which is an international body that defines the standards which governments can transpose into regulations for clinical trials involving human subjects. GCP enforces stringent guidelines on ethical aspects of a clinical study. High standards are required in terms of comprehensive documentation for clinical protocol, record keeping, training and equipment, including computers and software. Quality assurance and inspections ensure that these standards are achieved. GCP aims to ensure that the studies are scientifically authentic and that the clinical properties of the investigational product are properly documented. GCP also provides researchers and their study teams with the tools to protect human subjects and collect quality data.

As can be concluded from Table 1.2, GCP guidelines focus on the clear responsibilities of those who are involved in clinical research.

Table 1.2 GCP criteria and examples for applying these in a nuclear medicine field

GCP	Examples
Institutional review board/ethics committee	The responsibilities of the ethics committee are to
	Safeguard the rights, safety and well-being of trial subjects
	Review the qualifications of the investigator
	Review ongoing trials related to risk
Investigator	The investigator is responsible for
	Communication with the ethics committee regarding protocol, amendments and trial review
	Informed consent of trial subjects
	Records and reports, including safety and premature terminations or suspension of the trial
	Adequate resources for research
	Written procedures for generating data and keeping records
Sponsor	The sponsor is responsible for
	Access to records and safety information
	Adverse drug reaction reporting
	Monitoring and (internal) audit
	Having qualified individuals to make the trial design
	Investigator selection based on appropriate qualifications, knowledge and experience
Clinical trial protocol	The protocol contains general and background information, trial objectives and purpose, trial design, selection and withdrawal of subjects, treatment of subjects, assessment of efficacy and safety, use of statistics, direct access to source data and documents, QC and QA, ethics, data handling and record keeping, financing and insurance, as well as publication policy
	The protocol shall include compliance issues with legislations, e.g. reliable patient dosimetry according to the 2013/59 EURATOM Directive
Essential documents	Documents: trial protocol, informed consent, procedures, information, contracts or agreements, etc.
	Records are retained for at least 3 years after completion of the trial

1.2.2.3 ISO 9000 Family of Quality Management Systems Standards and ISO 9001

The ISO 9001 standards and business excellence models have similar purposes:

- To provide a model for the internal and external evaluation of the QMS
- To enable an organisation to identify its strengths and weaknesses and, thus, provide a basis for continuous improvement
- To obtain external recognition

The ISO 9000 family of QMS standards is designed to help organisations to ensure that they meet the needs of customers and other stakeholders by meeting the requirements related to a product or service. ISO 9001 provides the requirements for the QMS of organisations that wish to meet the standard.

ISO 9000 is based on eight quality management principles, all of which are fundamental to good business practices: customer focus, leadership, involvement of people, process approach, system approach to management, continual improvement, fact-based decision-making and mutually beneficial supplier relationships.

In 2012, a specific ISO 9001 for Healthcare Services (NEN-EN 15224) was released to translate the general terms of QMSs to the field of healthcare services, especially to the hospital environment. The ISO 9001 for Healthcare Services promotes a focus on the patient by emphasising patient centredness. Everything starts with the patient and the professional perspective, and real quality stems from the contact between the healthcare professional and the patient. In addition, this standard promotes the implementation of a risk-based approach to patient safety, which should be embedded in the QMS.

The 11 criteria of quality (appropriate, correct care; availability; continuity of care; effectiveness; efficiency; equity; evidence-/knowledge-based care; patient-centred care, including physical and psychological integrity; patient involvement; patient safety; and timeliness/accessibility) are suggested for use as tools for the organisation to describe the measurable quality characteristics of products and services delivered by the three primary processes of care, education and research, as Donabedian has suggested.(Donabedian 2005) By using the indicators associated with these quality characteristics and (clinical) risks, the QMS enables measurable improvement (Table 1.3).

1.2.2.4 EFQM Excellence Model

In 1988, 14 presidents of European multinationals took the initiative to launch a business excellence model: the European Foundation for Quality Management (EFQM) excellence model. National equivalents, such as the Dutch INK management model, are derived from the EFQM model. The EFQM model (see Fig. 1.2) shows that business results, customer results, people results and society results depend on actions taken in the five enabler areas: processes, products and services, partnerships and resources, people, and strategy and leadership.

Note that the results are framed more broadly than financial results, such as return on investment, profitability and sustainable financial growth. Excellent

Table 1.3 ISO criteria and examples for applying these in a nuclear medicine field

ISO criteria	Examples
The management and the QMS ("Act")	ThQMS is documented in a quality manual
	A quality policy with quality objectives is available
	Responsibilities, authorities and tasks are clearly defined
	(Top) Management reviews the QMS on a regular basis
The resources and the QMS ("Plan")	It is clear what resources (including infrastructure, work environment and personnel with the required competences) are needed to implement the QMS, to deliver quality products and services and to enhance customer satisfaction
The realisation of products and services ("Do")	Processes are planned, and risk assessments of clinical processes are worked out
	Requirements that apply to products/services are clear and are communicated with the customer
	The design of products and services meets the defined requirements
	Purchased, outsourced or subcontracted products are controlled, and suppliers are monitored
	Production and service provision are carried out under controlled conditions
	Measuring equipment is suitable and provides accurate data.
The measurement, analysis and improvement of quality ("Check")	Customer satisfaction is monitored
	An internal audit programme is implemented
	An approach to prevent or correct nonconformity (e.g. complaints) is applied

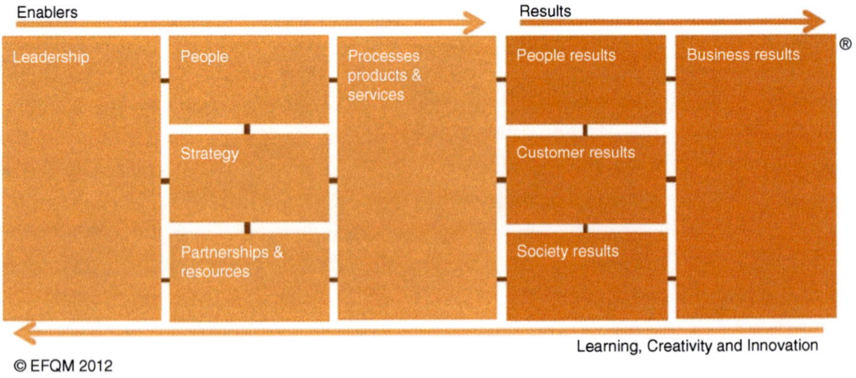

Fig. 1.2 EFQM excellence model. Actions in enabler areas lead to results and reviewing the results leads to learning, creativity and innovation

organisations have good customer results (e.g. value-added products and service excellence), people results (e.g. opportunities to grow, work–life balance and pride) and society results (e.g. brand reputation, ethical behaviour and transparent communication with the society). Hence, excellent organisations perform exceptionally well from a multistakeholder perspective. Furthermore, the model advocates a long-term focus and condemns a short-term focus on only bottom-line financial results.

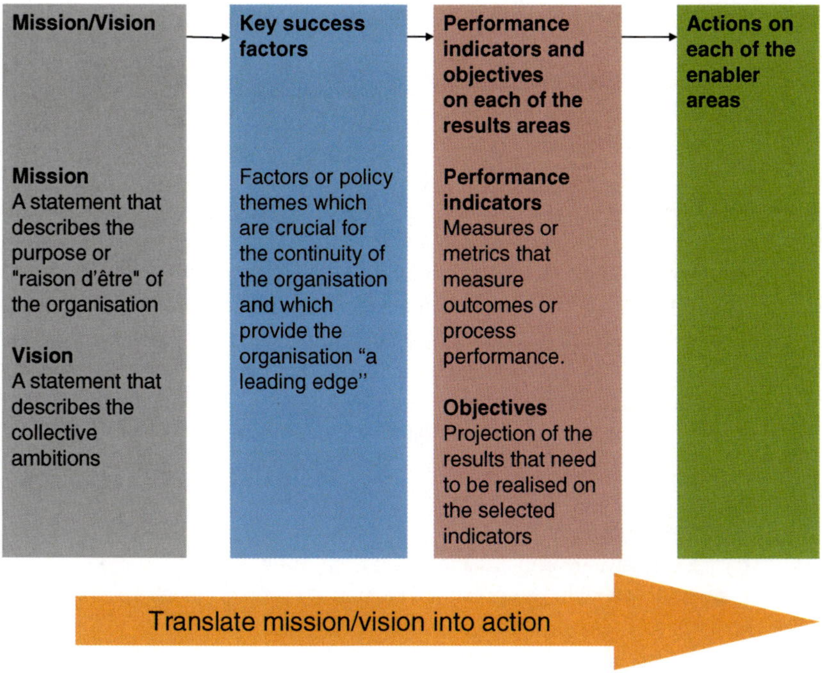

Fig. 1.3 Key concepts in performance management

There are two fundamentally different approaches to applying the EFQM excellence model. First, the model can be used for *continuous improvement*; this starts with elaborating on an analysis of improvement issues and actions in the enabler areas that have an impact on the results areas of the model and may end in writing a self-assessment application of 30–50 pages to apply for and be awarded with a three-, four- or five-star EFQM recognition. On average, two Dutch organisations per year are awarded with such a recognition (three, four or five stars). This implies that organisations that receive the recognition can be considered excellent organisations. In 2011, NMMI received a three-star recognition and is currently preparing a self-assessment document to apply for a four-star EFQM recognition. In the following section, we will reveal an outline of the EFQM criteria and provide examples of the evidence that NMMI applies these criteria.

Second, the model can be used for *management control* by applying the A3 approach (Doeleman et al. 2014). The A3 approach can be applied by drawing up an annual plan for the organisation on one A3-sized page. In such an annual plan, the mission, vision and key success factors are depicted. In addition, the organisation elaborates on the performance indicators of each of the results areas and on the actions in each enabler area that may impact the results. In Fig. 1.3, the meaning of and relationship between the key concepts in management control and performance management are depicted (Ahaus and Diepman 1998). In the following section, we will provide an example of the NMMI A3 annual plan, which illustrates examples of the mission, vision, key success factors, performance indicators and actions.

1.3 Quality Management at NMMI in UMCG

1.3.1 The Evolving Role of the Quality Management System

A QMS helps management to control the quality performance of the organisation. The system approach is simple: Say what you do, do what you say, show that you do what you say, and improve on it. This quality management philosophy is widely used—for example, the Deming quality improvement circle (plan–do–check–act).

The purpose of setting up and implementing a QMS can be to improve products or services; strengthen leadership, competences and working conditions of staff; harmonise management systems; reduce costs due to poor quality; and reduce the risk of adverse events (NEN-EN 15224, Health care services – quality management systems 2012b). When the quality improvement cycle is followed, the sustainability of what has been improved needs to be ensured within the organisation. An important precondition is the quality awareness of the healthcare worker, which is expressed by showing ownership and taking initiative and responsibility. The organisation should support this by defining standards and procedures to guide and support the working teams of the primary process and by implementing clear reporting relations.

In this section, we will show examples of the implementation of the QMS at NMMI. First, we will discuss what ISO 9001 (and its healthcare version) has brought. In addition, using examples, we will show how the EFQM excellence model is applied.

1.3.2 What Has ISO 9001 Brought?

ISO 9001 certification for quality management is a voluntary assessment that is regulated internationally and nationally. As discussed earlier, the ISO criteria focus specifically on the management cycle for quality improvement (plan, measure, analyse and report data).

Whilst the benefits of ISO 9001 are numerous, they can be categorised into one of three areas, which are also known as the 3 "C's" of ISO 9001: consistent service, customer satisfaction and continuous improvement (Metzcar). In the box below, we will discuss NMMI's journey in implementing ISO 9001. The box includes best practices and some lessons learned.

NMMI and ISO 9001

In 1997, NMMI in UMCG launched a project to implement a QMS to describe the processes of four service centres—the clinical laboratories, the hospital pharmacy, the Positron Emission Tomography (PET) Centre and the Department of Nuclear Medicine—and to accomplish the quality aims and sustain a method of working which meets the risks assessed. The search for a standard for QMSs and for implementation strategies offered several options: Dutch variants, such as the INK management model (the Dutch equivalent of the EFQM excellence model), the standards of the Netherlands Institute for

Accreditation in Health Care (NIAZ standards) and an international standard—the ISO 9001.

NMMI chose ISO 9001, and in 2000, NMMI was ISO 9001 certified. Quality improvement was accomplished based on data measured by key performance indicators. This required resources which were devoted to improvement, openness and collaboration. NMMI succeeded in engaging the professionals and motivating commitment to high standards of quality and continuous quality improvement.

In addition to patient care, scientific research and the education of healthcare professionals are also incorporated into the QMS. Explicitly, the "risks" associated with patient care and information security as aspects of the QMS are taken into account.

Best Practices of NMMI

- Quality policy with clear and measurable quality objectives related to key indicators
- Primary process of NMMI, which is "in control" by applying a set of indicators and conducting a regular management review
- A quality manual with protocols and SOPs
- List of risks with priority and the control of critical safety issues
- Patient centeredness within all primary processes, measured by patient satisfaction surveys
- Internal audits on the process of patient care

Lessons Learned

1. Before the start of the project, the QMS for the primary process was a book with instructions of which each person had his or her own interpretation. "SOPs" were implemented after the evaluation of the different interpretations. Now, the processes in the QMS handbook to direct the organisation and control the detailed primary processes fit perfectly. At first, the acceptance of the processes amongst the nuclear professionals was difficult, but their motivation improved when the effect was seen in process performance. A prospective risk assessment helped to include patient safety priorities in the improvement plans.
2. The combination of the different standards after harmonisation in the workplace helped the department to grow, developing a culture that focused on quality improvement.
3. Audits on chains of (care) pathways helped with getting the organisation to focus on patients and referring physicians.
4. Communication and collaboration with third parties regarding quality assurance/quality control was stimulating but also time-consuming.
5. The head of NMMI was a role model in this process of organisation development. However, including quality on the agenda of the board of directors was challenging in the beginning. This is a success factor, as the literature shows that it is positively associated with the effects of the certification and accreditation of the organisation's QMS (Shaw et al. 2014).

1.3.3 How EFQM Brought NMMI Further Along the Road to Excellence

The implementation of the ISO 9001 criteria has assisted NMMI to move to the next stage by helping it to improve and demonstrate its capabilities in a widely accepted framework. The embedding of the ISO 9001 framework in the NMMI QMS has assisted in its efforts to improve the organisation's effectiveness and efficiency. The next stage was applying a business excellence model such as the EFQM excellence model (or the Dutch equivalent, the INK management model).

In Sect. 1.2.2, the enabler and results areas of the EFQM excellence model were introduced. Moreover, we highlighted two different applications of the EFQM excellence model:

- By helping to improve organisational practices, capabilities and results, based on a self-assessment on the EFQM criteria
- By serving as a working tool for understanding and managing performance and for guiding annual planning—for instance, with the A3 approach.

As the quality management of an organisation matures, even if it is on the level of "sustainable success" and "excellent" performance, it remains important for the organisation to continue seeking ever-increasing effectiveness and efficiency gains.

First, we will discuss NMMI's journey with regard to applying the EFQM excellence model. Then, we will set out the EFQM criteria in a table and provide examples of the evidence NMMI reported in its 2015 self-assessment application. Finally, we will provide an example of NMMI's A3 annual plan.

NMMI and Business Excellence, Quality Improvement and EFQM

The business excellence models contain criteria that enable the comparative evaluation of organisational performance, and these are applicable to all activities and all interested parties ("stakeholders") of an organisation. Assessment criteria in business excellence models provide a basis for an organisation to compare its performance with that of other organisations. The combined use of the ISO 9001 standards and a business excellence model such as EFQM will give organisations the opportunity to broaden the application of the QMS as the scope of application of EFQM includes not only patients but also staff (including PhD students), referring physicians, hospital pharmacy, society and the board of directors.

The NMMI started a project to apply EFQM to improve its service level to the medical departments, to ensure that its reports were trustworthy and received in a timely manner and to ensure that its personnel were working in a safe environment and undertaking even more efficient processes.

Best Practices of NMMI

- An analysis of the expectations, needs and wishes of all stakeholders and the measurement of stakeholders' experiences in separate surveys amongst patients, referring physicians, employees, PhD students and the management of trends in stakeholder satisfaction
- The collaboration with other universities, hospitals and strategic partners, such as Siemens, which put NMMI in a leading position in the nuclear medicine field
- The contribution to society by writing books to disseminate scientific output, delivering presentations to congresses and educating students in the medical sciences

Lessons Learned

1. The role of the department manager is very important because he is personally involved in creating a culture of quality excellence.
2. The QMS (including safety management) of NMMI has been certified in all kinds of standards, and NMMI applies these criteria for many years. In addition, NMMI applies a quick yearly scan in the EFQM areas, followed by the application for EFQM recognition in 2011 and in the summer of 2015. By applying quality thinking for many years, it is in the "genes" of the NMMI.
3. The implementation of total quality management requires a vast investment in information technology (a documentation programme), extra equipment, personnel and education. It was important to think about the maintenance of up-to-date documentation, the maintenance of equipment, the measurement of stakeholders' experiences with questionnaires and the education needed to work with instruments such as internal auditing.
4. UMCG started a hospital-wide ISO 9001 initiative whilst NMMI started the application of the EFQM excellence model. There was a symbiosis of NMMI striving for excellence and UMCG as a whole striving for ISO 9001 certification.

In the following table, we list the main EFQM criteria and provide examples of the evidence derived from NMMI's self-assessment report. The EFQM self-assessment report is the source document for the external EFQM audit, which is an assessment that is done by EFQM auditors. It can be assessed whether NMMI can be awarded with a three-, four- or five-star recognition based on the score on a scale of 1–1,000 points. As discussed, NNMI received a three-star recognition in 2011 and is currently (2015) applying for a four-star recognition (Table 1.4).

Table 1.4 EFQM criteria and implemented practices at NMMI in UMCG

EFQM criteria	Examples of implemented practices ("evidence") at NMMI in UMCG
1. Leadership Excellent organisations have leaders who shape the future and make it happen, acting as role models for its values and ethics and inspiring trust at all times. They are flexible, enabling the organisation to anticipate and reach in a timely manner to ensure its ongoing success	The manager of the department fuels change processes within NMMI and promotes a culture with values such as transparency, trust, solution orientation, openness, professionalism and ownership. To reinforce ownership in NMMI's culture, the multi-intervention approach of TeamSTEPPS (Team Strategies and Tools to Enhance Performance and Patient Safety) is applied
	NMMI has been certified in the Dutch NTA safety management systems standard, ISO, GMP, UEMS/EBNM and EARL and has been awarded with a three-star INK (equivalent of EFQM) recognition. In addition there are peer reviews by the NVMBR (Dutch Society Medical Imaging and Radiotherapy), NVNG (Dutch Society of Nuclear Medicine) and NVKF (Dutch Society of Clinical Physicists). The manager of the department is the figurehead of the leading coalition of the UMCG regarding certification
	NMMI has various reporting systems to monitor the progress of performance improvement: a digital dashboard with the top nine key performance indicators, management reviews and quarterly reports based on the Balanced Scorecard
2. Strategy Excellent organisations implement their mission and vision by developing a stakeholder-focused strategy. Policies, plans, objectives and processes are developed and deployed to deliver the strategy	The mission of NMMI is based on UMCG's mission ("Building the Future of Health"). The mission and vision of NMMI are deployed in key success factors, key performance indicators, objectives and actions by drawing up an A3 annual plan and a 5-year plan. The key priorities are KLM: quality (in Dutch: Kwaliteit), linking with other modalities and molecular targeting
	NMMI collaborates with other universities (e.g. University of Twente for Knowledge of Technical Medicine, Applied Physics and Chemical Engineering) and with strategic partners, such as Siemens
	The staff is heavily involved in formulating the strategy of NMMI in "representative staff meetings"

Table 1.4 (continued)

EFQM criteria	Examples of implemented practices ("evidence") at NMMI in UMCG
3. People Excellent organisations value their people and create a culture that allows for the mutually beneficial achievement of organisational and personal goals. They develop the capabilities of their people and promote fairness and equality. They care for, communicate, reward and recognise in a way that motivates people, builds commitment and enables them to use their skills and knowledge for the benefit of the organisation	The employees prepare a portfolio for the yearly appraisal interviews, which are scheduled in the first half of the year. Hence, agreements on individual development (e.g. visiting congresses) can be included in the training and education plan and the budget. Talent development is promoted by task rotation (e.g. section coordinator)
	Effective communication is organised according to the New Year's speech of the manager of the department, department meetings, clinical lessons, PhD meetings, a buddy system for PhDs, etc. Excellent performance of employees is celebrated ("Wall of Fame"). The management of the department pays a great deal of attention to employees' non-work-related events
	The impact of the human resources policy is measured by an employee satisfaction survey and a PhD student survey. The progress in culture development (taking responsibility, calling on colleagues with respect to safe behaviour) is measured using the TeamSTEPPS monitoring tool
4. Partnerships and resources Excellent organisations plan and manage external partnerships, suppliers and internal resources to support their strategy, policies and the effective operation of processes. They ensure that they effectively manage their environmental and societal impact	Partners are referring physicians (e.g. oncology, neurology and internal medicine), other hospitals, the pharmaceutical industry and high-tech equipment manufacturers
	As part of management control, the department draws up an annual plan with a budget. For complex projects, a business case will be elaborated. In addition, the project budgets are discussed in research meetings. Examples of income increase (e.g. sales of radiopharmaceuticals) and cost reduction (e.g. lean six sigma project on the load factor of gamma cameras) are available
	The in-depth expertise and the unique equipment enable the development and production of tracers. There is a service level agreement with the Department of Instrumental Affairs/Medical Technical Devices on the technical management of the state-of-the-art equipment. The use of utilisation management software, which registers the use of imaging systems, is unique

(continued)

Table 1.4 (continued)

EFQM criteria	Examples of implemented practices ("evidence") at NMMI in UMCG
5. Processes, products and services Excellent organisations design, manage and improve processes, products and services to generate increasing value for customers and other stakeholders	A process architecture of primary, support and management processes has been worked out. Process owners have been found, processes are described, and process indicators are applied. The safety management system (which is certified) is integrated into the QMS. Safety management methods, such as prospective risk analysis, double-check on high-risk medication and Prisma analysis of incidents is applied. Dealing with radioactivity and the removal of radioactive waste receives much attention. The production of radiopharmaceuticals is according to GMP, and the production of scans is according to GCP. Both are integrated into one overarching QMS. The department is involved in the development of cross-departmental care pathways
	The management of the primary process "research" consists of appointing a research coordinator, supporting the PhDs (buddy system) and ensuring the integrity and storage of data
	Process improvement is promoted by walk-arounds from the patient's perspective
6. Customer results Excellent organisations achieve and sustain outstanding results that meet or exceed the needs and expectations of their customers	Every 3 years, a patient satisfaction survey is conducted. The department aims for higher than 90 % satisfaction scores on KPIs: information, treatment and care, planning and organisation and privacy and accommodation. The scores are at this 90 % satisfaction level. In addition, the department would like to receive continuous feedback; therefore, the Patient Perception Programme has been implemented. After the treatment of the patient, nine questions are asked, and the patients' answers provide direct feedback
	Since 2007, a satisfaction survey amongst referring physicians has been carried out every 3 years. The aim is again to obtain scores higher than 90 % on the 20 issues in the survey. The average is 88 %, and the scores on important aspects, such as collaboration, quality of the scans and the report and the expertise of nuclear medicine, are very high. Scores which are under 90 % (e.g. expertise of a referring physician and quality of information materials about diagnosis of, e.g., thyroid cancer) are targets for improvement
	Nine key performance indicators are selected to measure process indicators, such as waiting times

Table 1.4 (continued)

EFQM criteria	Examples of implemented practices ("evidence") at NMMI in UMCG
7. People results Excellent organisations achieve and sustain outstanding results that meet or exceed the needs and expectations of their people	Every 2 years, UMCG organises an employee satisfaction survey. Employees seem to be proud to work for NMMI. Yearly appraisal interviews, 360° feedback and TeamSTEPPS are examples of acting on the results of the survey
	The satisfaction survey amongst PhD students has led to improvements in their supervision (e.g. during the orientation period) and the working environment.
	The reduction of absenteeism is the result of promoting taking responsibility for not staying at home sick
8. Society results Excellent organisations achieve and sustain outstanding results that meet or exceed the needs and expectations of relevant stakeholders within society	The department is considered a role model within the nuclear medicine discipline at national and international levels; this is due to its quality management, control of radiation risk and economic impact because of industrial and academic collaboration
	The department shares with society by writing books to disseminate scientific output, delivering presentations to congresses and contributing to the education of students in the medical sciences
	Cost-effectiveness studies and treatment evaluations enable earlier diagnosis and more effective therapies
9. Business results Excellent organisations achieve and sustain outstanding results that meet or exceed the needs and expectations of their business stakeholders	The department realises its financial task-based budget. The shift of conventional diagnosis to PET scans is visible. The income stream from contract research is rising, and repeat projects show that NMMI's work is highly appreciated. The marketing of tracers may be a new example of NMMI's entrepreneurship
	The number of PhDs and scientific publications is growing year by year

Source: EFQM criteria: http://www.efqm.org/efqm-model/model-criteria

Below, NMMI's A3 annual plan is depicted. Imagine: the whole annual plan comprising mission, vision, key success factors, performance indicators, objectives and actions on one A3 page!

This sequence of mission, vision, key success factors, performance indicators, objectives and actions is the reading direction, which is depicted by the arrows in the A3 annual plan. By using different colours or numbers, the actions are connected with the key success factors, thereby enabling dialogue on what actions are needed the following year. During the year, the department is informed about the results on the selected indicators. When the results are below target, the department can have a dialogue on whether additional actions are needed (Fig. 1.4)

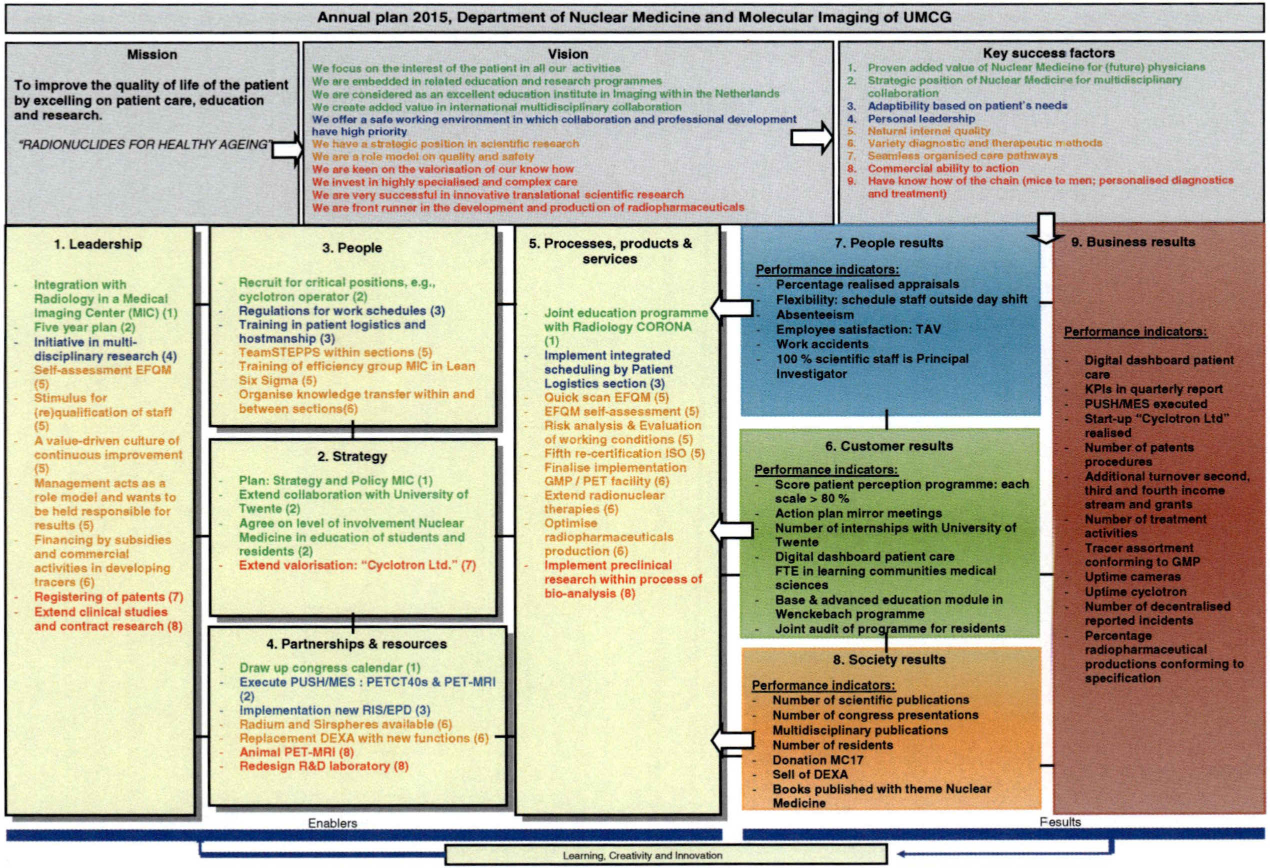

Fig. 1.4 Annual Plan 2015, Department of Nuclear Medicine and Molecular Imaging of UMCG

Conclusion

In this chapter, we described the standards, business excellence models and experiences of the NMMI in UMCG. We used the metaphors of a "road" and a "journey" to excellence. The beautiful quotes of Maraboli ("The *road* to success is always under construction") and Hemingway ("It is good to have an end to journey toward; but it is the *journey* that matters, in the end") remind us that after nearly 20 years of quality experience, NMMI is definitely intrinsically motivated to continue on this road, which is under continuous construction, as it is indeed the journey that matters.

References

Ahaus CTB, en Diepman FJ. Balanced scorecard & INK-managementmodel. 4th ed. Deventer: Kluwer; 1998, 2010.

De Vos FJ, De Decker M, Dierckx RA. The good laboratory practice and good clinical practice requirements for the production of radiopharmaceuticals in clinical research. Nucl Med Commun. 2005;26(7):575–9.

Doeleman H. Leiderschap in planning & control, Een onderzoek naar de onderbouwing, werking, implementatie en het effect van de A3 methodiek (Leadership in planning and control, a research study do the substrantiating, working mechanism, implementation and effect of the A3 methodology). Dissertation, VU University Amsterdam, March 2014. 2014.

Donabedian A. Quality in health care: whose responsibility is it? Am J Med Qual. 1993;8(2):32–6.

Donabedian A. Evaluating the quality of medical care. Milbank Q. 2005;83(4):691–729.

Institute of Medicine. Crossing the quality chasm: a new health system for the 21st century. Washington D.C.: National Academy Press; 2001.

ISO 9000:2005, Quality management systems – fundamentals and vocabulary, definition 3.1.1 quality.

ISO 9000:2005, Quality management systems – fundamentals and vocabulary, definition 0.2 quality management.

Metzcar W. The 3 C's of quality management and healthcare: ISO 9001.

NEN-EN-15224, Health care services – quality management systems. 2012.

NEN-EN-15224, Health care services – quality management systems. 2012, annex B.

Reeves C, Bednar D. Defining quality: alternatives and implications. Acad Manage Rev. 1994;19(3):419–45.

Shaw CD, Groene O, Botje D, Sunol R, Kutryba B, Klazinga N, Bruneau C, Hammer A, Wang A, Arah O, Wagner C, DUQuE Project Consortium. The effect of certification and accreditation on quality management in 4 clinical services in 73 European hospitals. Int J Qual Health Care. 2014;26 Suppl 1:100–7.

Internet Sources

Website EANM: http://www.eanm.org.

Website EFQM: http://www.efqm.org/efqm-model/model-criteria.

Website SNMMI: http://www.snmmi.org.

Wikipedia.

Good Clinical Practices in (Nuclear) Research

2

Herman Pieterse and Jan Pruim

Abstract

Nobody will deny that medical research should be conducted in an ethical and transparent way. Unfortunately, history shows that this has not been obvious all the time. It is generally known and accepted that for clinical research with medicinal products, it is required nowadays to conduct this research in compliance with the current Good Clinical Practice Guideline (ICH Harmonised Tripartite Guideline for Good Clinical Practice, Step 5, 1 May 1996 (CPMC 135/95) which became in operation as of January 1997). For all other interventional researches, it is an ethical and moral requirement to adjust the requirements of Good Clinical Practice to the most pragmatic approach in order to prove that the research has been conducted in such a way that always the safety, well-being, and privacy of participating subjects has been ensured and that the data collected are credible and reliable. The ICH GCP guideline is an international ethical and scientific quality standard for the design, conduct, collection of data, and reporting of clinical research in humans. This chapter describes the background, history, and principles of GCP. In detail the tasks and responsibilities of all parties involved in the conduct of clinical research will be elucidated. Also, peculiarities in relation to the use of radiopharmaceuticals will be elucidated.

H. Pieterse (✉)
Profess Medical Consultancy BV,
Paradijsvogel 31, Heerhugowaard 1704 WP, The Netherlands

Heymans Institute of Pharmacology, Ghent University,
De Pintelaan 185, Ghent B-9000, Belgium
e-mail: pieterse@profess.nl

J. Pruim
Department of Nuclear Medicine and Molecular Imaging, University Medical Center
Groningen, Hanzeplein 1, Groningen 9700 RB, The Netherlands

A.W.J.M. Glaudemans et al. (eds.), *Quality in Nuclear Medicine*,
DOI 10.1007/978-3-319-33531-5_2

Abbreviations

ALARA	As Low as Reasonably Achievable
CRA	Clinical Research Associate
DOH	Declaration of Helsinki
DSMB	Data Safety Monitoring Board
EMA	European Medicines Agency
EU	European Union
EudraCT	European Union Drug Regulatory Authorities Clinical Trials
FDA	Food and Drug Administration in the USA
GCP	Good Clinical Practice
IB	Investigator's Brochure
ICH	International Conference on Harmonisation of technical requirements for the Registration of Pharmaceuticals for Human Use
ICMJE	International Committee of Medical Journal Editors
ICRP	International Commission on Radiological Protection
PASS	Post Authorisation Safety Study
PRAC	Pharmacovigilance Risk Assessment Committee
SAE	Serious Adverse Event
SADE	Serious Adverse Device Effect
SOP	Standard Operating Procedure
SUSAR	Suspected Unexpected Serious Adverse Reaction
USADE	Unanticipated Serious Adverse Device Effect
WHO	World Health Organization

2.1 Origin of the GCP Regulations

2.1.1 Nuremberg Code

During World War II, a number of studies have been conducted which were even by standards of those days not ethically justified. Nazi investigators executed most of the studies, the notorious Dr. Mengele being the most well known. For instance, the German Air force wished to find an answer to the question which height is maximally safe for a pilot to jump out of a damaged airplane. To test this, a number of prisoners from Dachau concentration camp were placed in rooms where a low air pressure and low oxygen pressure were mimicked. The investigational team checked the vital signs of the prisoners under various conditions of lower air and oxygen pressure. Around 40 % of the subjects died. After World War II, a number of these "investigators" were prosecuted, sentenced to death, and executed in a process that is known as the "United States of America versus Karl Brandt et al." process.

After this trial, four American judges drafted a code that contained ten basic principles in ethical behavior when studies in humans are to be conducted. This ethical standard is known as the "Nuremberg Code" and contains the following rules:

1. Informed consent should be obtained without coercion.
2. The experiment should be useful and necessary.
3. Experiments in man should be based on preceding animal studies.
4. Physical and psychological suffering should be avoided.
5. Death or disability should never be the expected outcome of an experiment.
6. The extent of the risks should not exceed the human vested interests.
7. Subjects should be protected against the least chance of injury.
8. Only qualified persons should conduct medical research in humans.
9. Subjects should be free to withdraw from the study at any time.
10. The scientist should be prepared to stop the study at any moment.

Unfortunately, the Nuremberg Code could not prevent or stop the conduct of a long-lived experiment on – of all places – American soil, the so-called Tuskegee Syphilis Study. In 1932 an observational study was started in 399 black men with syphilis, in order to get more insight in the natural course of the disease. The subjects involved were not told the true nature of this study but simply told they had "bad blood." The study ran until 1972 (!). Because of the observational nature of the study, penicillin had been withheld to the participants, despite the fact that it is a good cure for syphilis. US governmental officials went to extreme lengths to insure that the men received no therapy from any source. Only in 1997, US President Bill Clinton apologized officially for the unethical conduct and the pains it had cost. Clearly, more measures were needed in order to prevent these kinds of missteps.

2.1.2 Declaration of Helsinki[1]

Another notorious case was the Softenon® (thalidomide) affair leading to phocomelia in newborns. In the 1950s, more than 10,000 deformed babies were born from mothers who were prescribed thalidomide during the first trimester of their pregnancy as a cure against a.o. nausea and morning sickness. From testimonials, it was evident that these mothers were not informed that thalidomide was not yet approved by the FDA, should therefore be considered an experimental moiety, and that the mothers had not given informed consent. This resulted in 1962 in the Declaration of Helsinki, drafted by the World Medical Association, where the basic principles of the Nuremberg Code were repeated and a number of other aspects were added. The Declaration of Helsinki makes a distinction between therapeutic and nontherapeutic research:

1. For therapeutic research, it is allowed under certain circumstances to include a subject in a study without informed consent.
2. A legal representative should justify the inclusion of a subject in a therapeutic of nontherapeutic trial.
3. Written informed consent is highly recommended.

[1]World Medical Association: Declaration of Helsinki. Adopted by the 18th WMA General Assembly, Helsinki, Finland, June 1964; last amended Fortaleza, Brazil October 2013.

2.1.3 The Development of the Good Clinical Practice Guideline

In the 1980s and the early 1990s, various countries were active to draw up codes, rules, and regulations for human research. In the UK, in 1986, the "Report on Good Clinical Research Practices" was published. In France, in the same period the "Bonnes Practiques Cliniques" were introduced, based on the Law Huriet that came into force in 1987. This Law Huriet is a penal law and describes the tasks and responsibilities of parties involved in research.

The first European Guideline for Good Clinical Practice originates from 1991. From this time on, it was obliged to conduct clinical research with nonregistered medicinal products in compliance with the Good Clinical Practice rules in all member states of the European Union.

Finally the "International Conference for the Harmonisation of Technical Requirements for the Registration of Pharmaceuticals for Human Use" was adopted in 1996, the ICH GCP guideline E6.[2] This guideline should be followed by the member states of the European Union, the USA, and Japan. At that time, these economic regions were the most important ones for research in the 1990s. Although emerging countries, like Brazil, Russia, India, China, and South Africa (BRICS), have published their own Good Clinical Practice Guidelines, these guidelines all fall back on the ICH GCP guideline for Good Clinical Research Practices.

In the European Union, the ICH GCP guideline has been enforced in law in 2001 on the basis of the Clinical Trial Directive. This Directive states that each interventional clinical study with a medicinal product should be conducted in compliance with ICH GCP. This Directive had to be transposed into national law in all 28 member states before May 2004. Most member states had the Directive transposed into national law by the deadline, but regrettably, the Netherlands postponed this until March 2006.

Good Clinical Practices should always be adopted for both medical care of patients and the initiation, preparation, conduct, analysis, and reporting of clinical research in humans. Some of the basic principles for the conduct of research in compliance with GCP are:

1. Always ensure the safety, well-being, rights, and privacy of the subject, and these should always prevail over interests of science and society.
2. The medical care given to, and medical decisions made on behalf of, subjects should always be the responsibility of a qualified physician or, when appropriate, of a qualified dentist.
3. Each individual involved in conducting a trial should be qualified by education, training, and experience to perform his or her respective task(s).
4. The data collected in the study should be credible and should have been collected in a reliable manner.

[2] http://www.ich.org/fileadmin/Public_Web_Site/ICH_Products/Guidelines/Efficacy/E6_R1/Step4/E6_R1__Guideline.pdf

5. All tasks and responsibilities for all involved parties are described completely and understandable in order to obtain full transparency and accountability for these tasks.

In the past, the safety of the participating subject was frequently violated. Legal jurisprudence[3] exists with respect to noncompliance with reporting safety aspects to the authorities.

In the USA, numerous studies have been proposed with a nonethical character. They are listed in the table below:

Year	Country of origin	Description of the GCP violations
1932–1972	USA	Tuskegee: 399 negroid men with syphilis were not treated for more than 30 years to study the natural course of the disease. 1997: apologies by President Clinton.
1996	USA	Yale University: N = 18 stabile schizophrenia patients became psychotic in an amphetamine provocation experiment
2001	USA	Biotech company requests permission to conduct a placebo-controlled study in children with a serious respiratory disease in Latin America
2001	USA	Nontherapeutic trial forbidden in children (lead poisoning in a study sponsored)

Apart from neglecting the patients' interests during clinical trials, there is also the issue of fraud, i.e., deliberately changing or faking data for the sake of the publication. Fraud also contains the omission of data that are displeasing to the researcher. For the Netherlands, the fraud case with a Dutch neurologist is notorious. In a clinical study with the objective to investigate the preventive effect of a compound for the treatment of cerebrovascular accidents, a neurologist included 438 patients. The data of all of these patients were proven to be fictitious. The neurologist was not convicted. More recently, a cardiologist who included patients in a noninterventional study without asking informed consent was convicted to 240 h community service. A professor in psychology who invented subjects for several studies, however, recently caused the greatest uproar. The university demoted him, and he himself decided to hand in his PhD title. However, the public prosecutor, who under Dutch law has the right to do so, refrained from prosecution because the psychologist had been punished enough by full exposure in the media.

Unfortunately, the common public often sees scientific misconduct and study risks as similar. This is incorrect. The two should be separated clearly. Scientific fraud in any form should be condemned completely and strongly. But there is no clinical trial with medical products that is without any risk. Those risks should be weighed against the benefits as accurate and fair as possible. For interventional

[3] Verzoek tot ontbinding arbeidsovereenkomst klokkenluider afgewezen. Conflict van plichten (Request to terminate employment whistleblower rejected. Conflict of duties (in Dutch)). Jurisprudentie Arbeidsrecht 25-02-2005, afl. 3, 257–263.

research, all involved parties should guarantee the accuracy and reliability. To this extent, and next to the investigator and his/her team, institutional review boards or independent regional ethics committees have been installed certifying that the sponsor of the study, and all others involved, should ensure that the study will be conducted correctly.

2.1.4 Conducting a Clinical Study in Compliance with GCP

As stated above, every person involved in a study bears the responsibility to conduct the study in compliance with the protocol and the rules and regulations as laid down in law. Both the investigator and his team and the sponsor or management of the hospital should obey basic rules for safety, accuracy, and reliability of the obtained data in all fairness according to plain common sense.

These basic rules are:

1. Always write down what you will agree with whom, for when!
2. Any agreement can be changed, but it is evident that it should be documented in order to avoid any misunderstanding in the future!
3. The design, review, and approval of standard essential documents (e.g., How to design a proper patient information folder?) should be described in a standard operational procedure (SOP). When the sponsor of a clinical study with medicinal products does not have any standard operational procedure embedded in a quality system, then it cannot be avoided in the near future that legal actions will be taken once the organization is sued for malpractice. This also holds true for clinical research with medical devices, food supplements, and other nutraceuticals or psychological experiments. Common sense dictates that any research should be done in compliance with the best practices for both scientific and ethical and moral reasons. To prove that credible data have been collected reliably, a risk-based quality control should be executed (i.e., risk-based monitoring).

   Any written quality system will be regarded as a bureaucratic burden by many, especially those working with it on an everyday basis. Although this is true, the burden can be made lighter when the procedures are simple, straightforward, checklist type, and easy to use. Also, the advantage of having checklists and instructions for a (limited) number of standard tasks is that the wheel is not invented over and over again. Moreover, essential steps in the process are not forgotten. That is the true essence of a simple yet complete quality system.
4. GCP is a set of standards, a quality system, that ensures an adequate protection for the participating subject concerning his or her safety, rights, well-being, and privacy. Moreover, by implementing GCP in the organization, the conduct of the study is such that adequate and appropriate data will be collected in a reliable manner.
5. Fore warned is fore armed: this means that everyone involved in clinical research or in patient care should think ahead and draft a quality system to describe the crucial tasks that should be done in the research process. Who within the organization is doing what, when, with whom, and how?

2.1.4.1 Phases

The clinical research process can be subdivided into three phases. First comes the preparation phase. In this phase, everything necessary to prepare the study is described: from study outline to study protocol, from patient information leaflet to informed consent form, from risk analysis to investigator's drug or device brochure, and from summary of product characteristics to investigational medicinal (or device) product dossier. Also the application for an ethics committee approval, resource management and workload calculations, and the drafting of a project plan and financing will be done in this phase.

Second comes the execution phase: who will do which tasks, how, by when, with whom, etc. Moreover, in this phase, you also describe in a monitor manual the extent of in-process quality control (monitoring) and how to report which adverse event to whom by when. It is recommended to describe any unanticipated situation in a project manual.

The last phase is the analysis and reporting phase: how to analyze the data will be described in a data management manual including instructions on how to collect and database the data and how to clean the data. For that purpose, a data validation plan will have to be drafted. The approach of the statistical analysis has been described in a statistical analysis plan that has been approved prior to the execution of the plan. The study report not only describes the results but also the process with an accurate account of all patients involved in the study (safety population, intention to treat population, and the per protocol population).

A number of supporting processes should also be described. In a quality manual, the business process will be described including the quality system and how to conduct quality assurance activities like auditing and improvement processes and how to survive a regulatory inspection. A definite part of the supporting documentation is the SOP on how to train, educate, and qualify personnel. If tasks will be delegated to third parties, then an SOP on how to select, qualify, and guide a third party is a prerequisite. And last but not least, clinical research is working with people and it is wise to prepare for the worst scenario. This means that a standard operational procedure on how to deal with suspicion for fraud or misconduct should be described.

The design and maintenance of a simple but effective quality system is an absolute condition to conduct the study in compliance with the regulatory requirements to ensure the public that the safety of participating subjects will be looked after and to ensure that everyone has performed his or her tasks as accurate as possible, honest, and fair.

We are well aware of the fact that performing research according to GCP results in extra "paperwork." And we realize that the GCP rules and regulations were drafted with mass production of medicines by pharmaceutical companies in mind. Normally, pharmaceutical companies and contract research organizations (CROs) have departments that deal with these issues, thereby reducing the burden to the individual researcher. Unfortunately, that is not the case in many hospitals. And a large part of the task comes down on the shoulders of the individual researcher. In itself that may never be an excuse not to comply to GCP, as it would mean breaking the law. But institutions and individual researchers should find ways to comply to the rules with a minimum effort. As we stated earlier in this paper that can be achieved by having simple and straightforward procedures of which checklists can be filled out in an easy way. With respect to nuclear medicine, it has to be realized that the chances of adverse events are very low, due to the low amount of substance injected and the limited number of preparations. Therefore, it is justified for the nuclear medicine world together with their hospital administrators to discuss with the authorities whether exceptions to the rules can be made, e.g., in toxicology testing. Never, however, to the principles of voluntary and knowledgeable participation.

2.2 The Independent Ethics Committee (IEC) or Institutional Review Board (IRB)

There is a principal difference between IECs and IRBs, the difference being that the IEC is a truly independent agency, whereas an IRB is situated in the same institution as the investigators. Consequently, the bylaws of the IRB should state explicitly complete independence. Up to a level that it may overrule the CEO/board of directors.

The IEC/IRB should ensure the rights, safety, and well-being of all participating subjects. Special attention should be given for research with vulnerable subjects. Vulnerable subjects[4] are individuals whose willingness to volunteer in a clinical trial may be unduly influenced by the expectation, whether justified or not, of benefits associated with participation or of a retaliatory response from senior members of a hierarchy in case of refusal to participate. Examples are members of a group with a hierarchical structure, such as medical, pharmacy, dental, and nursing students, subordinate hospital and laboratory personnel, employees of the pharmaceutical industry, members of the armed forces, and persons kept in detention. Other vulnerable subjects include patients with incurable diseases, persons in nursing homes, unemployed or impoverished persons, patients in emergency situations, ethnic minority groups, homeless persons, nomads, refugees, minors, and those incapable of giving consent.

2.2.1 Necessary Documents

Chapter 3 of the ICH GCP guideline describes which documents will be reviewed by the IEC in order to assess and approve the study proposal:

- Study protocol and amendments, if applicable
- Patient information leaflet and informed consent forms
- Recruitment material like advertisements and recruitment procedures

[4] See definition 1.61 in the ICH GCP guideline.

- Drug or device product brochure for the participating investigators and the IEC to learn about the current status of development of the study product
- Information on payment to the subject and compensation of costs, and if required by the IEC, the payment to the investigator. In the European Union, the Independent Ethics Committee should always assess the financial arrangements between the sponsor and the investigator(s)
- Qualification of participating investigators
- And a number of other documents as required by their application form

2.2.2 Approval of a Study Proposal

In the European Union, one leading accredited and qualified Independent Ethics Committee will assess a multicenter study per member state. This leading committee will assess the study protocol and the other essential documents as mentioned above. The assessment if positive is valid for all participating centers in that member state. Local ethics committees will give an opinion on the local feasibility of the investigator and his team, the facilities and equipment, and the capacity of the investigational team. This local feasibility assessment is an approval by the management board of the hospital. For the European Union, the leading Independent Ethics Committee should assess a study proposal within 60 calendar days for trials with medicinal products and within a reasonable period of 8 weeks for any study with another intervention.

The website of the regulatory authorities of the respective country should be checked to find specific information on the Independent Ethics Committee approval process, the timelines and conditions.

2.2.3 Content of an IEC Approval Letter

Normally, the approval letter contains not only the approval for the conduct of the study, it also contains some important information about the information the decision was based on. To the researcher, there are some issues to take extra into account:

- The date of the IEC approval is of vital importance. Any dosing with study medication should be done after the IEC approval has been issued. N.B. This should be documented.
- Always check the project number of the study that has been assigned by the IEC. An approval should give an overview of all assessed documents with a clear description of the version number and version date.
- If one of the members of the investigational team is also a member of the Independent Ethics Committee, then ensure that it has been documented that this person did not participate in the assessment of this study proposal.

2.2.4 Progress Reporting

The IEC is obliged to review the study at least yearly or more often depending upon the risks for the participating subjects. In practice this means that the IEC will send an email to the principal investigator/sponsor with the request to report the progress of the study. For studies with medicinal products, this is a requirement.

The principal researcher/sponsor is obliged to report all serious adverse events (SAEs) to the IEC unless for some expected events it has been agreed to waive this immediate reporting as documented in the study protocol. Any suspected (possibly or probably related to the intervention) but also any unexpected (not described in any product information) serious adverse reaction should be reported to the authorities within 15 calendar days. When the serious event is death or the patient arrived in a life-threatening situation, the reporting time is seven (7) calendar days. Adverse reactions from other studies in other countries can be submitted periodically. When the study takes longer than 1 year, a periodic safety update report (annual safety report) should be submitted to the regulatory authorities including the leading IEC. This will be a survey of all expected and unexpected serious adverse reactions.

The issue of unexpected serious adverse events needs some more clarification. Take, for instance, the situation in which an 80-year-old patient has consented to undergo a PET scan with a new radiotracer for dementia. Unfortunately, she falls off the couch and breaks a hip. Clearly, this is not related to the drug. But nevertheless, this is defined as an SAE, and it should be reported because you can only be sure that it is not related after a full analysis of the case. Who can tell ahead that the new solution, the new radiopharmaceutical was dissolved in, did not cause a temporary hypotension?

2.2.5 Composition and Functioning of an Independent Ethics Committee

As described in the ICH GCP guideline, an Independent Ethics Committee should consist at least of five members and secondly at least one member whose primary area of interest is in a nonscientific area and at least one member who is independent of the institution/trial site. In specific countries in the EU, the composition of an IEC has been specified. For instance, in the Netherlands a qualified and accredited Ethics Committee consists of one or more physicians, a pharmacist and a clinical pharmacologist, a lawyer, an expert in ethics, a methodologist, and a lay person. A member involved in the study proposal should not take part in the discussion and voting. The IEC should work with standard operational procedures. The Independent Ethics Committee documents all her activities. To learn about any specifications for Independent Ethics Committees in a specific country, surf the respective website of the hospital or regulatory authority.

2.3 The Investigator

In each investigation site, a principal investigator will be appointed who will bear the final responsibility for the study. This principal investigator is responsible for the correct conduct of the study. In a multicenter study, each site has one principal investigator. If the tasks are related to medical care, then a qualified physician or dentist should bear this responsibility. The principal investigator of the main study site often takes the role of coordinating investigator. This coordinating investigator bears the responsibility for the overall coordination of all principal investigators in all sites. The tasks of the coordinating investigator have been described prior to the start of the study.

2.3.1 Qualifications of an Investigator

The investigator should demonstrate that he/she has been qualified by education, training, and experience sufficiently in order to bear the responsibility for the proper conduct of a clinical trial. Moreover, the investigator should possess the relevant qualifications in compliance with local legal requirements.

These qualifications can be verified on the basis of an updated curriculum vitae (CV) that should be submitted to the IEC, the sponsor, and the competent regulatory authorities. This CV should be current, signed, and dated. A CV will only be updated when a person changes from function within the organization or changes to another organization. The changes in training and education will be documented in an up-to-date training record. In the near future, an updated CV, however, may not be enough. For instance, in the Netherlands the Union of Universities has decided that all researchers, whether new or experienced, should follow a special course on GCP and pass the subsequent examination, in order to qualify as principal investigator. A refresher course has to be followed after 4 years in order to get an update of the current rules and regulations. This refresher course is not followed by an exam.

The investigator should always be knowledgeable of the relevant legal regulatory requirements and should work according to predetermined standard operational procedures. These requirements are described extra in the current version of the Declaration of Helsinki.

Other members of the investigational staff should be qualified as well for the tasks delegated to them by the principal investigator. An instrument to document which tasks are assigned to a particular person is the "delegation log" or "signature sheet." The principal investigator should fill in this document in order to qualify the staff for their tasks. All members conducting tasks relevant for the study have to be put on the signature sheet and verify their assigned tasks by (short) signing it. In their CV and training records, their qualifications will be described.

The signature sheet is not required for general tasks, like a physician performing a general physical examination or a nurse drawing blood from a patient, but it should be for particular or specific tasks performed by any physician or nurse involved. This means that physicians including patients in your trial in the weekend should be qualified, and this should be documented.

The principal investigator delegating tasks should be aware of his responsibilities. Delegating tasks in medical care can only be done in compliance under three conditions:

1. The task can only be performed by an authorized (for some specific medical tasks) and competent person.
2. That person should have pronounced that he/she is competent to perform the task.
3. The responsible principal investigator should keep proper oversight (i.e., regular checking to verify if the tasks are conducted adequately).

2.3.2 Facilities Needed to Qualify for a GCP Study

According to ICH GCP, the investigator should have documented evidence of the availability of an adequate number of eligible subjects for the study, ample time to conduct the study, sufficiently qualified personnel, and adequate facilities.

The investigator should inform all personnel involved in the study sufficiently about the study protocol and the investigational products and should inform them in detail on their tasks and duties. In most cases, the investigator will arrange this training and information session together with the study monitor appointed by the sponsor of the study in a so-called "kickoff" meeting.

2.3.3 Emergency Care

A competent and registered physician or dentist in his or her role as an investigator bears the responsibility for the medical care of the subjects. This physician/dentist will take the medical decision. This person can delegate this medical task to another medical doctor keeping in mind the three conditions for delegation. The investigator as a physician should ensure that the subject gets the necessary medical care in case of serious adverse events, including clinically significant deviations of laboratory values. When the investigator is not medically qualified (e.g., psychologist or pharmacist), he or she should appoint a medically qualified person to bear this responsibility.

In nuclear medicine research, or drug research using nuclear medicine techniques, it is advisable to split the responsibilities between two medical doctors. The one doctor being responsible for all aspects of the (new) drug/compound administered, whereas the other doctor, most times the nuclear medicine physician, is responsible for all aspects of radiation safety.

2.3.4 Communicating with the IEC/IRB

In the early days, when submission to Independent Ethics Committees was simple, the investigator was the first contact with the Independent Ethics Committee. In the ICH GCP guideline, the investigator is still the one responsible to obtain the approval for the study. As described in the section Independent Ethics Committee, the investigator should ensure that the Independent Ethics Committee approval contains all references and conditions. Nowadays, the investigator will, together with representatives of the sponsor, submit all required documents and, if applicable, all amendments to the documents. The amendments are called substantial amendments when the amendments have a significant impact on:

1. The safety or physical or mental integrity of the subjects
2. The scientific value of the trial
3. The conduct or management of the trial
4. The quality or safety of any investigational medicinal product used in the trial

An Independent Ethics Committee in the European Union needs maximally 35 calendar days to arrive at a decision on the amendment.

When the amendment has no impact on these aspects, then the amendment is called a nonsubstantial or logistical or administrative amendment. For these nonsubstantial amendments, no prior IEC approval is required. These nonsubstantial amendments will be submitted for information purposes to the IEC. Examples of nonsubstantial amendments are the changing of telephone numbers, addresses, or textual improvements in a study protocol.

2.3.5 Is Compliance to the Study Protocol Required According to ICH GCP?

The investigator must conduct the study in compliance with the study protocol. This protocol has been signed by the investigator and sponsor to confirm the agreements made for this study.

The investigator can only deviate from the study protocol if the subject is in immediate risk for injury or to avoid such a situation. Other deviations can only be implemented after approval by the sponsor and the Independent Ethics Committee. Any deviations to avoid immediate danger, if required documented in an amendment, should be submitted to the Independent Ethics Committee and the competent regulatory authorities as soon as possible.

Deviations from a study protocol can be divided in deviations and violations. A protocol violation is an intended deviation from the study protocol and is a serious breach of the study protocol. Any subjects that do not comply with the inclusion and exclusion criteria are regarded as protocol violations. The statistician has to count for protocol violations in the study population differently. The worst-case scenario of a sponsor is that the investigator has so many protocol violations that not enough patients followed the whole study protocol resulting in a study that cannot be appropriately analyzed.

Note: any protocol deviation should be documented on a list!

2.3.6 Investigational Medicinal Product

2.3.6.1 What Is Required for Investigational Medicinal Products (IMPs)?

The investigator bears the responsibility for the handling and storage of IMPs on location. Certain tasks can be delegated to a competent pharmacist or other qualified person under supervision of the institution. For many countries, the responsibility for the handling and storage of medication lies with the pharmacist.

The investigator or the qualified person has to set up and maintain an administration of all IMPs, and this drug accountability administration should contain the following information:

1. The delivery and receipt of IMPs at the study location
2. The stock of the IMPs at the location
3. The use of IMPs by the subject
4. The return of IMPs from the subject
5. The return of IMPs to the sponsor

Note: the investigator should be able to demonstrate that the IMP has been stored in compliance with the storage conditions for the whole study period.

2.3.6.2 Should the Investigator Comply with the Randomization Procedure and Under Which Circumstances Should the Investigator Break the Study Code in a Double-Blind Study?

The investigator should always comply with the randomization procedure. The code can only be broken in accordance with the study protocol. In general, it means that breaking the code is only useful and allowed when knowledge of the IMP has a positive effect for the further treatment of the subject. Every break of the code should be documented immediately and should be explained.

In nuclear medicine, randomization between drug strategies or with placebo is rarely done. The latter being completely unethical in most cases as only half of the subjects would be exposed to radiation, or even worse, half of the subjects would be exposed to unnecessary radiation, violating the as low as reasonably achievable (ALARA, i.e., using the lowest possible dose in relation to the wanted/needed outcome, taking multiple factors, including societal and economical factors, into account) principle.

2.3.7 Informed Consent Procedure

An Independent Ethics Committee should approve all written information given to the study subject. This information should be amended when new important information becomes available. However, this new information should be relevant for the subject in order not to burden the subject with an extra informed consent procedure. Again, it is obvious that the Independent Ethics Committee should approve the new information before any action can be taken to the subject.

The patient information should be simple and understandable. The subject should have the opportunity to pose any questions, and the qualified staff should answer these questions adequately. The informed consent form should be signed and dated prior to the inclusion in the study (including any screening test) by the subject and the qualified member of the investigational staff who has explained the study, the tasks, and the obligations and conditions.

It is feasible that the subject keeps silent about certain personal conditions. The reason is that the subject wishes to maintain the good relationship with the physician/investigator. By requesting the subject to contact their general practitioner, the investigator is able to double-check any personal circumstances. This is a recommendation not an obligation. The subject has to give permission to contact the other caretaker.

Although a subject is not obliged to give his/her reason(s) for withdrawing prematurely from a trial, the investigator should make a reasonable effort to ascertain the reason(s) while fully respecting the subject's rights. If the reason is a logistical reason, then adequate measures can be taken. For example, when the effort to come to the hospital for drawing a blood sample is too much, then the nurse can go to the patient's home instead.

Drafting a patient information leaflet that is understandable for the average public is not easy. We advise to make a proposal and find any 12-year-old niece or nephew and ask her or him to underline any word they use but for which they do not know the meaning of the word. You will be amazed for which words they do not know the meaning.

If a subject is unable to read, then an impartial witness should be present during the whole informed consent procedure. This witness, not specified in detail in the ICH GCP guideline, should cosign and date the informed consent form as an attest.

The following information should be addressed in the patient information and consent form (Ref. ICH GCP 4.8.10):

(a) That the trial involves research.
(b) The purpose of the trial.
(c) The trial treatment(s) and the probability for random assignment to each treatment.
(d) The trial procedures to be followed, including all invasive procedures.
(e) The subject's responsibilities.
(f) Those aspects of the trial that are experimental.

(g) The reasonably foreseeable risks or inconveniences to the subject and, when applicable, to an embryo, fetus, or nursing infant.
(h) The reasonably expected benefits. When there is no intended clinical benefit to the subject, the subject should be made aware of this.
(i) The alternative procedure(s) or course(s) of treatment that may be available to the subject, and their important potential benefits and risks.
(j) The compensation and/or treatment available to the subject in the event of trial-related injury.
(k) The anticipated prorated payment, if any, to the subject for participating in the trial.
(l) The anticipated expenses, if any, to the subject for participating in the trial.
(m) That the subject's participation in the trial is voluntary and that the subject may refuse to participate or withdraw from the trial, at any time, without penalty or loss of benefits to which the subject is otherwise entitled.
(n) That the monitor(s), the auditor(s), the IRB/IEC, and the regulatory authority(ies) will be granted direct access to the subject's original medical records for verification of clinical trial procedures and/or data, without violating the confidentiality of the subject, to the extent permitted by the applicable laws and regulations and that, by signing a written informed consent form, the subject or the subject's legally acceptable representative is authorizing such access.
(o) That records identifying the subject will be kept confidential and, to the extent permitted by the applicable laws and/or regulations, will not be made publicly available. If the results of the trial are published, the subject's identity will remain confidential.
(p) That the subject or the subject's legally acceptable representative will be informed in a timely manner if information becomes available that may be relevant to the subject's willingness to continue participation in the trial.
(q) The person(s) to contact for further information regarding the trial and the rights of trial subjects and whom to contact in the event of trial-related injury.
(r) The foreseeable circumstances and/or reasons under which the subject's participation in the trial may be terminated.
(s) The expected duration of the subject's participation in the trial.
(t) The approximate number of subjects involved in the trial.

At 4.8.10.n.: Any third party not being the physician and his staff who is responsible for the medical care of the patient should ask permission from the subject to be able to inspect his medical files. This is true for any monitor, auditor, or member of the Independent Ethics Committee or regulatory authority but also for any other physician in the hospital who is not involved in the medical care of the patient. This is a privacy rule.

The subject should always get a signed copy of the informed consent form. This is also valid for any amended informed consent form.

Under Dutch law,[5] an extra person was introduced in the informed consent procedure, the so-called "independent" doctor or expert. This involves a (senior) physician or other expert not in any way involved in the study but knowledgeable about the topic to be studied. Potential participants can turn to this doctor to have questions answered, which for whatever reason they did not ask at the time of the explanation and signing of the informed consent form. In theory, this extra address looks promising; in practice, only few participants make use of the possibility. Also, the independence of the "independent doctor" can be questioned, as many are recruited from the direct vicinity of the principal investigator.

2.3.8 Nontherapeutic Trials

Nontherapeutic trials can only be conducted in subjects that can give informed consent themselves. There are exceptions when the following conditions are met:

1. The objectives of the trial cannot be met by means of a trial in subjects who can give informed consent personally.
2. The foreseeable risks to the subjects are low.
3. The negative impact on the subject's well-being is minimized and low.
4. Law does not prohibit the trial.
5. The approval/favorable opinion of the IRB/IEC is expressly sought on the inclusion of such subjects, and the written approval/favorable opinion covers this aspect.

In emergency situation, the legal representative of the subject should give informed consent. When this is not possible, then the specific situation and conditions should be documented in the study protocol.

Nontherapeutic trials can and will be conducted in nuclear medicine often, varying from the testing of a new diagnostic radiopharmaceutical to the testing of new equipment.

2.3.8.1 Informed Consent for Legally Restraint Subjects

Mentally handicapped persons, patients with degenerative diseases like Alzheimer's disease, coma patients, and patients who are in immediate danger when no actions will be taken, like patients with a threatening severe myocardial infarction, are legally restrained persons and cannot take an adequate decision to participate in a clinical study. For those persons, the legal representative can sign and date the informed consent. In most countries, there is a cascade of representatives who are allowed to sign for the subject. After the legal representative, an investigator should ask if written authorization (or affidavit) exists permitting that person to decide upon participation. Then the spouse or partner can take the decision, followed by the children of the subject with an age above 18 years, and last the siblings of the subject.

[5] Article 9 Medical Research in Human Subjects Act.

Prisoners need extra mentioning. By law, they are also legally restrained subjects, but in their case the consent of the legal representative is insufficient. The consent of the prisoner is paramount, but since a prison situation is not a normal situation and coercion from peers and/or guards often occurs within prison walls, we very much doubt the voluntariness of their decision. Therefore, studies, certainly nontherapeutic studies, should never be performed in a prison population.

2.3.9 Records and Reporting Requirements

All data from one patient as described in the study protocol will be recorded in the case report form (CRF) and delivered to the sponsor. The investigator should ensure the accuracy, completeness, legibility, and timeliness of the data reported to the sponsor in the CRFs and in all required reports. Moreover, the data recorded should be in compliance with the medical file of the patient and any other identified source documents like the X-ray, laboratory reports, and letters to other physicians.

Source documents should literally be what they are: the source of the data, meaning that they should be preserved for the time of the retention period. To put it bluntly: if you are stupid enough to write down data in the palm of your hand, you have a real problem for the next 15–20 years. Agreed, this is a joke, but it makes quite clear the importance of source data. In medical imaging, this raises an interesting question: what is considered the source? Is it the CT or PET scan image? Or is it the underlying data used for the reconstruction of the image ("list data")? The authors believe it is the latter, which will imply that these data may not be discarded after reconstruction but should be kept in the study archive for the length of time that is legally obliged. Also the reconstruction parameters should be noted and archived. We understand that this is contrary to the policy in many centers where the source data are discarded after the reconstruction has finished.

For both the manual and electronic data entry, a complete audit trail in the software should be present. This means that for all modifications, it can be traced back who has changed what when. For manual corrections, the original entry should always be readable, and any updating of the data should be initialed and dated and, if reasonable, an explanation of the modification. It is evident that the person who changes the data should have been qualified and authorized by the principal investigator. In practice, many computer systems and software, whether linked to our imaging machines or more general software, are missing such a tracking log. The unprotected "Excel" file is not according to GCP.

Upon request of either the monitor, auditor, or members of the IEC or regulatory authorities, the investigator should give direct access to the source documents of the subject. This agreement has been documented in a contract. However, the investigator and any other medical doctor should be aware of the fact that the patient decides who can have access in his or her medical file. The patient permits direct access by signing the informed consent. The statement of this subject is an integral and essential part of the informed consent.

The investigator should retain his records and all other essential documents according to ICH GCP until at least 2 years after the last approval of a marketing application in an ICH region and until there are no pending or contemplated marketing applications in an ICH region or at least 2 years have elapsed since the formal discontinuation of clinical development of the investigational product. These documents should be retained for a longer period, however, if required by the applicable regulatory requirements or by an agreement with the sponsor. It is the responsibility of the sponsor to inform the investigator/institution as to when these documents no longer need to be retained.

The retention period for essential documents in clinical research with medicinal products changes per regulation. It is not evident which retention period you should comply with. The consensus is about 20 years after completion of the study. Nowadays this retention period has been chosen in many countries. In general, we can state that problems with medicinal products always arrive approximately five to eleven years after introduction into the markets. It is useful and sensible to keep the data from clinical studies with medical products for a period of 15–20 years. The consensus is 20 years.

2.3.9.1 Progress Reporting

The investigator should report the progress of the study at least annually to the IEC. This can be a summary stating the following aspects:

1. Title of the study, start and finish (when preliminary stopped)
2. Reason for stopping the study, if applicable
3. Data first inclusion
4. Number of subjects included per country
5. Total number of subjects to be included
6. Number of subjects that should have been included according to the plan
7. Total number of subjects to be included according to the study protocol
8. Number of subjects who completed the study (per study group, if applicable)
9. Number of subjects who preliminary withdrew from the study
10. Overview of the reasons for withdrawal:
    (a) No efficacy
    (b) Adverse reactions
    (c) On personal request
    (d) Others, specify

Note: when the sponsor of the study is the pharmaceutical industry, the sponsor will provide this progress report.

2.3.10 Safety Reporting

The investigator should record all adverse events (as stated by the subject) in the CRF.

A serious adverse event (SAE) is defined as:
Any untoward medical occurrence that at any dose:

- Results in death
- Is life-threatening
- Requires inpatient hospitalization or prolongation of existing hospitalization
- Results in persistent or significant disability/incapacity
- Is a congenital anomaly/birth defect

SAEs should be reported to the sponsor of the study within 24 h. The investigator should not interpret the data; that is of latter concern. Although it could be feasible that the patient struggled over a marble causing such a hip injury that the patient needed to be hospitalized, it can never be excluded that the IMP should have been the root cause. Consequently, as an investigator, you should report SAEs to the sponsor without further delay. The sponsor is responsible for the assessment of relatedness and expectedness.

2.3.10.1 Annual Safety Reporting

The investigator should also submit once a year throughout the clinical trial and on request, a safety report of the medicinal product involved, to the CA. This report includes:

1. A list of all suspected (expected and unexpected) serious adverse reactions, including a table of all reported serious adverse reactions ordered per organ system for each study
2. A report involving the safety of the human subjects. This report consists of a full safety analysis and an evaluation of the balance between the efficacy and harmfulness of the medicinal product.

Normally, when the sponsor of the study is the pharmaceutical industry, the sponsor will provide this annual safety report.

2.3.10.2 Premature Temporarily or Final Stop of the Study

When the study ends prematurely or be put on hold temporarily, e.g., due to some unforeseen side effects, the investigator is under the obligation to report this to the management of the institution, the IEC, and the regulatory authorities for clinical studies with medicinal products in writing. Such a report should be issued within 15 calendar days. The reason for stopping the study (temporarily) should be mentioned explicitly. The investigator should also inform the subjects that participated in case a study has been stopped (prematurely), and they should be offered adequate follow-up for which the investigator is responsible.

2.4 The Sponsor

The actual sponsor of a clinical study with medicinal products is an individual, company, institution, or organization that takes responsibility for the initiation, management, and/or financing of a clinical trial.

When the study will be initiated by an institution (e.g., a hospital department), then the investigator is referred to as sponsor-investigator.[6] In such a case, the hospital board becomes responsible for the tasks of the sponsor and is also liable when the sponsor-investigator does not comply with the ICH GCP guideline. This kind of research is also referred to as investigator-initiated studies. Under normal circumstances, the contract between the employee/investigator and the hospital will cover all the aspects of good scientific conduct.

The sponsor should implement and maintain a system of quality control and quality assurance describing all processes in written predetermined standard operational procedures in order to ensure that the studies will be conducted and the data will be collected and reported in compliance with the study protocol, GCP, and relevant applicable regulatory requirements. The sponsor must also ensure that all involved parties will be granted direct access to all source documents for monitoring and auditing. The arrangements for direct access into the medical files of the subjects are documented in the written agreement between the sponsor and the investigator.

The sponsor is responsible for the hiring of qualified personnel for all trial-related tasks from the design of the study up to the reporting of the results. For medical tasks like the conduct of a physical examination, medical intervention, drawing blood, etc., then a medically qualified person should be hired to conduct these tasks. Performing the informed consent procedure is a task that can also be delegated to nonmedically qualified personnel. However, the principal investigator should realize that delegating this task should comply with the three conditions (i.e., person should be qualified, pronounce him/herself that they feel confident to perform the task, and the responsible investigator should keep a proper oversight).

The sponsor should select investigator and institution on the basis of predetermined selection criteria. All tasks in a clinical study will be allocated to qualified personnel. The sponsor is the responsible party to arrange for insurance when the patient gets injured.

The sponsor also is responsible for the approval of the study by the regulatory authorities. For the European Union, the sponsor should also apply for a specific European Drug Regulatory Affairs Clinical Trial Module (EUDRACT) number and to fill out the specific EUDRACT form. Within two years, this system will change due to the coming European Clinical Trial Regulation. A web portal is developed for all interventional studies with medicinal products in the European Union. Every application for such a study in Europe should use the web portal.

2.4.1 Delegation to a Contract Research Organization (CRO)?

A contract research organization (CRO) is a person or an organization (commercial, academic, or other) contracted by the sponsor to perform one or more of a

[6] An individual who both initiates and conducts, alone or with others, a clinical trial, and under whose immediate direction the investigational product is administered to, dispensed to, or used by a subject. The term does not include any person other than an individual (e.g., it does not include a corporation or an agency). The obligations of a sponsor-investigator include both those of a sponsor and those of an investigator. Ref. ICH GCP 1.

sponsor's trial-related duties and functions. Sponsors can delegate tasks to a CRO. It is one of the biggest misunderstandings in medical research that sponsors assume that with the transfer of the tasks also the responsibilities are transferred. This is incorrect. Under current rules, the sponsor can never transfer its responsibilities.

2.4.2 Arrangements for Trial Management, Data Handling, and Record Keeping

Depending upon the complexity of the study, the sponsor should appoint for the study a project manager and other personnel like the clinical research associate (CRA) or study monitor, data management personnel, and a biostatistician at a minimum. Data management personnel who will be authorized to change the data will be documented in a specific list. When a high-risk trial is to be executed, the sponsor may consider establishing an independent data monitoring committee (IDMC) to assess the progress of a clinical trial, including the safety data and the primary efficacy endpoints at intervals, and to recommend to the sponsor whether to continue, modify, or stop a trial. The IDMC should have written operating procedures and maintain written records of all its meetings.

When the sponsor is using electronic trial data handling and/or remote electronic trial data systems, the sponsor should (Ref. ICH GCP 5.5.3):

1. Ensure and document that the electronic data processing system conforms to the sponsor's established requirements for completeness, accuracy, reliability, and consistent intended performance (i.e., validation).[7]
2. Maintain SOPs for using these systems.
3. Ensure that the systems are designed to permit data changes in such a way that the data changes are documented and that there is no deletion of entered data (i.e., maintain an audit trail, data trail, edit trail).
4. Maintain a security system that prevents unauthorized access to the data.
5. Maintain a list of the individuals who are authorized to make data.
6. Maintain adequate backup of the data.
7. Safeguard the blinding, if any (e.g., maintain the blinding during data entry and processing).

The sponsor should keep all sponsor-relevant essential documents for the same retention period as described for the investigator.

[7] Any data handling software in these kind of trials should be validated. In the USA, this means that the software should comply with the FDA regulations described in 21 CFR Part 11 on electronic records and electronic signatures.

2.4.3 Investigational Medicinal Products (IMPs) and the Tasks of the Sponsor

It is the sponsor's responsibility that sufficient data are available concerning the safety and efficacy of the investigational product to justify administration to humans. Moreover, the sponsor should adapt the investigator's drug brochure (IB) when new important information becomes available at least annually. Also, the sponsor should ensure that the IMPs will be manufactured in compliance with the current good manufacturing practice guideline (GMP). The IMPs should be coded and labeled in such a manner that the blinding will be kept in case the protocol demands blinding. The labeling should conform the regulatory requirements. It has to be emphasized that radiopharmaceuticals by law are to be treated as any other pharmaceutical.

The labeling of IMPs should at least contain the following information:[8]

(a) Name, address, and telephone number of the sponsor, contract research organization, or investigator (the main contact for information on the product, clinical trial, and emergency unblinding)
(b) Pharmaceutical dosage form, route of administration, quantity of dosage units, and in the case of open trials, the name/identifier and strength/potency
(c) The batch and/or code number to identify the contents and packaging operation
(d) A trial reference code allowing identification of the trial, site, investigator, and sponsor if not given elsewhere
(e) The trial subject identification number/treatment number and, where relevant, the visit number
(f) The name of the investigator (if not included in (a) or (d))
(g) Directions for use (reference may be made to a leaflet or other explanatory document intended for the trial subject or person administering the product)
(h) "For clinical trial use only" or similar wording
(i) The storage conditions
(j) Period of use (use by date, expiry date, or re-test date as applicable), in month/year format and in a manner that avoids any ambiguity
(k) "Keep out of reach of children" except when the product is for use in trials where the product is not taken home by subjects

The sponsor should determine all conditions for the IMP like the storage conditions, stability data for the expiry date, solvents in case of dry powder for injection, etc.

The sponsor should ensure that IMP can be identified quickly when the product has to be identified in case of an emergency and should also take measure that breaking the code of the blinding invisibly is not possible.

[8] Annex 13 to the EC Guide for Good Manufacturing Practice, III/3004/91, 1 July 1997 revised per 3 February 2010. http://ec.europa.eu/health/files/eudralex/vol-4/2009_06_annex13.pdf.

The sponsor is responsible for the delivery and handling of the IMP to the investigator. This should not take place before the sponsor has obtained all required essential regulatory documents (e.g., approval letter of the IEC). The sponsor should keep an administration of the whole trail of the IMP (transport, receipt, distribution to the hospitals, return, and destruction).

The sponsor should ensure that written procedures exist with instructions for the investigator for the handling and storing of the IMP at the investigator site and how to document all these activities. The sponsor should keep a system for the return of the IMP and for reuse of the IMP when this is pharmaceutically allowed and the return of unused IMP. The sponsor should ensure the stability of the IMP during the whole period of use. Moreover, the sponsor should take care that enough stock is available of the IMP and should also be able to determine the product specifications again, if deemed necessary. A registration of all samples for analyses and specifications of each batch should be retained.

2.4.4 What Should the Sponsor Do to Ensure Direct Access in the Medical Files of the Subjects?

The sponsor should verify and ensure that the investigator and the hospital have agreed in writing that direct access into all medical source documentation relevant for the clinical study has been arranged for monitoring, auditing, and inspection by either members of the IEC or inspectors of the regulatory authorities. The sponsor should verify if every participating subject has given permission to direct access in his/her medical files in the informed consent form. This permission of the subjects makes monitoring, auditing, and inspection of the source documents possible.

2.4.5 Which Safety Information of the IMP Should Be Made Available by the Sponsor?

The sponsor should continuously evaluate the safety of the IMP. Besides that, the sponsor should inform both the investigators and the IEC/IRB and the regulatory authorities immediately when new relevant information (this refers to information that negatively can influence the safety, rights, and well-being of participating subjects) on the safety of the product becomes available.

2.4.6 Reporting of Adverse Drug Reactions

Adverse events, whether or not related to the administered formulation, are a case for concern and should be reported. Depending on the severity of the findings, these reports should be reported within a certain time frame. The following definitions are being used:

2.4.6.1 Adverse Event (AE)

An adverse event is any untoward medical occurrence in a patient or clinical trial subject who is administered a medicinal product but which does not necessarily have a causal relationship with this treatment. For instance, a subject participating in a long-running trial into a new drug against dementia is scheduled to undergo hip replacement surgery. This surgery is then considered an adverse event, unrelated.

2.4.6.2 Adverse Reaction (AR)

Adverse reactions are all untoward and unintended responses to an IMP related to any dose administered. All adverse events, judged by either the investigator or the sponsor, that are suspected of having a reasonable causal relationship to an IMP qualify as adverse reaction. The causality assessment given by the investigator cannot and should not be downgraded by the sponsor. For example, our patient did not only undergo the hip replacement; it was also found out that she is suffering from a low blood pressure. Since it can be reasonably assumed that there is a possible relation between drug and hypotension, this finding qualifies as an adverse reaction.

2.4.6.3 Unexpected Adverse Reaction

An unexpected adverse reaction is an adverse reaction, the nature or severity of which is not consistent with the applicable product information (e.g., investigator's brochure for an unapproved IMP or summary of product characteristics (SPC) for an authorized medicinal product).

2.4.6.4 Serious AE or Serious AR

To stay with our example, the patient develops a myocardial infarction and is hospitalized. At this stage, we cannot tell whether this is related or unrelated, but according to the criteria given below, it is classified as serious: a serious adverse event is any untoward medical occurrence or effect that at any dose:

- Results in death
- Is life-threatening (at the time of the event)
- Requires hospitalization or prolongation of existing inpatients' hospitalization
- Results in persistent or significant disability or incapacity
- Is a congenital anomaly or birth defect
- Is a new event of the trial likely to affect the safety of the subjects, such as an unexpected outcome of an adverse reaction, lack of efficacy of an IMP used for the treatment of a life-threatening disease, post study event, etc.

Suspected and unsuspected serious adverse events/reactions (SUSARs) should be reported to the sponsor promptly by the investigator that encountered the event. The sponsor should expedite the report of those adverse reactions that are both serious and unexpected to the other investigators involved in the trial, the IEC/IRB and the competent regulatory authorities, and also the competent authorities in other member states where the IMP is subject of a clinical trial run by the same sponsor. Expedited reporting means not later than 15 days after the sponsor obtained first knowledge of the adverse reactions. For fatal or life-threatening cases, the maximal term is 7 days for a preliminary report with another 8 days for completion of the report.

In addition, the sponsor should submit periodically (at least annually) an overview of all safety (an overview of all SAEs, suspected serious adverse drug reactions, and the suspected unexpected serious adverse reactions) reporting to the authorities in compliance with the applicable national requirements. This safety report will also be used to update the investigator's brochure annually.

In case of a multinational trial with an authorized medicinal product with different legal product information (summary of the product characteristics or SPCs), the sponsor must select one of the SPCs as reference document in order to be able to judge the expectedness. The reference document to be used should be a part of the investigator's brochure; it should be attached in the clinical trial application and mentioned in the covering letter.

Also SUSARs that occur in another trial with the same IMP conducted by the same sponsor, within or outside the European Economic Area (EEA: the European Union, Norway, Iceland, and Liechtenstein), should be reported as well as SUSARs related to comparators (including placebo).

2.4.7 SUSARs in Blinded Trials

In nuclear medicine, blinded trials are unlikely. Nevertheless, we feel that it is important to at least summarize the prerequisites in case of SUSARs in a blinded trial. Basic is that codes should be broken prior to reporting but only for the specific patient experiencing the SUSAR. It is also recommended that, when possible and appropriate, the blind be maintained for persons, such as biometrics personnel responsible for data analysis and interpretation of results at the study's conclusion. Especially in trials in patients with a high morbidity and/or mortality disease state, it is recommended that an independent Data and Safety Monitoring Board (DSMB) be in charge of the decision to unblind single SUSAR cases.

2.4.8 Electronic Reporting of SUSARs

Nowadays, within the EU, reporting is done electronically. Sponsors should send their SUSARs to the EudraVigilance Clinical Trial Module (EVCTM) at the EMA, the EC, and the competent regulatory authorities. For reporting SUSARs occurring in nonindustry-sponsored trials, it will be possible to report SUSARs to the EudraVigilance Clinical Trial Module using the eSUSAR form. For investigator-initiated studies with IMPs, most regulatory authorities in the European Union have implemented a simplified reporting module for SUSAR reporting. Surf to the website of the relevant regulatory authority for details. After completion of the eSUSAR form, the regulatory authorities will transmit the report forward to EudraVigilance CT thereafter.

2.4.9 Monitoring

Monitoring is the act of overseeing the progress of a clinical trial and of ensuring that it is conducted, recorded, and reported in accordance with the protocol, standard operating procedures (SOPs), GCP, and the applicable regulatory requirement(s). The sponsor should appoint monitors who have been educated appropriately, who possess sufficient medical and scientific knowledge in order to monitor the study adequately. These qualifications should be documented.

The sponsor should ensure that the study will be monitored adequately. The extent and the kind of monitoring depend entirely on the complexity of the study. Risk-based monitoring is the approach to this subject. This means that when the patients are more at risk or the procedure are more complex another extent of monitoring will take place. A site that performs below the predetermined standard is also monitored more frequently. At the end, both the investigational site and the monitor will deliver good-quality data collected reliably.

The monitor will perform the following tasks (Ref. ICH GCP 5.18):

1. Acting as the main line of communication between the sponsor and the investigator.
2. Verifying that the investigator has adequate qualifications and resources and these remain adequate throughout the trial period and that the staff and facilities, including laboratories and equipment, are adequate to safely and properly conduct the trial and these remain adequate throughout the trial period.
3. Verifying, for the investigational product(s):
   (a) That storage times and conditions are acceptable and that supplies are sufficient throughout the trial
   (b) That the investigational product(s) are supplied only to subjects who are eligible to receive it and at the protocol specified dose(s)
   (c) That subjects are provided with necessary instruction on properly using, handling, storing, and returning the investigational product(s)
   (d) That the receipt, use, and return of the investigational product(s) at the trial sites are controlled and documented adequately
   (e) That the disposition of unused investigational product(s) at the trial sites complies with applicable regulatory requirement(s) and is in accordance with the sponsor's authorized procedures
4. Verifying that the investigator follows the approved protocol and all approved amendment(s), if any.
5. Verifying that written informed consent was obtained before each subject's participation in the trial.
6. Ensuring that the investigator receives the current investigator's brochure, all documents, and all trial supplies needed to conduct the trial properly and to comply with the applicable regulatory requirement(s).
7. Ensuring that the investigator and the investigator's trial staff are adequately informed about the trial.

8. Verifying that the investigator and the investigator's trial staff are performing the specified trial functions, in accordance with the protocol and any other written agreement between the sponsor and the investigator/institution, and have not delegated these functions to unauthorized individuals.
9. Verifying that the investigator is enrolling only eligible subjects.
10. Reporting the subject recruitment rate.
11. Verifying that source data/documents and other trial records are accurate, complete, kept up-to-date, and maintained.
12. Verifying that the investigator provides all the required reports, notifications, applications, and submissions, and that these documents are accurate, complete, timely, legible, dated, and identify the trial.
13. Checking the accuracy and completeness of the CRF entries, source data/documents, and other trial-related records against each other. The monitor specifically should verify that:
    (a) The data required by the protocol are reported accurately on the CRFs and are consistent with the source data/documents.
    (b) Any dose and/or therapy modifications are well documented for each of the trial subjects.
    (c) Adverse events, concomitant medications, and intercurrent illnesses are reported in accordance with the protocol on the CRFs.
    (d) Visits that the subjects fail to make, tests that are not conducted, and examinations that are not performed are clearly reported as such on the CRFs.
    (e) All withdrawals and dropouts of enrolled subjects from the trial are reported and explained on the CRFs.
14. Informing the investigator of any CRF entry error, omission, or illegibility. The monitor should ensure that appropriate corrections, additions, or deletions are made, dated, explained (if necessary), and initialed by the investigator or by a member of the investigator's trial staff who is authorized to initial CRF changes for the investigator. This authorization should be documented.
15. Determining whether all adverse events (AEs) are appropriately reported within the time periods required by GCP, the ICH Guidance for Clinical Safety Data Management: definitions and standards for expedited reporting, the protocol, the IRB/IEC, the sponsor, and the applicable regulatory requirement(s).
16. Determining whether the investigator is maintaining the essential documents.
17. Communicating deviations from the protocol, SOPs, GCP, and the applicable regulatory requirements to the investigator and taking appropriate action designed to prevent recurrence of the detected deviations.

The monitoring of a study needs to be planned beforehand and described in a monitor manual. This manual should contain the following information:

1. Introduction
    (a) Short summary of the trial
    (b) Describe the objective of the monitoring process.

2. Study team
   (a) List members of the study team (data management, statistician, coinvestigators, research nurses). Refer to the list of principal investigators, for multicenter trials.
3. Monitor Training:
   (a) Describe study-specific training for the monitor.
4. Monitoring method
   (a) Describe in general terms the monitoring method (telephone contacts, visits, etc.) Describe the role of the monitor in the selection and qualification of investigators, the initiation of the trial, the frequency of monitoring, and the close-out visit.
5. Reporting monitor visits
   (a) Refer to the templates for reporting the selection, initiation, monitor, and close-out visit. Describe who will review these reports and provide feedback to the monitor.
6. Trial master file
   (a) Describe the role of the monitor concerning the setup and verification of the trial master file and, for multicenter trials, the investigator files.
   (b) Describe which forms have been designed for the trial and the location on the computer where these forms can be found.
7. Verification of source documents
   (a) Describe the extent of verification of source documents. Describe which source documents will be verified 100 % for all patients.
   (b) Describe what to do when source documents are incomplete.
   (c) Describe what to do when source documents are not consistent with data in the CRF
8. Verification of CRFs
   (a) Describe details with respect to the verification of CRFs. Describe which cross-checks must be performed.
9. Collection of CRFs
   (a) Describe whether copies will be made of completed CRFs.
10. Queries from data management
    (a) Describe the procedure for handling data management queries.
11. Overviews
    (a) Describe which overviews will be kept on the computer, the update frequency, quality control, and printing of these overviews.

Reporting of each monitor visit should take place, and appropriate actions must be taken when the investigational team does not comply with the agreed protocol, procedures, GCP, and other applicable regulatory requirements. If the investigational site repeatedly breeches the agreements, i.e., serious noncompliance exists, then this should be reported to the regulatory authorities of the country where the study is conducted and to the applicable Ethics Committee.

From the above, it can be learned that monitoring is a "conditio sine qua non" (a condition without which it does not exist) for clinical research. Not only when new (radio)pharmaceutical drugs are involved but in virtually any clinical research. At this moment, industry-driven research is well monitored, often by independent monitoring companies. But monitoring in hospital-driven research is less well developed, unfortunately. In order to improve transparency and quality of the process, we would urgently advise the hospital authorities to arrange a proper monitoring system within their hospital.

2.4.10 Auditing

The sponsor determines if auditing is necessary. The sponsor needs to draft a quality policy describing how the quality assurance system will be conducted. In this policy, the sponsor should describe how the quality in the clinical studies will be ensured. One of the means to check this is to arrange for audits. Both on-site clinical audits at the investigator's site and laboratory audits of the organization supporting the study and organization and system audits at the offices of the sponsor or CRO. For studies with medicinal products, the audit certificate demonstrating that an audit of this study has taken place, by whom, when, and how is an integral part of the clinical study report that has to be submitted to the regulatory authorities.

2.4.11 Inspection

When a competent regulatory authority will start an official investigation to verify if the clinical study has been conducted in compliance with the study protocol, GCP, and the applicable regulatory requirements, then we refer to this event as an inspection. The inspectors will investigate the documentation of the study (trial master file and all investigator files), the facilities and used equipment, and all other sources that refer to this clinical study. They will also plan various interviews with the involved parties. The inspection can take place at the investigator site or at the offices of the sponsor, CRO, or both.

2.5 Noncompliance to GCP

If an investigator or members of his/her staff do not follow guidances, instructions, procedures, and the study protocol, then the sponsor should take appropriate measure to ensure compliance.

If the investigator seriously, repeatedly, and persistently does not comply with the rules and appropriate measures were already taken, then the participation of this site should be ended, and the regulatory authorities should be informed. Thereafter, the sponsor informs both this investigator and the IEC and the regulatory authorities that the participation of this site has been suspended or ended.

The sponsor ensures that a proper clinical study report will be written and sent to the competent regulatory authorities as required by law. The sponsor takes care that all investigators follow the guidelines for the conduct of the study.

It should be realized that noncompliance with GCP rules and regulations is a felony in many countries, certainly in the countries of the EU.

2.6 Clinical Investigations with Medical Devices

Rules and regulations for medical devices, i.e., a wide range of products from simple bandages to the most sophisticated life-supporting or diagnostic products, require that clinical evidence should be present to proof that the medical device is safe, independent of their risk classification. Within the European Union, the so-called Medical Device Directive (MDD) was originally launched in 1993 with the aim of harmonizing the laws in the different member states and was revised in 2007. In this directive, medical devices are divided in three risk classifications, Class Ia, Im, IIa, IIb, or III.[9] Article 11 of the MDD states that procedures should be implemented by the manufacturer to demonstrate that their products (equipment or prostheses) should comply to the European directives in order to apply for the CE certification in order that the public should be reassured that the product complies with the directive with respect to the properties, functions or proposed use and will be subdivided in one of the four risk classes:

Table medical device risk classification

Class I	Devices with a low risk Sterile devices (Class Is) Devices in Class I with a measuring function (Class Im)
Class II(a) en Class II(b)	Devices with an intermediate risk
Class III	Devices with a high risk

A part of the clinical evidence is a critical evaluation of existing relevant literature and a survey of the clinical data of an equivalent product and all nonpublished data. This analysis is a part of the clinical evaluation report that should be submitted to the notified body responsible for the assessment of the product. When the clinical evaluation report cannot substantiate that the product is safe and complies therefore to the European essential safety requirements then a new prospective trial with the new product should be initiated.

A medical device that formally has been approved for the European market bears a CE label (Conformité Européenne), which signifies that the competent regulatory authority of that European member state approved the conformity assessment of the product conducted by the notified body. For Class I medical devices (no risk to the patient, e.g., a hospital bed), the product can be self-certified by the manufacturer.

[9]Annex IX of the Medical Device Directive. http://ec.europa.eu/health/medical-devices/index_en.htm.

For certain types of medical devices, a prospective controlled trial is required if the product will be submitted to a regulatory authority for market approval, and the product can influence the safety and well-being of the user:

1. High risk or critical medical devices (active implantable, Class III devices, implantable or long-term invasive devices of Class IIa or IIb, devices that can support body function)
2. New devices or new technologies where components, materials, functions, mechanisms of action, or the technology are not known and for which no precedent exists with respect to the performance of this product in literature
3. Devices using new materials or components used in another way or elsewhere in the body or another application and has never been used in another medical device
4. Devices with existing (known) materials or components used in another way, in another application or elsewhere in the body
5. Existing devices who have been modified in such a manner that the modification could have an big impact on the clinical safety and performance of the medical device
6. Well-known certified medical devices for new indications, new applications, or a new claim
7. Devices that will be used much longer than anticipated at the beginning

The study with non-CE-certified medical devices should be conducted in compliance with the ISO standard 14155 and the general principles of Good Clinical Practice including the Declaration of Helsinki. Studies with devices that are not yet placed on the market are by definitions intervention studies and have to be submitted to an Ethics Committee for assessment. The study has also to be submitted to the regulatory authorities for assessment.

The reporting of incidents with medical devices in studies to the authorities can be summarized as follows. For pre-CE studies, SAEs and serious adverse device effects (SADEs) should be reported within 7 calendar days and within 2 calendar days for serious unexpected adverse device effects (USADEs). Events that have taken place outside the European Union, Turkey, and Switzerland do not need to be reported.

Normally, nuclear medicine physicians and clinical physicists working in clinical practice will limit their activities to checking whether the CE certification has been issued, as applying for the certification is the task of the manufacturer. However, in case the device is used for different purposes as the original CE certification was issued, or in case of a beta-site testing environment (in cooperation with the manufacturer), the above given rules apply.

2.6.1 Radiopharmaceuticals

From a legal point of view, there is no difference between "normal" pharmaceuticals and radiopharmaceuticals.[10] The distinction simply is not made. Consequently,

[10] Directive 2001/83/EC. *Off J Eur Union* 2001;L(311):67–128.

studies with radiopharmaceuticals are subject to the rules and regulations described above. Despite the fact that adverse events are unlikely to occur because of the low amounts of substance administered. For example, in 30 years of worldwide clinical positron emission tomography, only one case report with an adverse event has been described. This concerns a case of ^{18}F-DOPA, which was administered too fast in a patient with a carcinoid. The patient subsequently developed a carcinoid crisis. After changing the protocol for administration, the event was never seen again.[11]

In contrast to the low pharmaceutical risks, one has to take the justification of using radioactivity into account and adhere to the so-called as low as reasonably achievable (ALARA) principle. By law there are no limitations to the use of radioactivity to a patient, provided it is applied for diagnosis and/or treatment of the illness. In healthy volunteers, however, the International Commission on Radiological Protection (ICRP) has set limitations.[12] In publication number 62 of the ICRP (ICRP-62), the risks associated with radiation exposure are divided into three categories:

Level of risk	Category	Detriment[a]	Corresponding effective dose (mSv)	Level of societal benefit
"Trivial"	I	< Approximately 10^{-6}	<0.1	"Minor"
"Minor to intermediate"	IIa	Approximately 10^{-5}	0.1–1.0	"Intermediate to moderate"
	IIb	Approximately 10^{-4}	1–10	
"Moderate"	III	> Approximately 10^{-3}	>10	"Substantial"

[a]Detriment = total damage for adults [= sum of all fatal cancers + weighed average of nonfatal cancers + risk of serious genetic diseases in the next generation(s)]. For children, the detriment is set to be approximately 2–3 times that of adults; for adults >50 yrs the detriment is set to be 10–20 % that of adults

The question is what category is acceptable in healthy volunteers, if acceptable at all. Generally, in our experience, the idea is that an exposure to the max of category II (10 mSv) is the maximum acceptable exposure in healthy volunteers. However, each investigator will also have to proof to the judging Ethics Committee that the use of radioactivity cannot be avoided.

Some Ethics Committees have argued that a patient, irrespective of the underlying disease or age, should be treated as a healthy volunteer in case he or she is entered in a clinical study, and therefore the same limitations, i.e., 10 mSv, apply. We tend to disagree with this opinion, as it does not take into account the risks of the disease of the patient, which will be much more life-threatening than the use of radioactivity. Already in 1990, Holm related the radiation dose to the negative effects of chemotherapy and proved that the detrimental effects of chemotherapy are

[11] Koopmans KP, Brouwers AH, De Hooge MN, et al. Carcinoid Crisis After Injection of 6-18 F-Fluorodihydroxyphenylalanine in a Patient with Metastatic Carcinoid. *J Nucl Med* 2005; 46:1240–1243.

[12] ICRP Publication 62. *Radiological Protection in Biomedical Research. International Commission on Radiological Protection*. Oxford, Pergamon Press 1993.

comparable to those of radiotherapy and also that the effects of extra diagnostic procedures are negligible.[13] Also, the ICRP-62 suggests us that the age of the patient should be taken into account, with increased risks in children (which therefore are preferably excluded from participation) but also reduced risks at an older age. These risks should then be compared to the life expectancy of the patients. For example, the overall survival for non-small cell lung cancer is around 49 % after 5 years in stage Ia patients but around 1 % in stage IV patients.[14]

2.7 Production of PET Radiopharmaceuticals

The past few years, a hefty discussion has been going on between the authorities, the pharmaceutical industries, and PET centers with a cyclotron on-site that produce their own radiopharmaceuticals. The initial outcome of this discussion is that PET centers were to be equated with the pharmaceutical industry in terms of provisions and legislation, despite the fact that they produce small quantities of PET radiopharmaceuticals for in-house use and despite the special nature of radiopharmaceuticals. This became a real hurdle in the implementation of new radiopharmaceutical developments into the clinic. Despite initiatives from the field to counteract these developments, this has only led to limited success. In Regulation (EU) No 536/2014 on clinical trials, which focuses on patient safety and reasonable and proportionate risk assessments, several exceptions for radiopharmaceuticals were introduced, such as no need to hold an authorization for manufacture or hold of radiopharmaceuticals used as diagnostic IMPs when carried out in hospitals or simplified labeling of radio pharmaceuticals.[15,16]

Conclusions

Nuclear medicine departments involved in clinical research are by law obliged to adhere to ICH GCP guidelines. Irrespective whether they are the sponsor of the trial or whether they are just supporting in performing the study.

GCP asks a thorough documentation of data in order to ascertain the reliability and transparency of the study. This asks a quality system that centers can fall back to.

The use of radiopharmaceuticals should make every investigator ask himself or herself again and again whether the use of radioactivity is valid in the specific study and specific patient group or volunteer group.

[13] Holm LE. Cancer occurring after radiotherapy and chemotherapy. *Int J Radiat Oncol Biol Physics* 1990;19(5):1303–1308.

[14] www.cancer.org

[15] Regulation (EU) No 536/2014. *Off J Eur Union* 2014;L(158):1–76.

[16] Decristoforo C, Penuelas I, Elsinga P, et al. Radiopharmaceuticals are specials, but is this recognized? The possible impact of the new Clinical Trials Regulation on the preparation of radiopharmaceuticals. *Eur J Nucl Med Molec Imaging* 2014;41:2005–2007.

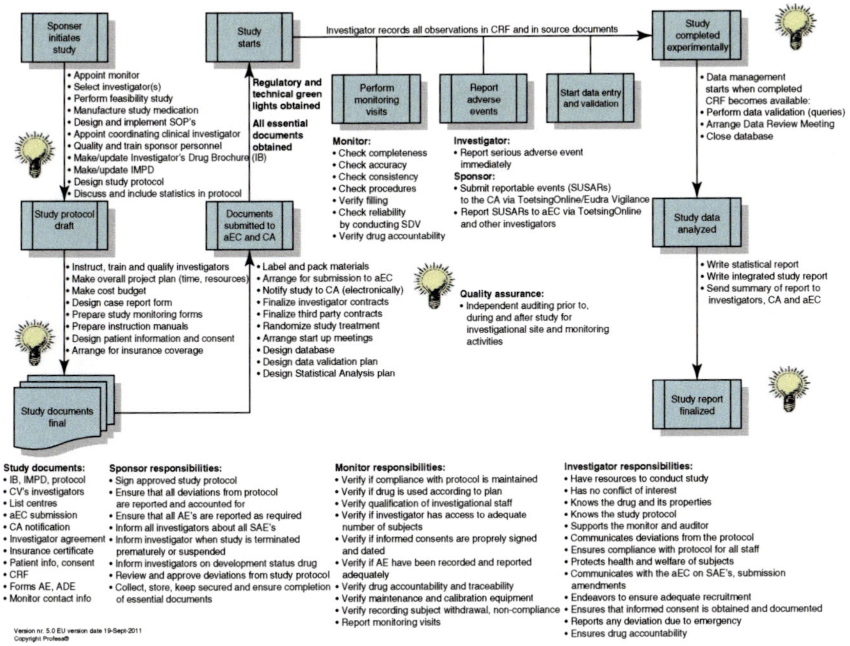
Sponser initiates study
• Appoint monitor
• Select investigator(s)
• Perform feasibility study
• Manufacture study medication
• Design and implement SOP's
• Appoint coordinating clinical investigator
• Quality and train sponsor personnel
• Make/update Investigator's Drug Brochure (IB)
• Make/update IMPD
• Design study protocol
• Discuss and include statistics in protocol
Study protocol draft
• Instruct, train and qualify investigators
• Make overall project plan (time, resources)
• Make cost budget
• Design case report form
• Prepare study monitoring forms
• Prepare instruction manuals
• Design patient information and consent
• Arrange for insurance coverage
Study documents final
Documents submitted to aEC and CA
• Label and pack materials
• Arrange for submission to aEC
• Notify study to CA (electronically)
• Finalize investigator contracts
• Finalize third party contracts
• Randomize study treatment
• Arrange start up meetings
• Design database
• Design data validation plan
• Design Statistical Analysis plan
Regulatory and technical green lights obtained
All essential documents obtained
Study starts
Investigator records all observations in CRF and in source documents
Perform monitoring visits
Report adverse events
Start data entry and validation
Monitor:
• Check completeness
• Check accuracy
• Check consistency
• Check procedures
• Verify filling
• Check reliability by conducting SDV
• Verify drug accountability
Investigator:
• Report serious adverse event immediately
Sponsor:
• Submit reportable events (SUSARs) to the CA via ToetsingOnline/Eudra Vigilance
• Report SUSARs to aEC via ToetsingOnline and other investigators
Quality assurance:
• Independent auditing prior to, during and after study for investigational site and monitoring activities
Study completed experimentally
• Data management starts when completed CRF becomes available:
• Perform data validation (queries)
• Arrange Data Review Meeting
• Close database
Study data analyzed
• Write statistical report
• Write integrated study report
• Send summary of report to investigators, CA and aEC
Study report finalized
Study documents:
• IB, IMPD, protocol
• CV's investigators
• List centres
• aEC submission
• CA notification
• Investigator agreement
• Insurance certificate
• Patient info, consent
• CRF
• Forms AE, ADE
• Monitor contact info
Sponsor responsibilities:
• Sign approved study protocol
• Ensure that all deviations from protocol are reported and accounted for
• Ensure that all AE's are reported as required
• Inform all investigators about all SAE's
• Inform investigator when study is terminated prematurely or suspended
• Inform investigators on development status drug
• Review and approve deviations from study protocol
• Collect, store, keep secured and ensure completion of essential documents
Monitor responsibilities:
• Verify if compliance with protocol is maintained
• Verify if drug is used according to plan
• Verify qualification of investigational staff
• Verify if investigator has access to adequate number of subjects
• Verify if informed consents are proprely signed and dated
• Verify if AE have been recorded and reported adequately
• Verify drug accountability and traceability
• Verify maintenance and calibration equipment
• Verify recording subject withdrawal, non-compliance
• Report monitoring visits
Investigator responsibilities:
• Have resources to conduct study
• Has no conflict of interest
• Knows the drug and its properties
• Knows the study protocol
• Supports the monitor and auditor
• Communicates deviations from the protocol
• Ensures compliance with protocol for all staff
• Protects health and welfare of subjects
• Communicates with the aEC on SAE's, submission amendments
• Endeavors to ensure adequate recruitment
• Ensures that informed consent is obtained and documented
• Reports any deviation due to emergency
• Ensures drug accountability
Version nr. 5.0 EU version date 19-Sept-2011
Copyright Profess®

The Added Value of Good Manufacturing Practices (GMP) in the Production of Radiopharmaceuticals

3

Edwin Gerrits, Herman J. Woerdenbag, Gert Luurtsema, Marjolijn N. Lub-de Hooge, and Hendrikus H. Boersma

Abstract

Manufacturers of medicinal products including radiopharmaceuticals have to follow regulations from their governmental organizations as well as professional societies to ensure built-in quality combined with patient safety issues. This chapter is a concise review of Good Manufacturing Practices (GMP) with a special focus on the production of radiopharmaceuticals. Furthermore, attention is given to the added value of GMP as a tool for providing more insights and awareness. Working under GMP conditions leads to potentially faster problem solving in daily practice, as compared to the "skills-only"-based approach. The latter had been a mainstay for a long time but is being more and more replaced by a "skills-based and oversight approach" nowadays.

E. Gerrits
Department of Clinical Pharmacy and Pharmacology, University of Groningen, University Medical Center Groningen, Groningen, The Netherlands

Department of Pharmaceutical Technology and Biopharmacy, University of Groningen, Groningen, The Netherlands

H.J. Woerdenbag
Department of Pharmaceutical Technology and Biopharmacy, University of Groningen, Groningen, The Netherlands

G. Luurtsema
Department of Nuclear Medicine and Molecular Imaging, University of Groningen, University Medical Center Groningen, Groningen, The Netherlands

M.N.L.-d. Hooge • H.H. Boersma (✉)
Department of Clinical Pharmacy and Pharmacology, University of Groningen, University Medical Center Groningen, Groningen, The Netherlands

Department of Nuclear Medicine and Molecular Imaging, University of Groningen, University Medical Center Groningen, Groningen, The Netherlands
e-mail: h.h.boersma@umcg.nl

A.W.J.M. Glaudemans et al. (eds.), *Quality in Nuclear Medicine*,
DOI 10.1007/978-3-319-33531-5_3

"If it is not documented, it is not done"

3.1 Introduction

For a consumer, it is usually difficult to judge whether a drug product will work, is safe enough to use, or, in the worst case, might inflict harm. Therefore, quality assurance (QA) is an indispensable aspect in the production of (radio)pharmaceuticals. QA can be considered as the sum of organized arrangements with the objective of ensuring that products will be of the quality required for their intended use. For the production of pharmaceuticals, Good Manufacturing Practices (GMP) are an important aspect of QA. According to the European Medicines Agency (EMA), GMP is defined as "that part of quality assurance which ensures that products are consistently produced and controlled to the quality standards appropriate to their intended use" (EMA website, visited October 2014). GMP guidelines must ensure that a product is suitable for use and that it contains the ingredients as indicated and possesses the strength it claims to have (EMA website, no year indicated). GMP guidelines contain minimal and concise requirements for the methods, facilities, and controls used in manufacturing, processing, and packing of a drug product.

Working according to GMP requires full discipline from all personnel, especially from those that are not familiar with the legislations and the documentation describing the incorporation and implementation of GMP guidelines in the working environment. The aim of the current chapter is to evaluate the added value of GMP in the production of radiopharmaceuticals in a hospital setting. First, an introduction into GMP is given. Second, guidelines applicable to the small-scale radiopharmacy are presented. Third, the importance of GMP and its added value for the quality of radiopharmaceuticals are underlined and discussed.

3.2 An Introduction into Good Manufacturing Practices (GMP)

GMP consists of a set of guidelines which, when translated into procedures and implemented by manufacturers for therapeutic goods, should ensure that the products manufactured under these conditions possess the required quality. GMP primarily aims to diminish the risks inherent to any pharmaceutical production, such as contamination and mix-ups.

The World Health Organization (WHO) recently compiled an important report on the specifications of pharmaceutical preparations. In Annex 2 of this report, the basic requirements for GMP are summarized as follows (WHO-GMP 2014):

(a) *All manufacturing processes are clearly defined, systematically reviewed in the light of experience, and shown to be capable of consistently manufacturing pharmaceutical products of the required quality that comply with their specifications.*

(b) *Qualification and validation are performed.*
(c) *All necessary resources are provided, including:*
  (i) *Sufficient appropriately qualified and trained personnel*
  (ii) *Adequate premises and space*
  (iii) *Suitable equipment and services*
  (iv) *Appropriate materials, containers, and labels*
  (v) *Approved procedures and instructions*
  (vi) *Suitable storage and transport*
  (vii) *Adequate personnel, laboratories, and equipment for in-process controls*
(d) *Instructions and procedures are written in clear and unambiguous language, specifically applicable to the facilities provided.*
(e) *Procedures are carried out correctly and personnel are trained to do so.*
(f) *Records are made (manually and/or by recording instruments) during manufacture to show that all the steps required by the defined procedures and instructions have in fact been taken and that the quantity and quality of the product are as expected. Any significant deviations are fully recorded and investigated with the objective of determining the root cause and appropriate corrective and preventive action is implemented.*
(g) *Records covering manufacture and distribution, which enable the complete history of a batch to be traced, are retained in a comprehensible and accessible form.*
(h) *The proper storage and distribution of the products minimizes any risk to their quality and takes account of good distribution practices (GDP).*
(i) *A system is available to recall any batch of product from sale or supply.*
(j) *Complaints about marketed products are examined, the causes of quality defects investigated, and appropriate measures taken in respect of the defective products to prevent recurrence.*

3.3 Guidelines for Radiopharmaceuticals

Throughout the world, the production of radiopharmaceuticals varies greatly, depending on the level of expertise, available equipment, and size of the organization. In recent years, it has become more apparent that (inter)national regulatory agencies for radiopharmaceutical legislation started to collaborate to achieve a global-wide applicable set of documents for the implementation of GMP guidelines. Specific guidelines regarding radiopharmaceuticals are described in a dedicated GMP Annex (Annex 3). All GMP guidelines and related documents are published online in the Eudralex, a web-based compendium of European pharmaceutical legislation (Eudralex, EU-GMP, website visited October 2014). Annex 3 covers various aspects, including the importance of quality assurance in the manufacturing of radiopharmaceuticals in relation to their particular characteristics, such as low volumes, the occasional administration of the product before quality testing is completed, and the use of hot cells. Furthermore it addresses all general topics of GMP (documentation, personnel, premises and equipment, documentation, production, quality control, and distribution) that of course also apply for radiopharmaceuticals.

The drawback of the GMP documents is that they focus mainly on industrial, large-scale production and that they are difficult to apply as such for preparations that are performed on a smaller scale in, for example, hospital pharmacies or nuclear medicine centers. To overcome this gap, several sets of guidelines have been drawn up recently, based on "conventional" GMP, focusing mainly on the production of radiopharmaceuticals in a clinical setting, thereby also giving more guidance to GMP in a smaller setting. The Radiopharmacy Committee of the European Association of Nuclear Medicine published the "Guidelines on Current Good Radiopharmacy Practices (cGRPP) in the preparation of radiopharmaceuticals" (Guidelines on cGRPP 2007). The Pharmaceutical Inspection Convention / Pharmaceutical Inspection Co-operation Scheme (PIC/S) in addition provided a number of useful references for quality assurance into the production of radiopharmaceuticals in the small-scale setting. These guidelines are found in the document "PIC/S Guide to good practices for the preparation of medicinal products in healthcare establishments" (PIC/S 2008). Finally, the International Atomic Energy Agency published "Operational Guidance on Hospital Radiopharmacy: A safe and Effective approach" (IAEA 2008). In this document, essential details are provided ensuring the use of a safe and effective approach in the hospital radiopharmacy. The application and interpretation of all available guidelines to relevant topics are elaborated below (Guidelines on cGRPP 2007; Elsinga et al. 2010; PIC/S 2008; IAEA 2008).

3.3.1 Personnel and Resources

All personnel should be appropriately trained (and maintained well trained) in all aspects of quality assurance in which they are involved. As radiopharmaceuticals are mainly administered by intravenous injection, personnel should have knowledge and skills of applying aseptic techniques. An important focus also lies with radiation protection. Moreover, a main challenge is to optimize the air pressure in the radiopharmaceutical production cleanroom complex. The latter in order to comply with both GMP and nuclear energy laws at the same time. Training concerning the safe handling of radioactive products should be given to all personnel employed in areas where radioactive products are handled. With approved personnel dosimeters, which are regularly checked and their readings recorded, personnel should be controlled for radiation exposure (Guidelines on cGRPP 2007; Elsinga et al. 2010). Additionally, radiopharmacy staff should receive training in (inter)national legislation related to ionizing radiation regulations (Guidelines on cGRPP, 2007; Elsinga et al. 2010; PIC/S 2008; IAEA 2008). Furthermore, these rules are to be followed by cleaning staff and technical maintenance staff in a similar way, certainly when these individuals work in a sophisticated environment with hot cell containing cleanrooms and (dedicated) synthesis modules, e.g., for the production of small PET molecules.

3.3.2 Quality Assurance

Most radionuclides are short living and thus pose additional implications on the quality assurance system, due to their short half-life and rapid decay. When preparing or synthesizing radiopharmaceuticals in a small-scale radiopharmacy, a full QA system should be in place. This system must cover preparation methods and should assure that sufficient quality is implemented in the production of PET radionuclides by incorporating the principles of GMP, cGRPP, and an appropriate risk assessment. In the European Union (EU), a difference is made between GMP part II (production of the molecule) and manufacturing of the final product (GMP part I). In many cases, this opens the opportunity to operate under less strict conditions before the purification step and final formulation of the final radiopharmaceutical, for which the regular GMP guidelines apply (Eudralex, EU-GMP, website visited October 2014). Before a product can be released, a rapid but strict QA system should be applied, requiring short communication links and immediate follow-up. All documents of the QA system should be filed to monitor its effectiveness and to oversee the preparation operations in the course of time (Guidelines on cGRPP 2007; Elsinga et al. 2010; PIC/S 2008; IAEA 2008).

3.3.3 Equipment and Facilities

In small-scale radiopharmacy units, premises should be designed in such a way that minimal risk of causing contamination of materials and products is assured. Adequate measures should also be taken to protect the operator from the materials being handled, to avoid the spread of radioactivity, and to prevent microbiological contamination from controlled areas. Working under negative pressure is a proven method to protect the operator and environment from contamination with radioactivity. Executing the production in a lead-shielded compartment, the hot cell, is another method to protect both operator and environment. Suitable shielding of the hot cells according to the energy and type of emission of the radionuclide should be taken into account. Ideally, the hot cells where synthesis takes place should operate under grade C (according to GMP) environment. An adjacent grade A LAF work bench and/or a grade A/B hot cell used for dispensing should be present, while the whole system should be located in a room meeting grade C level. In an optimal setting, adjacent technical rooms meet at least grade D level.

Although a properly designed area in a room can be used for several different purposes in the small-scale radiopharmacy, an appropriate level of consciousness and awareness is always required to prevent possible contamination and mix-ups. Therefore, the use of disposables for most synthesis processes is to be advocated in order to prevent contamination partially.

The aseptic working area should comply with appropriate environmental requirements to be suitable for the preparation of injectable materials. All surfaces, such as walls, floors, and ceilings, should be made in such a way that they can be easily cleaned, disinfected, and, in case of radioactive spill, decontaminated. The workstation and the environment should be monitored on a regular basis for microbiological contamination by using settle plates, particle counters, and/or swabs, during entire preparation procedures or during selected critical steps. Cleaning duties may only be performed by staff who has received documented training regarding relevant elements according to GMP.

All equipment used in the (automated) production of radiopharmaceuticals must be exclusively reserved for this purpose and should be properly installed, maintained, and validated. For final purification, preparative HPLC columns or other chromatography methods are in use. Calibration procedures should be executed regularly, usually following the recommendation of the supplier, unless the responsible person determines that a different frequency is preferred. In all cases, standard operational procedures (SOPs) are available. Measuring radioactivity in the working areas is an important safety aspect in the production of radiopharmaceuticals. Dose calibrators used for this purpose require a background activity check each time they are used, in order to compensate for the everyday present radiation in the environment.

Before entering a production facility, a gowning area should be in place, restricted to authorized personnel only. All operators must wear clothes dedicated to the process and grade of the work area. It should be worn in such a way that it protects the product from contamination from human sources and protects the operator from being contaminated by the environment (Guidelines on cGRPP 2007; Elsinga et al. 2010; PIC/S 2008; IAEA 2008).

3.3.4 Documentation

A good and reliable documentation system is an essential component of each QA system. Detailed control of record-keeping of each produced batch of radiopharmaceuticals is required and should comply with GMP guidelines. Every relevant step in the entire process is documented, either in written form or electronically. This includes, but is not limited to, written specifications of materials, production protocols, QC procedures, SOPs, and maintenance. All documents should be drafted, reviewed, approved, and distributed according to written procedures. Records should be kept and archived for a sufficiently long period to meet legal requirements. All deviations and changes made are documented as well (Guidelines on cGRPP 2007; Elsinga et al. 2010; PIC/S 2008; IAEA 2008).

3.3.5 Production and Process Controls

To ensure the consistent preparation of a radiopharmaceutical, production and process controls should meet the applicable quality standards, including but not limited to written production and process control records, master and batch production, control records, and validation of the production process. Deviations and changes to the production protocol should be carefully documented in order to establish a corrective or action-orientated environment and to timely identify atypical trends. Microbiological control on aseptic processing and sterilizing filtration should guarantee the lack of microbial and endotoxin contamination of radiopharmaceuticals. As aseptic conditions may also be compromised by an environmental deviation, microbial testing of the workstation should be performed regularly as well. Circumstances may force to an increased monitoring frequency, such as detected deviations and changes or interventions in the environment (Guidelines on cGRPP 2007; Elsinga et al. 2010; PIC/S 2008; IAEA 2008).

3.3.6 Laboratory Controls

Each laboratory should be designed for its appropriate use, including but not limited to sampling and testing procedures for in-process controls. Laboratory control (QC) methods, such as HPLC, UPLC, and thin layer chromatography, should be sufficiently sensitive, specific, accurate, and reproducible and should be validated if the method is not described by a pharmacopeia. All materials used in the laboratory should be adequately controlled and labeled to unambiguously indicate their identity and composition. The responsible person, usually the qualified person or the head of production, should ensure that the laboratory has a comprehensive knowledge of microbiology and that microbiological quality assurance systems are regularly reviewed. Equipment must be routinely inspected, maintained, and calibrated. Off-site testing facilities should be regularly audited (Guidelines on cGRPP 2007; Elsinga et al. 2010; PIC/S 2008).

3.3.7 Labeling and Packaging

To protect a product from alteration or damage during storage, handling, distribution, and use, it should be shipped and packaged in appropriate containers. Shelf life and storage conditions are indicated on the label. Labels will preferably be prepared in advance, because of the rapid radiation decline. Ideally, labels are generated using a computerized system. The labels undergo a final check to verify if the product is filled out correctly and completely before the labels are put on the containers (Guidelines on cGRPP 2007; Elsinga et al. 2010).

3.3.8 Complaint Handling

Complaint handling should be performed by a designated individual, responsible for the entire conduct, from collecting information of the drug production to completing the investigation of the involved radiopharmaceutical. All steps in the complaint handling procedure should follow a documented route. Also a suitable procedure should be available to directly and effectively recall an already finished product. A recalled radiopharmaceutical should not be destroyed but stored as a retention sample for analysis until the root cause investigation is performed (Guidelines on cGRPP 2007; Elsinga et al. 2010; PIC/S 2008; IAEA 2008).

3.3.9 Self-Inspection

A self-inspection will ameliorate the quality assurance system when conducted in an independent, detailed way by competent people. Generally, in 3 years, the total contents of GMP should be covered by all executed self-inspections. An inspection of the QA system should be performed at least once a year. Ideally, the premises should be inspected twice a year. Personnel inspections should be random; however, when new personnel is trained and found capable of working independently, additional internal personnel inspections can be performed (Guidelines on cGRPP 2007; Elsinga et al. 2010; PIC/S 2008; IAEA 2008).

3.4 Importance of Guidelines for Radiopharmaceutical Production

Considering the limited time between production of a radiopharmaceutical and its administration to patients, staff has to be confident that the preparation is reliably completed according to the best practices. Although Annex 3 of the GMP is a good guidance for the industrial production, it is hard to apply it directly to the small-scale setting of the manufacture of radiopharmaceuticals (Eudralex, EU-GMP, website visited October 2014). Therefore, several agencies drafted up GMP-derived guidelines that are more tailor made to the small-scale radiopharmacy setting in hospitals (Guidelines on cGRPP 2007; Elsinga et al. 2010; PIC/S 2008; IAEA 2008; Poli et al. 2012; Dechrostoforo and Peňnuelas 2005; Duatti and Bhonsle 2013). Following these GMP-derived guidelines (and always with the general GMP in mind), production facilities are better suited to produce radiopharmaceuticals in a hospital setting. It ensures that personnel is properly trained which in turn will lead to fewer errors, less waste, and a more efficient company performance.

Given the short half-life of commonly used radiopharmaceuticals (e.g., $T_{1/2}$ of ^{11}carbon is 20.4 min), a rapid quality control is needed before a product can be released. According to the requirements of the guidelines, production lines should be short, thereby reducing the time needed for QC. This should ensure that the product is sufficiently radioactive at the time it is administered to the patient.

By using a well-established documentation system, it can be assured that deviations, change controls, and risk assessments are drawn up and that follow-up measures are taken accordingly. This facilitates a critical self-reflection and elicits that mistakes are prevented in an early stage rather than found in later steps of production.

Working according to GMP-derived guidelines not only ensures a better in-house procedure and thus a more reliable product for the patient but can also be favorable in the cooperation with the pharmaceutical industry. Recently, the pharmaceutical industry became more involved in the small-scale production of radiopharmaceuticals. By meeting the requirements of GMP-derived guidelines, high quality can also be achieved in a small-scale setting.

Next to built-in quality of a product, GMP has great value for the regular maintenance of a facility. It creates awareness of many pitfalls in the facility system, and as a result, more problems can and will be solved. When we compare current daily practice of the (radio)pharmacist with the situation two decades ago, a shift from skills-based pharmacist to skills- and quality-based pharmacist is seen. Initially, the only possible conclusion was that "something went wrong." There was no insight in what could be a possible root cause, simply because of the lack of (documented) information. Even when information was available, e.g., caused by the repetitive character of a failure, there was generally a lack of oversight on the entire situation of the radiopharmaceutical facility. The latter has often been an additional complication and has hampered proper problem solving. So, implementation of GMP-derived guidelines will, on top of incorporated safety, lead to more awareness, insights, and an oversight in the situation of a GMP facility at a certain moment.

In conclusion, measuring up to GMP-derived guidelines ensures that quality is not only tested in finished products but rather is built in by design in every single step in a production process, thereby safeguarding the patient and the operator as well as leading to a better maintenance of the operated GMP facility.

References

Decristoforo C, Peñnuelas I. Towards a harmonized radiopharmaceutical regulatory framework in Europe? Q J Nucl Med Mol Imaging. 2005;53:394–401.

Duatti A, Bhonsle U. Strengthening radiopharmacy practice in IAEA member states. Semin Nucl Med. 2013;43:188–94.

Elsinga P, Todde S, Penuelas I, Meyer G, Farstad B, Faivre-Chauvet A, Mikolajczak R, Wester G, Gmeiner-Stopar T, Decristoforo C. Guidance on current good radiopharmacy practice (cGRPP) for the small-scale preparation of radiopharmaceuticals. Eur J Nucl Med Mol Imaging. 2010;37:1049–62.

EMA website (Good-manufacturing-practice and good-distribution-practice compliance). http://www.ema.europa.eu/ema/index.jsp?curl=pages/regulation/document_listing/documentlisting_000154.jsp. Website visited Oct 2014.

Eudralex – volume 4. Good manufacturing practice (GMP) Guidelines. European Commission. http://ec.europa.eu/health/documents/eudralex/vol-4/index_en.htm. Website visited Oct 2014.

Guidelines on current good radiopharmacy practice (cGRPP) in the preparation of radiopharmaceuticals. cGRPP-guidelines version 2, march 2007. http://www.eanm.org/publications/guidelines/gl_radioph_cgrpp.pdf. Website visited Oct 2014.

IAEA. Operational guidance on hospital radiopharmacy a safe and effective approach. International Atomic Energy Agency; 2008, ISBN 9201067089, 9789201067081.

PIC/S. Pharmaceutical Inspection Convention/Pharmaceutical Inspection Cooperation Scheme: PIC/S guide to good practices for the preparation of medicinal products in healthcare establishments – PE 010-1 Into force on 1 Oct 2008. http://www.picscheme.org/pdf/23_pe0103-revisedgppguide.pdf.

Poli M, Petroni D, Pardini S, Salvadori PA, Menichetti L. Implementation of a quality assurance system according to GMP and ISO 9001:2008 standard for radiopharmaceutical production in a public research centre. Accred Qual Assur. 2012;17:341–8.

WHO-GMP. WHO good manufacturing practices for pharmaceutical products: main principles. In: WHO Expert Committee on specifications for pharmaceutical preparations. Forty-eighth report. Geneva: World Health Organization; 2014, Annex 2 (WHO Technical Report Series, No. 986).

KEW/Euratom (In Europe and Internationally)

4

Emmy I.M. Meijne

4.1 Introduction

Radioactivity is a natural phenomenon, and ionizing radiation and radioactive substances have many beneficial applications, ranging from power generation to uses in medicine, industry, and agriculture. At the same time, ionizing radiation is a cause of concern because the exposure of the human body may cause health detriment.

In normal situations, doses are very low so that there are no clinically observable tissue effects. There is, however, still possible late effect, in particular cancer. It is assumed that there is no dose threshold for this so-called stochastic effect: any exposure, however small, can be the cause of cancer later in life. It is further assumed that the probability of occurrence of cancer is proportional to the dose.

This has led to the establishment of an approach in radiation protection based on the three principles: justification, optimization, and dose limitation.

1. Justification: an act or action is only justified when the social benefits of the act (e.g., health benefits or economic gain) surpass the disadvantages (increased radiation exposure). An act that is not justified is prohibited.
2. Optimization: radiation exposure should be kept as low as reasonably achievable (ALARA), economic and social aspects taken into account (ALARA principle).
3. Dose limits: to ensure that people are not exposed to unacceptable high radiation exposures dose limits for the public and workers who may not be exceeded. The dose limits are such that deterministic effects are avoided and the risk of stochastic effects remains limited.

E.I.M. Meijne
Manager Radiation Safety, University Medical Center Groningen, Groningen, The Netherlands
e-mail: e.m.i.meije@umcg.nl

A.W.J.M. Glaudemans et al. (eds.), *Quality in Nuclear Medicine*,
DOI 10.1007/978-3-319-33531-5_4

Based on these principles that were established many decades ago by the International Commission on Radiological Protection (ICRP), a system of radiation protection has been build that forms the fundament of all legislation regulating ionizing radiation.

4.2 International Organizations

Regulating radiation safety is a responsibility of national authorities. It was however acknowledged at an early stage that radiation risks may transcend national borders and that international cooperation serves to promote and enhance safety globally. The creation of an international body to both regulate and promote the peaceful use of atomic energy was first proposed in 1953 by Eisenhower, president of the United States, in his Atoms for Peace address to the UN General Assembly. International collaboration between national authorities with regard to the radiation safety on a worldwide level started in 1957 with the establishment of the International Atomic Energy Agency (IAEA) (29th of July) and on a European level by the establishment of the European Atomic Energy Community (Euratom) (Treaty of Rome: 25th of march 1957). Both organizations have published a large number of safety standards and directives that have been used by national authorities to establish their national legislation. The safety standards established by the IAEA and Euratom are in turn based on recommendations and scientific data published by the ICRP and the United Nations Scientific Committee on the Effects of Atomic Radiation (UNSCEAR).

4.2.1 International Atomic Energy Agency (IAEA)

The IAEA is an independent, intergovernmental, science and technology-based organization with more than 2000 staff members. The principle objective of the IAEA is "to accelerate and enlarge the contribution of atomic energy to peace, health and prosperity throughout the world." The programs of the IAEA not only encourage the development of the peaceful applications of nuclear technology but also promote nuclear security and safety (including radiation protection in medicine) and the exchange and training of scientists and experts. The IAEA is authorized to establish or adopt safety standards and to provide for the application of these standards. Some safety standards are developed in cooperation with other bodies in the United Nations system or other specialized agencies, including the Food and Agriculture Organization of the United Nations (FAO), the United Nations Environment Program (UNEP), the International Labor Organization (ILO), the Organization for Economic Co-operation and Development (OECD) Nuclear Energy Agency (NEA), the Pan American Health Organization, and the World Health Organization (WHO). In 2013, 195 States were members of the IAEA.

4.2.2 European Atomic Energy Community (Euratom)

Euratom is an international organization that is legally distinct from the European Union (EU), but has the same members. It was established by the Euratom Treaty on 25 March 1957 alongside the European Economic Community (EEC) by six of the current Member States (Belgium, Germany, France, Italy, Luxembourg, and the Netherlands). Although most other European communities merged to form the European Union, the nuclear program has maintained a legally distinct nature from the European Union. The Euratom Treaty establishing the European Atomic Energy Community (Euratom) was initially created to coordinate the research programs for the peaceful use of nuclear energy and to establish uniform safety standards between European Member States. Over the years, the role of medicine in radiation protection has increased. At present, the overall population exposure due to medical procedures hugely exceeds any other man-made exposure. The protection of the patients and other individuals exposed in medical practice has therefore become one of a main priority task for the European Commission under the Health and Safety Chapter of the Euratom Treaty. Today Euratom acts in several areas connected with atomic energy, including research, the drawing-up of safety standards, and the peaceful uses of nuclear energy.

4.2.3 International Commission on Radiological Protection (ICRP)

The ICRP is an independent international nonprofit organization that provides recommendations and guidance on radiation protection. The members of ICRP are leading scientists and policy makers in the field of radiological protection. The ICRP was established in 1928 by the International Society of Radiology (ISR) to respond to the growing concerns about the effects of ionizing radiation that were observed in the medical community. At the time it was called the International X-ray and Radium Protection Committee (IXRPC). To be able to better take account of uses of radiation outside the medical area, the IXRPC was later restructured and in 1950 ICRP was given its present name. Since its establishment, ICRP has developed and elaborated a system of radiological protection that is used worldwide as the common basis for radiological protection standards, legislation, guidelines, and practice.

ICRP is comprised of a main commission, five standing committees (on radiation effects (Com. 1), doses from radiation exposure (Com. 2), protection in medicine (Com. 3), application of the commission recommendations (Com. 4), and the protection of the environment (Com. 5)), and a series of task groups and working parties. The scope of committee 3 not only includes medical exposures (primarily to patients but also occupational exposures to healthcare staff and members of the public resulting from the use of radiation in medical practices.

ICRP works closely together with the International Commission on Radiation Units and Measurements (ICRU) and has official relationships with UNSCEAR, WHO, and the IAEA. In addition ICRP works with a large number of other organizations which includes the European Commission. Originally the ICRP published its recommendations and advice as papers in various scientific journals in the fields of medicine and physics. Since 1977 the ICRP has its own series of publications in the shape of a scientific journal, the Annals of the ICRP (publications applicable to medical exposure are listed in Appendix IV). Legislation in most countries adheres closely to ICRP recommendations. The International Basic Safety Standards (IAEA) are based heavily on the ICRP recommendations, and European legislation has always followed the recommendation of ICRP.

4.2.4 United Nations Scientific Committee on the Effects of Atomic Radiation (UNSCEAR)

UNSCEAR was set up by resolution of the United Nations General Assembly in 1955. More than 25 countries provide scientists to serve as members of the committee which holds formal meetings annually. The organization has no power to set radiation standards nor to make recommendations. It was established solely to "define precisely the present exposure of the population of the world to ionizing radiation." Since its institution, UNSCEAR has issued 21 major publications. These reports are highly regarded as principal sources of authoritative information. Governments and organizations throughout the world, including ICRP, rely on the Committee's estimates as the scientific basis for evaluating radiation risk and for establishing protective measures.

4.3 IAEA Safety Standards and Their Application

Article III.6 of the IAEA statute authorizes the Agency to establish or adopt safety standards.

ARTICLE III: Functions

A. The Agency is authorized:

6. To establish or adopt, in consultation and, where appropriate, in collaboration with the competent organs of the United Nations and with the specialized agencies concerned, standards of safety for protection of health and minimization of danger to life and property (including such standards for labour conditions), and to provide for the application of these standards to its own operation as well as to the operations making use of materials, services, equipment, facilities, and information made available by the Agency or at its request or under its control or supervision; and to provide for the application of these standards, at the request of the parties, to operations under any bilateral or multilateral arrangements, or, at the request of a State, to any of that State's activities in the field of atomic energy;

The IAEA started its safety standards program in 1958. The safety standards published by the IAEA reflect an international consensus on what constitutes a high level of safety for the protection of people and the environment from harmful effects of ionizing radiation. The publications by means of which the IAEA establishes its safety standards are issued in the IAEA Safety Standards Series. They are approved by the IAEA Board of Governors. The series covers nuclear safety, radiation safety, transport safety and waste safety. There are three publication categories in the Safety Standard Series: (1) safety fundamentals, 2) safety requirements, and 3) safety guides.

1. Safety fundamentals
   Safety fundamentals present the fundamental safety objective and principles of protection and safety and provide the basis and rationale for the safety requirements.
2. Safety requirements
   The safety requirements establish the requirements that must be met to ensure the protection of people and the environment, both now and in the future. The requirements are governed by the objective and principles of the safety fundamentals. If the requirements are not met, measures must be taken to reach or restore the required level of safety.
3. Safety guides
   Safety guides provide recommendations and guidance on how to comply with the safety requirements. The safety guides present international good practices, and increasingly they reflect best practices that help users striving to achieve high levels of safety.
   The coherence and hierarchy of the IAEA safety standards are given in Fig. 4.1.

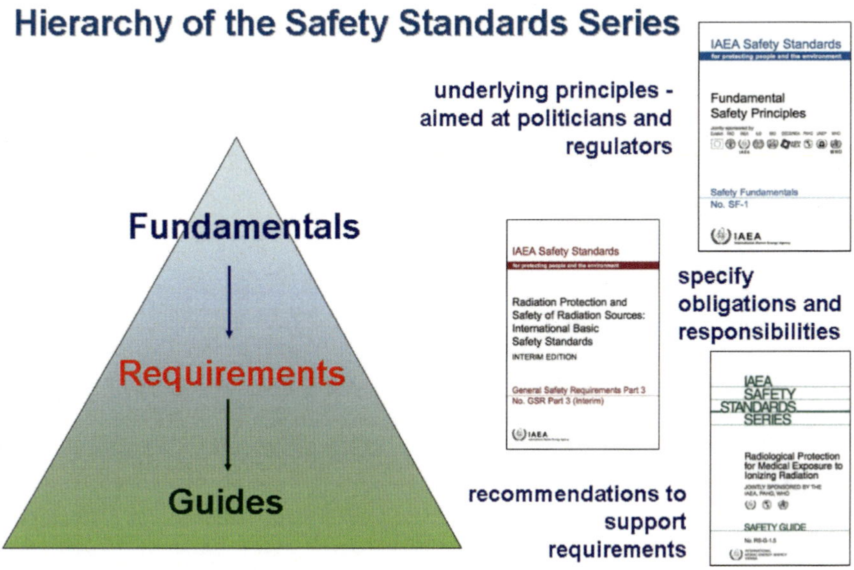

Fig. 4.1 Hierarchy of the IAEA Safety standards publication Series

Fundamental safety objectives and safety principles are the bases of the IAEA's safety standards and its safety-related program. The fundamental safety objective of the IAEA is to "protect people and the environment from the harmful effects of ionizing radiation."

Ten safety principles have been formulated, on the basis of which the safety requirements are developed and safety measures have to be implemented. The ten safety principles form a set that is applicable in its entirety.

1. Responsibility for safety: The prime responsibility for safety must rest with the person or organization responsible for facilities and activities that give rise to radiation risks.
2. Role of government: An effective legal and governmental framework for safety, including an independent regulatory body, must be established and sustained.
3. Leadership and management for safety: Effective leadership and management for safety must be established and sustained in organizations concerned with, and facilities and activities that give rise to, radiation risks.
4. Justification of facilities and activities: Facilities and activities that give rise to radiation risks must yield an overall benefit.
5. Optimization of protection: Protection must be optimized to provide the highest level of safety that can reasonably be achieved.
6. Limitation of risks to individuals: Measures for controlling radiation risks must ensure that no individual bears an unacceptable risk of harm.
7. Protection of present and future generations: People and the environment, present and future, must be protected against radiation risks.
8. Prevention of accidents: All practical efforts must be made to prevent and mitigate nuclear or radiation accidents.
9. Emergency preparedness and response: Arrangements must be made for emergency preparedness and response for nuclear or radiation incidents.
10. Protective actions to reduce existing or unregulated radiation risks: Protective actions to reduce existing or unregulated radiation risks must be justified and optimized.

The three general principles of radiation protection (justification, optimization of protection, and the application of dose limits) are expressed in safety principles 4, 5, 6, and 10.

In addition to the safety standard, the IAEA has published a large number of lower level documents. Reports on safety and protection in nuclear activities are issued as safety reports, which provide practical examples and detailed methods that can be used in support of the safety standards. Other safety-related IAEA publications are issued as radiological assessment reports, technical reports, and TECDOCs. The IAEA also issues reports on radiological accidents, training manuals and practical manuals, and other special safety-related publications. Examples of these reports are shown in Fig. 4.2. An overview of all IAEA publications can be found on the website of the IAEA (http://www.iaea.org/Publications/).

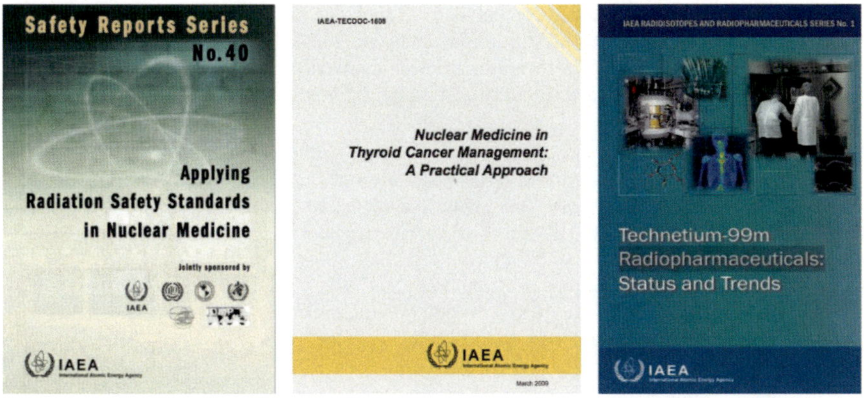

Fig. 4.2 Examples of IAEA documents that provide guidance and technical information for the implementation of the safety standards

The IAEA's statute makes the safety standards binding on the IAEA in relation to its own operations and also on States in relation to IAEA-assisted operations. They also form the basis for the IAEA's safety review services. For individual Member States, the International BSS are nonbinding in nature. They, however, provide support to States in meeting their obligations under general principles of international laws. The IAEA safety standards are intended to apply primarily to new buildings and activities and therefore might not be fully met by older existing facilities. Individual States have to take this into account when establishing legislation.

4.4 Radiation Protection System of Euratom

The Euratom Treaty forms the regulatory basis for Euratom. Euratom's competence to regulate in the field of health protection against ionizing radiation is explicitly recognized in Title I Article 2b. The requirements for radiation protection are laid down in Title II Chapter 3 "Health and Safety," Articles 30–39 of the Euratom Treaty.

TITLE I – The tasks of the Community

Article 2
In order to perform its task, the Community shall, as provided in this Treaty:
b. establish uniform safety standards to protect the health of workers and of the general public and ensure that they are applied;

TITLE II – Provisions for the encouragement of progress in the field of nuclear energy

CHAPTER 3 HEALTH AND SAFETY
Article 30
Basic standards shall be laid down within the Community for the protection of the health of workers and the general public against the dangers arising from ionizing radiations. The expression "basic standards" means:

a. maximum permissible doses compatible with adequate safety;
b. maximum permissible levels of exposure and contamination;
c. the fundamental principles governing the health surveillance of workers.

Article 31
The basic standards shall be worked out by the Commission after it has obtained the opinion of a group of persons appointed by the Scientific and Technical Committee from among scientific experts, and in particular public health experts, in the Member States. The Commission shall obtain the opinion of the Economic and Social Committee on these basic standards.

After consulting the European Parliament the Council shall, on a proposal from the Commission, which shall forward to it the opinions obtained from these Committees, establish the basic standards; the Council shall act by a qualified majority.

There are three basic types of EU legislation: regulations, directives, and decisions.

1. Regulations: Regulations are the most direct form of EU law – as soon as they are passed, they have binding legal force throughout every Member State, on a par with national laws. National governments do not have to take action themselves to implement EU regulations. A regulation is similar to a national law with the difference that it is applicable in all EU countries.
2. Directives: Directives set out general rules to be transferred into national law by each country as they deem appropriate. EU directives lay down certain end results that must be achieved in every Member State. National authorities have to adapt their laws to meet these goals, but are free to decide how to do so. Directives may concern one or more Member States, or all of them. Each directive specifies the date by which the national laws must be adapted. Directives are used to bring different national laws into line with each other.
3. Decisions: A decision only deals with a particular issue and specifically mentioned persons or organizations. Decisions are EU laws relating to specific cases. They can require authorities and individuals in Member States to either do something or stop doing something and can also confer rights on them. EU decisions are fully binding.

In addition to legislation, Euratom has published recommendations and reports (radiation protection series) that can be used as guidance for the implementation of binding legislation. These publications are nonbinding in nature. A list of publications relevant to medical exposure is given in Appendix III.

After the Euratom Treaty entered into force, a comprehensive set of legislation establishing basic safety standards has been enacted on the basis of Article 31 of the Treaty of which the Basic Safety Standards (BSS) Directive forms the main pillar. The first European BSS Directive was adopted in 1958. Council Directive 96/29/Euratom laying down basic safety standards for the protection of the health of workers and the general public against the dangers arising from ionizing radiation (Euratom BSS Directive) of 13 May 1996 is the basis for existing legislation of European Member States.

Other directives based on Article 31 of the Euratom Treaty that have relevance for medical practices are:

- Council Directive 90/641/Euratom of 4 December 1990 on the operational protection of outside workers exposed to the risk of ionizing radiation during their activities in controlled areas (Outside Workers Directive)
- Council Regulation 1493/93/Euratom of 8 June 1993 on shipments of radioactive substances between Member States
- Council Directive 97/43/Euratom of 30 June 1997 on health protection of individuals against the dangers of ionizing radiation in relation to medical exposure, repealing Directive 84/466/Euratom of 3 September 1984 (Medical Directive)
- Council Directive 2003/122/Euratom of 22 December 2003 on the control of high-activity sealed radioactive sources and orphan sources (HASS Directive)

The Euratom BSS Directive 96/29 has recently been revised. The revision was launched by the European Commission after the publication of new recommendations by the ICRP in 2007 (ICRP Publication 103). The revision also involved a simplification of the European legislation on radiation protection by merging directive BSS Directive 96/29 with four other Euratom directives including the Medical Directive 97/43/Euratom. In this way the revision made it possible to extend the requirements of the European BSS to medical exposure, public information, outside workers exposure, and high-activity sealed sources. In addition the requirements of the former BSS Directive and of Medical Directive were upgraded to the latest scientific knowledge and regulatory experience. The revised European BSS Directive allows better integration of the protection of patients with the protection of medical staff and the management of effluents and radioactive waste from nuclear medicine. The Commission adopted the Proposal for a Council Directive laying down BSS for protection against the dangers arising from exposure to ionizing radiation in May 2012. On the 5th of December 2013, the new directive was adopted by the Council. The different chapters and the main changes in the revised directive compared to the former directive, as published in the explanatory memorandum, are described in Appendix I. Regulations with regard to the protection of patients are given in chapter VII. The text of the Articles in this chapter is cited Appendix II.

Although the European Commission cooperated with the IAEA on the revision of the International BSS, they were not referred to or incorporated in the revised European legislation. Incorporation was not considered feasible because the language of the International BSS does not conform to EU legal drafting rules. In addition the international requirements are sometimes far too detailed and go beyond the idea of "basic" standards in the Euratom Treaty. The requirements of the Euratom BSS also need to take into account internal market rules. On the other hand, the International BSS allow for the fact that countries throughout the world, with different levels of regulatory and technological infrastructure, must be able to comply with them. The European legislation is more ambitious at that point. Euratom is bound by the Treaty to establish uniform basic safety standards. The revised Euratom BSS therefore varies from the International BSS. Nevertheless, the Commission pursues the largest possible coherence between Euratom and international standards. The revised Euratom BSS is binding for all Members States and has to be incorporated in the national legislation within 4 years after its publication.

4.5 National Legislation (The Netherlands)

Regulating radiation safety is the responsibility of a national authority. As a Member State of the European Union and Euratom, the Netherlands are obliged to implement the requirement in the Euratom Council Directives into national legislation.

4.5.1 Nuclear Energy Act

The Nuclear Energy Act (Kernenergiewet) is the most important law in the field of radiation protection in the Netherlands. All practices and work activities involving ionizing radiation are regulated by this law. The Nuclear Energy Act is a framework, which aims to protect people and the environment against the dangers of ionizing radiation, and the law also aims to promote the peaceful use of nuclear energy. In addition, the nuclear energy can be characterized as an integral sector law since the law also regulates aspects of environmental management, occupational safety, patient protection, transport, and physical security.

In addition to the law itself, there are a number of decrees and ministerial guidelines that are enacted on the basis of this law. The Nuclear Energy Act dates from 1963, but only became effective in 1970 to its fullest extent. The law contains about 90 articles in which the competences of the national government are described. In addition, there are opportunities for further legislation and a system of permits included. From the viewpoint of radiation protection, Articles 29 and 34 are the most relevant. These articles give regulations regarding the manufacture, transport, possession, and use of radioactive substances (art. 29) and regulations regarding the use of ionizing radiation-emitting devices (art. 34). The Nuclear Energy Act further gives a formal framework for (the system) permits. The law itself contains few concrete standards. Substantive information about the rules that apply in practice is given in underlying decrees and ministerial guidelines. Other laws that apply to working with radiation in the Netherlands are laws that deal with procedures for authorization and notifications and environmental protection ("algemene wet bestuursrecht," "wet milieubeheer" en de "wet op de beroepen in de individuele gezondheidszorg (BIG)").

4.5.2 Radiation Protection Decree

The most important decree under the Nuclear Energy Act is the Radiation Protection Decree (Besluit Stralingsbescherming (Bs)) which also contains the implementation of the Euratom Council Directives. The current Dutch legislation originates in a number of Council Directives of the European Union/Euratom, i.e., Council Directive 96/29, Council Directive 97/43, and Council Directive 2003/122. It has recently been revised. The revised Bs came into force on January 1, 2014 but is still based on the 1996 Euratom BSS.

The Bs contains an elaboration of the provisions that are prescribed by the European Union to Member States. The Bs provides the basic principles for radiation protection, the system of notifications and authorizations for the use of ionizing radiation, the general rules for expertise and instruction, specific rules for population, workers and patients exposure to radiation and use of resources and interventions. Also, the licensing of radioactive sources and devices is elaborated in the Bs. The Bs serves as a definition decree for the remainder regulations and also formalizes for the Netherlands by international and European regulations a prescribed three-stage system of justification, optimization, and dose limitation. Because the radiation protection policy covers several domains, the political responsibility rests with several ministers: occupational exposure is the responsibility of the Minister of Social Affairs and Employment (Social Affairs), medical applications of radiation and radiation protection of patients are the responsibility of the Minister of Health , Welfare and Sport (VWS), and the protection of the population and environment are the responsibility of the Minister of Economic Affairs , Agriculture and Innovation (EL& I).

The Radiation Protection Decree is aimed at everyone who applies ionizing radiation (individuals, organizations, as well as companies). In addition to the Radiation Protection Decree, there are a number of other decrees that contain regulations concerning a specific topic (e.g., transport). The decrees in the Netherlands with relevance to medical facilities and their coherence with ministerial guidelines are shown in Fig. 4.3.

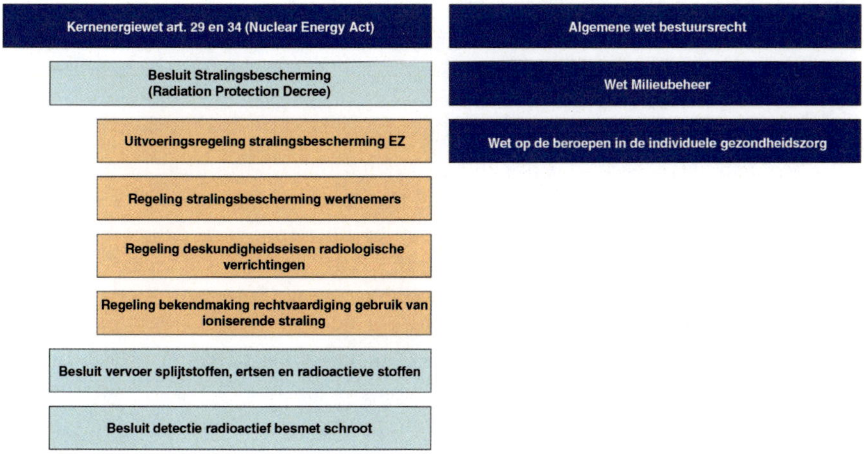

Fig. 4.3 Legislation regulating radiation protection in the Netherlands

4.5.3 Ministerial Guidelines

Ministerial guidelines (ministeriële regelingen) contain specific technical and practical information on how to comply to the more general provision given in the Radiation Protection Decrees.

Appendices

Appendix I: Outline of the Revised BSS Directive

The recast of the five directives yields a voluminous single directive, with over 100 articles and numerous annexes. The different chapters and the main changes in each chapter as published by the Euratom are listed below. Regulations with regard to the protection of patients are given in chapter VII. This chapter includes ten Articles that are listed in Appendix II.

Chapter I: Subject Matter and Scope

This chapter defines the scope of the new directive (general purpose of the directive across different categories of exposure and different exposure situations and specific purposes resulting from integration of the requirements for high-activity sealed radioactive sources and for public information and the exclusion of noncontrollable exposures). The scope is broadened to include the exposure of space crew to cosmic radiation, domestic exposure to radon gas in indoor air, external exposure to gamma radiation from building materials, and the protection of the environment beyond environmental pathways leading to human exposure.

Chapter II: Definitions

This chapter includes all definitions given in the earlier directives, with some adjustments to resolve inconsistencies as well as to adjust to the new terminology introduced in ICRP Publication 103 and in the draft International Basic Safety Standards.

Chapter III: System of Radiation Protection

This title includes the general principles of radiation protection: justification, optimization, and dose limitation. It explains the more prominent role of dose constraints and reference levels in the process of optimization, with Annex I giving the bands of reference levels proposed by the ICRP for existing and emergency exposure situations. The dose limits are not modified, except for a uniform definition of the annual occupational dose limit (no averaging over 5 years) and a lower organ dose limit for the lens of the eye, as recommended by the ICRP. The new directive no longer includes the technical measurements entering into the definition of the effective dose and other factors entering into the assessment of doses, but refers to ICRP Publication 103 for this purpose. In addition, the directive no longer includes the long lists of radionuclide-specific dose coefficients (doses per unit intake by ingestion or inhalation), but will refer to a forthcoming consolidated publication of the ICRP which can be downloaded free of charge.

Chapter IV: Requirements for Radiation Protection Education, Training, and Information

This chapter brings together the miscellaneous requirements governing education and training in the different directives and includes provisions for recognition of the "Radiation Protection Expert" and "Medical Physics Expert."

Chapter V: Justification and Regulatory Control of Practices

The application of the principle of justification remains a national responsibility. Specific attention is given to the justification of practices involving the deliberate exposure of humans for nonmedical imaging (e.g., security screening in airports).

The regime for regulatory control is now presented as a three-tier system (notification, registration, licensing), replacing the earlier two-tier system of reporting and "prior authorization." A more detailed list of which types of practice are subject to either registration or licensing is given. As part of the concept of a "graded approach" to regulatory control, there is explicit provision for the specific exemption of practices (from notification and from authorization) at national level. The default values for exemption on the basis of activity concentrations are now taken from IAEA Safety Guide RS-G-1.7. The same default values apply to release from regulatory control (clearance levels), but allow for specific values in European guidance. Member States will be allowed to keep default clearance levels in current national legislation and to keep the existing exemption values for moderate amounts of material. Details of exemption criteria and exemption and clearance levels are given in Annex VI.

This chapter also includes more precise requirements on the information to be provided with a license application (the issuing of discharge authorizations for radioactive airborne or liquid effluent is covered in Chapter VIII).

Chapter VI: Protection of Workers, Apprentices, and Students

This title includes, with little amendment, the provisions on occupational exposure in Directive 96/29/Euratom. It also includes the specific requirements in the Outside Workers Directive and introduces a clear allocation of responsibilities between the employer and the undertaking where the practice is conducted. The data system for individual radiological monitoring of exposed workers and the minimum set of data to be communicated for outside workers has been updated in the light of recommendations by HERCA.

No distinction is made between the management of occupational exposures in NORM industries and other practices, but the former will benefit from a graded regulatory approach on the basis of prevailing exposures and their potential to increase with time.

This chapter now covers occupational exposure in all exposure situations, which provides more explicit protection for emergency workers as well as for workers exposed to high levels of indoor radon in their workplace.

Chapter VII: Protection of Patients and Other Individuals Subjected to Medical Exposure

This chapter includes the relevant requirements from the Medical Directive, but strengthens them, in particular with regard to:

- The application of the justification principle
- Information to patients on the health risks and benefits
- Information on doses
- Diagnostic reference levels
- Involvement of the Medical Physics Expert
- Prevention of accidental and unintended medical exposures

Chapter VIII: Protection of Members of the Public

This chapter includes the public exposure requirements in Directive 96/29/Euratom, with more explicit consideration of the issuing of discharge authorizations for radioactive effluent (also with reference to Commission Recommendation 2004/2/Euratom).

The section on emergency exposure situations includes the requirements of the Public Information Directive.

The section on existing exposure situations addresses indoor exposure to radon, with a somewhat lower maximum reference level for existing dwellings than in Commission Recommendation 90/143/Euratom, in line with ICRP and WHO recommendations. It also includes requirements for the classification of building materials on the basis of a radioactivity index and a uniform reference level for the annual dose resulting from residence in a building constructed with such materials.

Chapter IX: Protection of the Environment

This chapter, in line with the broader scope of the directive as in the International Basic Safety Standards, aims to provide a means to demonstrate compliance with environmental criteria. While the ICRP has published a methodology for dose assessment for biota, a publication on the application of criteria is still awaited. Pending such further guidance, it is up to national authorities to assess the doses to representative animals and plants in terms of protection of the ecosystem.

Appropriate technical measures also need to be taken to avoid the environmental consequences of an accidental release and to monitor existing levels of radioactivity in the environment, from the perspectives of both environmental protection and human health.

Chapter X: Requirements for Regulatory Control

This chapter includes all the responsibilities of the regulatory authorities in all exposure situations. A clear structure is provided by the following sections:

- Institutional infrastructure
- Control of sealed radioactive sources (with Annexes II, XII, XIII, XIV, XV incorporating different aspects of the directive on high-activity sealed radioactive sources)

- Orphan sources (with new requirements with regard to metal contamination)
- Emergency exposure situations (establishment of an emergency management system and international cooperation, while requirements for the protection of workers and members of the public in an emergency exposure situation are addressed in Chapters V and VIII, respectively)
- Existing exposure situations (general provisions for the management of contaminated areas, radon action plan)
- System of enforcement (inspection program and response to deficiencies)

The first section on "institutional infrastructure" calls for a clear definition of the responsibilities of different authorities. The Commission is to receive periodically updated information and publish this in the Official Journal. This section also defines the responsibilities of the "Radiation Protection Expert," the "Radiation Protection Officer" (in the current BSS these concepts were merged within the function of "Qualified Expert"), and the "Medical Physics Expert."

Chapter XI: Final Provisions

The transposition of the new directive into national law should not require a major legislative effort, so a 2-year transposition deadline is deemed sufficient. Specific new features, such as the protection of the environment, can be transposed later.

In line with the Euratom Treaty, the Basic Standards are to be uniformly applied in the Member States, though without prejudice to those requirements for which flexibility is clear from the wording of the text. However, dose limits, default exemption values, the reference level for building materials, etc. are explicitly intended for uniform transposition and application.

Appendix II: Regulation for the Protection of Patients in European Legislation

The revised BSS Directive yields over 100 articles divided over eleven chapters and numerous annexes. Regulations with regard to the protection of patients are given in Chapter VII. The Articles in this chapter, as described in the "Proposal for a Council Directive laying down basic safety standards against the dangers arising from exposure to ionizing radiation" (com(2012)242), are given below.

The full text of the directive can be found on the website of European Commission (http://ec.europa.eu/energy/nuclear/radiation_protection/doc/2012_com_242.pdf).

Chapter VII: Protection of Patients and Other Individuals Subjected to Medical Exposure

Article 54: Justification

1. Medical exposure shall show a sufficient net benefit, weighing the total potential diagnostic or therapeutic benefits it produces, including the direct benefits to health or well-being of an individual and the benefits to society, against the

individual detriment that the exposure might cause, taking into account the efficacy, benefits and risks of available alternative techniques having the same objective but involving no or less exposure to ionising radiation.

Account shall also be taken of the individual detriment from the exposure of the medical radiological staff and other individuals.

(a) all new types of practices involving medical exposure shall be justified in advance before being generally adopted;

existing types of practices involving medical exposure shall be reviewed whenever new, important evidence about their efficacy or consequences is acquired;

all individual medical exposures shall be justified in advance taking into account the specific objectives of the exposure and the characteristics of the individual involved.

If a type of practice involving a medical exposure is not justified in general, a specific individual exposure of this type may be justified in special circumstances, to be evaluated on a case-by-case basis and documented.

The referrer and the practitioner shall seek, where practicable, to obtain previous diagnostic information or medical records relevant to the planned exposure and consider these data to avoid unnecessary exposure.

In particular the following requirements shall be applied:

2. Medical exposure for biomedical and medical research shall be examined by an ethics committee, set up in accordance with national procedures and/or by the competent authorities;
3. Specific justification for medical radiological procedures to be performed as part of a health screening programme shall be carried out by the health authority in conjunction with appropriate professional bodies.
4. The exposure of carers and comforters shall show a sufficient net benefit, taking into account the direct health benefits to a patient, the benefits to the carer / comforter and the detriment that the exposure might cause.
5. Any medical radiological procedure on an asymptomatic individual, to be performed for the early detection of disease, shall be part of a health screening programme, or shall require specific documented justification for that individual by the practitioner, in consultation with the referrer, following guidelines from relevant professional bodies and competent authorities. Special attention shall be given to the provision of information to the patients, as required by Article 56(3).
6. If an exposure cannot be justified in accordance with paragraphs 1 to 5, it shall be prohibited.

Article 55: Optimisation

1. All doses due to medical exposure for radiodiagnostic and interventional radiology purposes shall be kept as low as reasonably achievable consistent with obtaining the required imaging information, taking into account economic and social factors.

   For all medical exposure of individuals for radiotherapeutic purposes, exposures of target volumes shall be individually planned, taking into account that doses of non-target volumes and tissues shall be as low as reasonably achievable and consistent with the intended radiotherapeutic purpose of the exposure.

2. Member States shall ensure the establishment, regular review and use of diagnostic reference levels for radiodiagnostic examinations, and when appropriate, for interventional radiology procedures, and the availability of guidance for this purpose.
3. Member States shall ensure that for each biomedical and medical research project:
   (a) the individuals concerned participate voluntarily;
   these individuals are informed about the risks of exposure;
   a dose constraint is established for individuals for whom no direct medical benefit is expected from exposure;
   in the case of patients who voluntarily accept to undergo an experimental diagnostic or therapeutic practice and who are expected to receive a diagnostic or therapeutic benefit from this practice, the dose levels concerned shall be considered on an individual basis by the practitioner and/or referrer.
4. The optimisation shall include the selection of equipment, the consistent production of adequate diagnostic information or therapeutic outcomes, the practical aspects of medical exposure procedures, quality assurance, and the assessment and evaluation of patient and staff doses or administered activities, taking into account economic and social factors.
5. Member States shall ensure that:
   (a) dose constraints are established for the exposure of carers and comforters;
   appropriate guidance is established for the exposure of carers and comforters;
6. Member States shall ensure that in the case of a patient undergoing treatment or diagnosis with radionuclides, the practitioner or the undertaking, as appropriate, provides the patient or legal guardian with written instructions with a view to restricting doses to persons in contact with the patient as far as reasonably achievable and providing information on the risks of ionising radiation.

These instructions shall be handed out before leaving the hospital or clinic or a similar institution.

Article 56: Responsibilities

1. The referrer and the practitioner shall be involved in the justification process as specified by Member States.
2. Member States shall ensure that any medical exposure takes place under the clinical responsibility of a practitioner.
3. The practitioner shall ensure that the patient or legal guardian is provided with adequate information relating to the benefits and risks associated with the radiation dose from the medical exposure to enable informed consent. Similar information as well as relevant guidance in accordance with Article 55(5)(b) shall be given to carers and comforters.
4. Practical aspects of medical exposure procedures may be delegated by the undertaking or the practitioner, as appropriate, to one or more individuals entitled to act in this respect in a recognised field of specialisation.

Article 57: Procedures

1. Written protocols for every type of standard medical radiological procedure shall be established for each equipment.
2. Member States shall ensure that referral guidelines for medical imaging, taking into account the radiation doses, are available to the referrers.
3. In medical radiological practices, a medical physics expert shall be appropriately involved, the level of involvement being commensurate with the radiological risk posed by the practice. In particular:
   (a) in radiotherapeutic practices other than standardised therapeutic nuclear medicine practices, a medical physics expert shall be closely involved;
   in standardised therapeutical nuclear medicine practices as well as in radiodiagnostic and interventional radiology practices, a medical physics expert shall be involved;
   for other simple radiodiagnostic procedures, a medical physics expert shall be involved, as appropriate, for consultation and advice on matters relating to radiation protection concerning medical exposure.
4. Clinical audits shall be carried out in accordance with national procedures.
5. Member States shall ensure that appropriate local reviews are undertaken whenever diagnostic reference levels are consistently exceeded and that corrective action is taken where appropriate.

Article 58: Training

Member States shall ensure that training and recognition requirements, as laid down in Articles 15, 19 and 81, are met for the practitioner, the medical physics expert and the individuals referred to in Article 56(4).

Article 59: Equipment

1. Member States shall take such steps as they consider necessary with a view to avoiding unnecessary proliferation of medical radiological equipment.
2. Member States shall ensure that:
   (a) all medical radiological equipment in use is kept under strict surveillance regarding radiation protection;
   an up-to-date inventory of medical radiological equipment for each medical radiological installation is available to the competent authorities;
   appropriate quality assurance programmes and dose or administered activity assessments are implemented by the undertaking; and
   acceptance testing, involving the medical physics expert, is carried out before the first use of the equipment for clinical purposes, and performance testing is carried out thereafter on a regular basis, and after any major maintenance procedure.
3. Competent authorities shall take steps to ensure that the necessary measures are taken by the undertaking to improve inadequate or defective features of medical radiological equipment. They shall also adopt specific criteria for the acceptability of equipment in order to indicate when appropriate corrective action is necessary, including, if appropriate, taking the equipment out of service.

4. The use of fluoroscopy equipment without a device to control the dose rate, or without an image intensifier or equivalent device, shall be prohibited.
5. Any equipment used for interventional radiology and computed tomography shall have a device or a feature informing the practitioner of the quantity of radiation produced by the equipment during the medical radiological procedure. Any other medical radiodiagnostic equipment brought into use after this Directive has entered into force shall have such a device or a feature or equivalent means of determining the quantity of radiation produced. The radiation dose shall form part of the report on the examination.

Article 60: Special practices

1. Member States shall ensure that appropriate medical radiological equipment, practical techniques and ancillary equipment are used for medical exposure
   (a) of children;
   as part of a health screening programme;
   involving high doses to the patient, such as interventional radiology, computed tomography or radiotherapy.
   Special attention shall be given to quality assurance programmes and the assessment of dose or administered activity, as mentioned in Article 59(2)(c), for these practices.
2. Member States shall ensure that practitioners and those individuals referred to in Article 56(4) who perform the exposures referred to in paragraph 1 of this Article obtain appropriate training in these medical radiological practices as required by Article 19.

Article 61: Special protection during pregnancy and breastfeeding

1. In the case of a woman of childbearing age, the referrer and the practitioner shall inquire as specified by Member States whether she is pregnant or breastfeeding, if relevant.

   If pregnancy cannot be excluded, depending on the type of medical exposure, in particular if abdominal and pelvic regions are involved, special attention shall be given to the justification, particularly the urgency, and to the optimisation of the medical exposure, taking into account the exposure both of the expectant mother and the unborn child.
2. In the case of breastfeeding women, in nuclear medicine, depending on the type of medical examination or treatment, special attention shall be given to the justification, particularly the urgency, and to the optimisation of the medical exposure, taking into account the exposure both of the mother and the child.
3. Without prejudice to paragraphs 1 and 2, Member States shall take measures to increase the awareness of women to whom this Article applies, such as public notices in appropriate places.

Article 62: Accidental and unintended exposures

Member States shall ensure that:

(a) all reasonable steps are taken to minimizse the probability and magnitude of accidental or unintended exposures of patients from all medical radiological procedures, taking into account economic and social factors;

for radiotherapeutic practices the quality assurance programme includes a study of the risk of accidental or unintended exposures;
for all medical exposures the undertaking implements a system for the registration and analysis of events involving or potentially involving accidental or unintended exposures;
the undertaking declares as soon as possible to the competent authorities the occurrence of significant events as defined by the authorities, including the results of the investigation and the corrective measures to avoid such events. The competent authorities shall share this information with the competent authorities for post-market surveillance established in Council Directive 93/42/EEC concerning medical devices;
arrangements are made to inform the referrer, the practitioner and the patient about an unintended or accidental exposure.

Article 63: Estimates of population doses

Member States shall ensure that the distribution of individual dose estimates from medical exposure is determined and shall take into account the age distribution and the gender of the exposed population.

Appendix III: Medical Guidance Documents Published by Euratom

Since 1976 the European Commission has published a large number of publications covering a wide range of issues relating to ionizing radiation and radiation protection (radiation protection series). A complete list can be found on the website of Euratom (http://ec.europe.eu/energy/nuclear/radiation_protection/publications_en.htm). The following radiation protection publications dealing with medical exposures have been issued in the past decade or so and are expected to still have relevance today:

RP 172 Cone beam CT for dental and maxillofacial radiology – evidence-based guidelines
RP 162 Criteria for acceptability of medical radiological equipment used in diagnostic radiology, nuclear medicine, and radiotherapy
RP 159 European Commission guidelines on clinical audit
RP 158 EU Scientific Seminar 2008 – Emerging evidence for radiation induced circulatory diseases
RP 154 European guidance on estimating population doses from medical X-ray procedures and annexes
RP 149 EU Scientific Seminar 2003, medical overexposures
RP 136 European guidelines on radiation protection in dental radiology
RP 131 Effects of in utero exposure to ionizing radiation during the early phases of pregnancy
RP 130 Medicolegal exposures, exposures with ionizing radiation without medical indication proceedings of the International Symposium, Dublin, 4–6 September 2002

RP 119	Multimedia and audiovisual radiation protection training in interventional radiology
RP 116	Guidelines on education and training in radiation protection for medical exposures (in the process of update)
RP 109	Guidance on diagnostic reference levels (DRLs) for medical exposures
RP 102	Proceedings of the workshop "Implementation of the Medical Exposure Directive (97/43/EURATOM)" – Madrid on 27 April 1998
RP 100	Guidance for protection of unborn children and infants irradiated due to parental medical exposures
RP 99	Guidance on medical exposures in medical and biomedical research
RP 97	Radiation protection following iodine-131 therapy (exposures due to outpatients or discharged inpatients)

Appendix IV: Guidance Documents Published by ICRP

Since 1928 the ICRP has published a large number of publications covering a wide range of issues relating to ionizing radiation and radiation protection (Annals of the ICRP). Publications dealing with specific aspects of radiological protection in medicine that were published in the last years are listed below. A complete overview of the published documents and additional information can be found on the website of the ICRP (http://www.icrp.org/publications.asp).

ICRP, Khong P-L, Ringertz H, Donoghue V, Frush D, Rehani M, Appelgate K, Sanchez R. Radiological protection in paediatric diagnostic and interventional radiology. ICRP Publication 121. Ann ICRP. 2013;42(2).

ICRP, Cousins C, Miller DL, Bernardi G, Rehani MM, Schofield P, Vaño E, Einstein AJ, Geiger B, Heintz P, Padovani R, Sim K-H. Radiological Protection in Cardiology. ICRP Publication 120. Ann ICRP. 2013;42(1).

ICRP, Stewart FA, Akleyev AV, Hauer-Jensen M, Hendry JH, Kleiman NJ, MacVittie TJ, Aleman BM, Edgar AB, Mabuchi K, Muirhead CR, Shore RE, Wallace WH. ICRP Statement on Tissue Reactions / Early and Late Effects of Radiation in Normal Tissues and Organs – Threshold Doses for Tissue Reactions in a Radiation Protection Context. ICRP Publication 118. Ann ICRP. 2012;41(1/2).

ICRP, Rehani MM, Ciraj-Bjelac O, Vaño E, Miller DL, Walsh S, Giordano BD, Persliden J. Radiological Protection in Fluoroscopically Guided Procedures outside the Imaging Department. ICRP Publication 117. Ann. ICRP. 2010;40(6).

ICRP, Petoussi-Henss N, Bolch WE, Eckerman KF, Endo A, Hertel N, Hunt J, Pelliccioni M, Schlattl H, Zankl M. Conversion Coefficients for Radiological Protection Quantities for External Radiation Exposures. ICRP Publication 116, Ann ICRP. 2010;40(2–5).

ICRP, Vaño E, Rosenstein M, Liniecki J, Rehani M, Martin CJ, Vetter RJ. Education and Training in Radiological Protection for Diagnostic and Interventional Procedures. ICRP Publication 113. Ann ICRP. 2009;39 (5).

ICRP. Adult Reference Computational Phantoms. ICRP Publication 110. Ann ICRP. 2009;39(2).

ICRP. Nuclear Decay Data for Dosimetric Calculations. ICRP Publication 107. Ann ICRP. 2008;38(3).

ICRP. Radiation Dose to Patients from Radiopharmaceuticals – Addendum 3 to ICRP 53. ICRP Publication 106. Ann ICRP. 2008;38 (1–2).

ICRP. Radiological Protection in Medicine. ICRP Publication 105. Ann ICRP. 2007:37(6).

ICRP. 2007 Recommendations of the International Commission on Radiological Protection (Users Edition). ICRP Publication 103 (Users Edition). Ann ICRP. 2007;37(2–4).

ICRP. Managing Patient Dose in Multi-Detector Computed Tomography (MDCT). ICRP Publication 102. Ann ICRP. 2007;37(1).

5 Vertebrate Animals Used for Experimental and Other Scientific Purposes: Principles and Practice for Legislation and Protection

Miriam van der Meulen-Frank, Jan-Bas Prins, Barry-Lee Waarts, and Wiebe Hofstra

5.1 General Introduction

In all medical disciplines, extensive research is required before physiological and pathological mechanisms are understood and treatments are effective and safe for use in human patients.

Vertebrate animals are often found in the toolbox of the scientist, but the use of vertebrate animals cannot be regarded as common practice. This chapter is guiding the reader through the background of legislation and the principles behind laboratory animal science and legislation to create awareness and a basic level of knowledge in this field. Several aspects of the European legislation are addressed in detail, but the principles have been accepted worldwide, and they have influenced the legislation in many countries, driven by moral obligation and public concern.

M. van der Meulen-Frank (✉)
Animal Welfare Officer, University of Groningen, Research Building 3218, room 2.23, A. Deusinglaan 1, 9713 AV Groningen, The Netherlands
e-mail: m.van.der.meulen-frank@umcg.nl

J.-B. Prins
Director, Central Animal Facility, Leiden University Medical Center, Postzone T-07, PO Box 9600, 2300 RC Leiden, The Netherlands

B.-L. Waarts
Biosafety Officer, University Medical Center Groningen, UMC-Staff Safety and Permits, Hanzeplein 1, 9713 GZ Groningen, The Netherlands

W. Hofstra
Biosafety Officer, Central Animal Facility, University Medical Center Groningen, Building 3218, room 2.19, A. Deusinglaan 1, 9713 AV Groningen, The Netherlands

A.W.J.M. Glaudemans et al. (eds.), *Quality in Nuclear Medicine*,
DOI 10.1007/978-3-319-33531-5_5

5.2 Part I. Legislation: Summary of EU Legislation

The regulation concerning the protection of animals used for scientific purposes in Europe consists mainly of two documents. The first is the European Convention for the protection of vertebrate animals used for experimental and other scientific purposes, European Treaty Series 123 (ETS 123) at the level of the Council of Europe (1986). The second is at the level of the European Union (EU): The European Directive 2010/63/EU on the protection of animals used for scientific purposes (The European Parliament and the Council of the European Union 2010). Both documents ensure tight regulation of the housing, care, and use of animals for scientific purposes especially within the European Union. Appendix A of ETS 123 contains recommendations on housing, environmental enrichment, and care (Council of Europe 2006).

The legislation is complemented with recommendations and guidelines produced by pan-European operating expert organisations, such as ESLAV (European Society for Laboratory Animal Veterinarians), ECLAM (European College for Laboratory Animal Medicine), and FELASA (Federation of European Laboratory Animal Science Associations).

A compilation of the legislation on the protection of animals for scientific purposes effective in different parts of the world has been published recently (Guillén 2013). This summary of EU legislation focuses on the European Directive 2010/63/EU rather than on ETS123, also because Appendix A of ETS123 has been incorporated in 2010/63/EU as Annex III.

5.2.1 The European Directive 2010/63/EU

The Directive was published on the 22nd of September 2010. It marked the end of a process of revision of its predecessor Directive 86/609/EEC. The objectives of the European Commission (EC) with 2010/63/EU were to improve animal welfare; to implement the principles of replacement, reduction, and refinement (the 3Rs) (Russell and Burch 1959); and to create a level playing field across the EU. The member states of the EU (MSs) were granted a transition period until November 2012 to transpose the Directive into national legislation, which had to be in place no later than January 1, 2013 (EC transposition score board 2014). The level playing field is supported by the fact that the Directive does not allow MSs to include stricter measures into their national legislation except for those that were already in force on the 9th of November 2010 and of which the EC had been notified.

The Directive consists of two main parts and eight annexes. The first part consists of a body of 56 recitals in which the intentions of the Directive are described. The second part consists of the 66 articles of the Directive divided into six chapters: (1) General provisions, (2) Provisions on the use of certain animals in procedures, (3) Procedures, (4) Authorisation, (5) Avoidance of duplication and alternative approaches, and (6) Final provisions. Four out of the eight annexes list elements referred to in articles of the Directive (Annexes I, II, V, VI). The other annexes provide information on (1) requirements for the establishments and for the care and accommodation of animals (Annex III), (2) methods of killing animals (Annex IV), (3) duties and tasks of the union reference laboratory (Annex VII), and (4) severity classification of procedures (Annex VIII). By including Annex III, the EC has incorporated provisions of ETS 123 Appendix A into EU legislation which demands compliance.

5.2.2 The Directive and the Implementation in National Legislations

The Directive should be regarded as a legislative framework that needs to be filled in by secondary legislation in the MSs. The EC previewed the drafting of deviating secondary legislations by MSs jeopardising the principle of a "level playing field" across the EU at the same time. Therefore, the EC took the initiative to publish a "questions and answers" document intended as guidance to assist member states and others affected by the Directive to arrive at a common understanding in the Directive (http://ec.europa.eu/environment/chemicals/lab_animals/pdf/qa.pdf). The EC established Expert Working Groups (EWGs) on different topics to draft proposals for the MSs on which consensus was regarded essential. They included EWGs on education and training, genetically altered animals, nontechnical project summaries, inspection and enforcement, project evaluation and retrospective assessment, severity assessment, and statistical reporting. Their progress reports and the consensus documents are published on the European Commission's website (http://ec.europa.eu/environment/chemicals/lab_animals).

5.2.3 The Scope of 2010/63/EU

The scope provides the user of animals for scientific purposes clarity when the Directive applies, what it wants to stimulate and achieve, and for whom it is applicable. It lays down rules on the replacement and reduction for the use of animals in procedures[1] and the refinement of the breeding, accommodation, care, and use of animals in procedures; the origin, breeding, marking, care and accommodation, and killing of animals; the operation of breeders, suppliers, and users; and the evaluation and authorisation of projects involving the use of animals in procedures (2010/63/EU: Article 1.1). The Directive applies where animals are used or intended to be used in procedures or bred specifically so that their organs or tissues may be used for

[1] Procedure means any use, invasive or noninvasive, of an animal for experimental or other scientific purposes, with known or unknown outcome, or educational purposes, which may cause the animal a level of pain, suffering, distress, or lasting harm equivalent to, or higher than, that caused by the introduction of a needle in accordance with good veterinary practice. This includes any course of action intended, or liable, to result in the birth or hatching of an animal or the creation and maintenance of a genetically modified animal line in which such condition but excludes the killing of animals solely for the use of their organs or tissues (2010/63/EU: Article 3.1).

scientific procedures. The elimination of pain, suffering, distress, or lasting harm by the successful use of anesthesia, analgesia, or other methods does not exclude the use of an animal in procedures from the scope of the Directive (2010/63/EU: Article 1.2). The Directive applies to the following animals: live nonhuman vertebrate animals, including independently feeding larval forms and fetal forms of mammals as from the last third of their normal development, and live cephalopods (2010/63/EU: Article 1.3). In Article 1(EC transposition score board 2014) of the Directive, situations are summed up where the Directive does not apply. They include nonexperimental agricultural and clinical veterinary practices, among others.

The aim is to replace and reduce the use of animals in procedures and to refine the breeding, accommodation, care, and use of animals in procedures. However, the European Commission does recognise that the use of live animals continues to be necessary to protect human and animal health and the environment. However, it also states that the Directive represents an important step toward achieving the final goal of full replacement of procedures on live animals for scientific and educational purposes as soon as it is scientifically possible to do so. To that end, it seeks to facilitate and promote the advancement of alternative approaches. It also seeks to ensure a high level of protection for animals that still need to be used in procedures (2010/63/EU: recital 10).

5.2.4 2010/63/EU: Updates and New Provisions

2010/63/EU calls for a mandatory project evaluation including an ethical review and project authorisation. Project proposals will have to be presented to an impartial review committee for ethical review after which an authorisation has to be obtained from the competent authority (CA). It is not sufficient just to perform a prospective severity assessment. Also after termination of the project, a (retrospective) severity evaluation needs to be performed and reported.

MSs should publish nontechnical project summaries subject to safeguarding intellectual property and not containing information that is traceable to individuals. The nontechnical project summary has to include information on the objectives of the project, including the predicted harm and benefits, the number and types of animals to be used, and a demonstration of compliance with the requirements of the 3Rs.

MSs will have to ensure that each breeder, supplier, and user set up an animal welfare body with tasks as specified in Article 27 of the Directive. They include 1. advising the staff dealing with animals on matters related to the welfare of animals, in relation to their acquisition, accommodation, care, and use; 2. advising the staff on the application of the requirement of replacement, reduction, and refinement and to keep them informed of technical and scientific developments concerning the application of that requirement; 3. establish and review internal operational processes as regard monitoring, reporting, and follow-up in relation to the welfare of animals housed or used in the establishment; 4. to follow the development and outcome of projects, taking into account the effect on the animals used, and to identify and advise as regards elements that further contribute to replacement, reduction, and refinement; and 5. to advise on rehoming schemes, including the appropriate socialisation of the animals to be rehomed.

5.2.5 Categories of Staff and Education and Training Requirements

The Directive defines four functions as listed in Article 23(The European Parliament and the Council of the European Union 2010): (a) carrying out procedures on animals, (b) designing procedures and projects, (c) taking care of animals, and (d) killing animals. The Directive goes on to define specific requirements for each of these functions. Persons carrying out function (b) are required to have received instruction in a scientific discipline relevant to the work being undertaken and should have species-specific knowledge. Staff carrying out function (a), (c), or (d) should be supervised in the performance of their tasks until they have demonstrated the requisite competence. Furthermore, MSs must ensure that each breeder, supplier, and user have one or several persons on site who are responsible for overseeing the welfare and care of animals in the establishment and that the staff people dealing with animals have access to information specific to the species housed in the establishment, and they are responsible for ensuring that the staff people are adequately educated, competent, continuously trained and that they are supervised until they have demonstrated the requisite competence (2010/63/EU: Article 24(Council of Europe 1986)). Especially the inclusion of continuing professional development (CPD) deserves special attention. CPD programs will provide the necessary platforms to also keep competence, knowledge, and skills abreast with progress and new developments over time.

Education and training are matters of the MSs par excellence. Especially as free movement of persons within the EU is dependent on a "level playing field" among MSs. The EC has called for an EWG to develop a common education and training framework to fulfill the requirements under the Directive. These are not considered to be binding; however, they may be adopted by the member states in accordance with the advisory procedure referred to in Article 56 (The European Parliament and the Council of the European Union 2010) of the Directive (2010/63/EU: Article 23(Guillén 2013)). The EWG's consensus document describes a modular training structure and learning outcome approach that is flexible. Learning outcomes are the specific intentions of a training program or module, written in specific terms. The learning outcomes deal with output rather than processes and help to define the skills and knowledge that module participants should be able to demonstrate by the time these learning outcomes are assessed. They describe what a student should know, understand, or be able to do at the end of that module (http://ec.europa.eu/environment/chemicals/lab_animals/pdf/Endorsed_E-T.pdf).

5.2.6 Conclusion Part I

The European/EU legislative framework in place today puts the 3Rs center stage and provides conditions to optimally protect the welfare of animals used in scientific procedures and to create a level playing field among EU's member states.

5.3 Part II. The Principles: Replacement, Reduction, and Refinement, 3Rs

Over the last centuries, knowledge of anatomy, physiology, and biochemistry of man and animals has increased tremendously. The use of animals for research purposes has been developed over centuries because of man's search for knowledge, health, food, and safety, and animals seem to model many (human) characteristics in a satisfactory way.

This knowledge has also influenced the attitude of man toward animals in the modern western society. With the increase of evidence that animals are sentient creatures, we have a moral obligation to respect all animals and consider their suffering and memory. This moral obligation is leading us to replace live animals in procedures by other methods not entailing the use of live animals, although the use of live animals still continues to be necessary to protect human and animal health and the environment. In addition, and equally important, it is widely recognised that the most humane possible treatment of experimental animals is actually a prerequisite for successful animal experiments. Good science, both fundamental and applied, and good animal health are not competitors but allies.

For research in the field of nuclear medicine and as for all other fields where animals are used for scientific and educational purposes, this cannot go unnoticed. The EU Directive 2010/63/EU means an important step toward achieving the final goal of full replacement of procedures on live vertebrate animals *for scientific and educational purposes* as soon as it is scientifically feasible to do so. To that end, it seeks to create awareness and promotes the advancement of alternative approaches (recital (Balls 2013) Directive 2010/63/EU). The European Commission and the member states shall contribute to the development and validation of procedures which could provide the same or higher levels of information as those obtained by using animals but which do not involve the use of animals or use fewer animals or involve less painful procedures (Art. 47 Directive 2010).

The EU directive is also designed as a framework for the sharing of knowledge, e.g. managing public databases and information systems, and for promoting the route from development through validation and the use or application of alternative methods.

What are the three Rs? The three Rs are also referred to as *alternative methods* in animal experiments.

In 1959, William M.S. Russell and Rex L. Burch published "The principles of humane experimental technique" in which they classified humane techniques under the headings of *replacement*, *reduction*, and *refinement,* the three Rs or 3Rs.

They restricted their book to vertebrate animals, making it a fundamental document for the contemporary European directive. They introduced the word "distress" to cover any kind of unpleasant event or suffering like pain, fear, and stress. The driving forces for the development of the 3R principles were observations of both extreme unpleasantness *and* very large numbers of animals and a combined estimate of the two.

Despite the ever-increasing knowledge, we often lack criteria for the existence of distress in nonhuman vertebrates, and we must fall back on analogy with effects of a given symptom, treatment, or stimulus upon man. Analogy exists when the key factors are present in two compared systems. If a procedure causes distress in man and the key factors are present both in man and in the experimental animal, the same kind and level of distress is expected in the animal.

The choice of a model should follow a stepwise approach, including the search for alternatives, the 3Rs. An ethical assessment is finally conducted for each animal experiment. Under all circumstances, the consideration of methods without using animals is the first step taken. If no such methods are available, it should be considered how pain, suffering, and lasting harm can be minimised in the proposed experiment and how the number of animals used can be reduced without loss of information. In the majority of research projects in the field of biomedical research, a smart combination of replacement, reduction, and refinement alternative methods is applied. The contribution of each may vary largely, depending on the field of research and the effort spent on developing alternative methods.

5.3.1 Replacement

Russell and Burch developed different approaches to replacement. They distinguished between *absolute replacement*, in which vertebrate animals are not required at all, and *relative replacement*, where animals are still required but are not exposed to distress of procedures at all. In the *relative replacement* group, they included "non-recovery experiments on living and intact, but completely anaesthetised animals" and "experiments where animals are still required, but only to furnish preparations after being painlessly killed" (Art. 47 Directive 2010). In the EU directive, procedures which are performed entirely under general anesthesia from which the animal shall not recover consciousness will be classified as "non-recovery" being a separate class, not linked to any level of discomfort.

When a scientifically satisfactory method or testing strategy, not entailing the use of live animals, exists, then the use of animals for the same purpose is prohibited (9, Art. 4.3).

Other classifications of replacement are less common although many experiments are conducted with methods covered by at least one of these classifications: partial vs. total replacement and direct vs. indirect replacement (Balls 2013).

In experiments with *partial replacement*, animals are exposed to a procedure or treatment, and, after sacrificing the animal, its cells, tissues, or organs are subject to in vitro experiments. In *total replacement*, all experiments are performed in vitro on cells, tissues, or organs without being subject to any treatment or procedure prior to death. The numbers of animals used for such in vitro experiments are not shown in the European statistical reviews as they are in the Dutch reviews.

Results of a *direct replacement* technique are directly comparable to results obtained from the animal procedure, requiring a two-step extrapolation, from replacement technique to animal to goal species, whereas the results of an *indirect replacement* technique relate to the goal species without intermediate extrapolation. These replacement techniques are more advanced.

In vitro techniques may suffice for the first steps in tracer development: affinity for target cells requires a cell line of the target cells, appropriate media to bring tracer and cells together, and methods for analysis. For pharmacodynamics and pharmacokinetics, a more advanced system is required. Animal experiments for pharmacodynamics can be classified as experiments with partial replacement because it requires the in vivo administration of the tracer, but distribution of the tracer is measured in separate organs, after sacrificing the animal. Data for pharmacokinetics are obtained by imaging anesthetised animals at several timepoints. This does not contribute to the replacement alternative, but reduction may be involved.

5.3.2 Reduction

The number of animals used in projects is reduced to a minimum without compromising the objectives of the project. The European directive repeatedly lays emphasis on this: e.g. the numbers of animals used may be reduced by resorting to other methods, such as the elimination of unnecessary duplication or by (regulatory) testing or by implementing testing strategies, such as the use of in vitro and other methods that would reduce and refine the use of animals (9, recital, Art. 4.2 Directive 2010/63/EU).

Reduction was seen by Russell and Burch as the "R" which was *most obviously, immediately and universally advantageous in terms of efficiency* (Russell WMS n.d.). It can be defined as the use of fewer animals to obtain a particular level of information or obtain more information with a given number of animals so that fewer animals are used overall (Balls 2009). The accuracy of an experiment depends on the *number of samples (animals) per experimental group, the variation in response to the treatment, and the quality of the experimental design and collection of data for the experiment*, i.e. the right choice of strategies in the planning and performance of the research project (Art. 47 Directive 2010).

The first, and most essential, step in the planning of any experimental program is a clear identification of the objectives of the program. However, the objectives of a single experiment must be defined within the context of the overall strategy of which it is typically only a small brick (Das et al. 2009).

To get the best results, many experiments benefit from standardisation of parameters other than those selected in the experimental design, variation of which would disturb and influence the research data in an uncontrolled way. Standardisation is achieved by minimising the (interindividual) variation in each parameter ("noise") and maximising any effect on the parameter from a treatment ("signal"). Standardisation and randomisation are considerations that need proper attention when planning an experiment.

The psychosomatic condition of experimental animals is probably a neglected subject in the development of efficient technique in animal experiments. The importance becomes clear when the strong influence of the interaction between the brain and body on the results obtained is considered. Standardisation of this interaction contributes strongly to the quality of these results. Standardisation of animal care and experimental techniques plays an integral part of this. Proper housing conditions and the application of enrichment are among the basic requirements enforced through legislation. Environmental enrichment contributes to the well-being of the animals. Enrichment, i.e. offering more than basic materials and elements, contributes to refinement and extends the range of activities available to the animal and increases their coping activities (9, Art. 33.1). This contributes to refinement first and secondly to reduction.

In addition, the use of a heterogeneous stock is not the best way to obtain a wide inductive base for better extrapolation to the heterogeneous human/animal population but by choosing several different homogeneous samples or by using a set of selected pure lines or preferably F1 crossbreds offering the possibility of making a relatively precise estimate of the error instead. Models capable of *discriminating* between compounds of a given dose level and correctly predicting effects in humans are valuable models, independent of their level of fidelity (Festing 2009).

If all animals in a cage get the same treatment, not the animal but the cage is the experimental unit. To address each animal as an independent experimental unit, animals of different treatment groups are housed in mixed social groups or, when necessary, singly housed. Proper randomisation of the experimental units must be achieved and bias be excluded whenever possible. The distribution of cages among the rack and in the animal holding room may also influence the outcome of the experiment (Das et al. 2009).

Furthermore, a consideration of the available facilities and the feasibility of the experimental procedures in the context of the design needs attention, for example, the maximum capacity of the cages and available time required for and sequence of the treatments.

In an existing research field or program, group sizes should be calculated by selecting the appropriate statistical test and feeding the test with relevant figures of previous experiments. If intermediate loss of animals or unsuitable data are expected, an adequate number of animals need to be added.

Whenever the training of personnel can reduce the intermediate loss of animals and the adequacy of data, proper education and training should be provided to fulfill moral and legal requirements.

A full research data set also includes data of the individual animal (strain (inbred or outbred), sex, body weight, etc.), food and water, environment, health status, staff involved in procedures, transport, etc.

With a strategic, long-term approach for future reduction and refinement, sufficient details are included in the (scientific) publication. Unfortunately, it is still common practice to include only a limited description of "material and methods" in publications, thus hampering the repeatability of experiments.

The term reuse is used when an animal is used again in an experiment after completion of one series of procedures for another experiment, i.e. when the objectives of the experiments could have been met by the use of an unused animal (9, Art. 16). The ability to reuse animals is critical to the implementation of the reduction and refinement of procedures (Art. 47 Directive 2010).

Regulations and guidelines on equipment and facilities are brief and general, but the 3Rs and the design of the facility including the equipment installed are not separate entities, and specifically for the behavioral needs of animals, the facilities should provide a suitable environment.

5.3.3 Refinement

Breeding of animals, the accommodation, their care, and methods used in procedures can eliminate or reduce to a minimum any possible discomfort to the animals like pain, suffering, distress, or lasting harm (9, Art. 4.3). Refinement means that all appropriate methods should be provided to prevent, limit, or reduce any suffering to the animal, either by administration of suitable painkillers, anesthesia, special care (food, temperature-controlled (micro-)environment, fluid therapy, etc.) or early abatement of the procedure which is the source of suffering. Any method selected should be compatible with the purpose of the procedure.

When a non-animal alternative is not available, reduction and refinement should always be implemented. The detailed explanation of reduction has already unveiled the close relationship between reduction and refinement.

A prerequisite for fulfilling the requirement of refinement is that personnel is skilled in all procedures. Directive 2010/63/EU emphasises the importance of training, supervision, and competence of personnel. Member states shall publish minimum requirements with regard to training, not only for obtaining but also for maintaining (continuing professional development, CPD) and demonstrating the requisite competence.

Refinements are also found in the requirements for separate housing of species that are incompatible (e.g. predator and prey) and availability of special purpose procedure rooms for situations where, from an animal's well-being point of view, it is undesirable to carry out the procedures or observations in the holding rooms, e.g. if these procedures may cause distress to other animals present in the holding room.

Pilot studies are a useful tool, both for reduction and refinement. Pilot studies may prevent the waste of animals and resources by revealing deficiencies in the design of a proposed experiment or procedure, allowing these to be addressed before time and resources are expended on large-scale studies. They may provide information about variability under the existing experimental conditions and indicate whether or how this might be controlled. Their value for refinement is in providing vital information on the severity of proposed procedures or treatments and directed toward development of refinement. Severe effects should be avoided for ethical reasons and because they may evoke responses from the animals that invalidate the experimental results (Das et al. 2009). In case of an uneventful pilot study, the results may contribute to the large-scale study, and it can serve as a confirmation of the initial experimental design, which is not a waste of animals.

In nuclear medicine, the capacity of small animal equipment, PET, SPECT, CT, or MRI forces the researcher into a lengthy time schedule. The first series of animals may serve as a pilot group allowing for adjustment in the coming series.

Humane Endpoints The suffering of animals is effected by the duration and severity of the manipulations and its effects on the animal. Based on the principle of refinement, this suffering shall be kept to the minimum. It requires the detection of sources of discomfort before starting the experiments. All methods available are used to reach the experimental goal already in an early stage and monitor animals on an appropriate level to discover unexpected discomfort and alleviate or stop suffering. Reduction in time span, frequency of unpleasant events, or intensity means a big improvement in reducing the level of suffering.

A humane endpoint can be considered as a possible refinement alternative for those experiments that involve pain and discomfort for the animals. A humane endpoint can be defined as "the earliest indicator in an animal experiment of (potential) pain and/or distress that, within the context of moral justification and scientific endpoints to be met, can be used to avoid or limit pain and/or distress by taking actions such as humanely killing or terminating or alleviating the pain and distress."

A humane endpoint should be balanced against the scientific endpoints to be met and should never be beyond the scientific endpoint or beyond the level of moral justification (Website humane-endpoints.info).

The animal welfare body (AWB) plays a crucial role in overseeing the conduction of animal experiments. The AWB is similar to the Institutional Animal Care and Use Committee (IACUC) in the USA, although there may be significant differences. The AWB tasks have to do with oversight and the review process including to "advise the staff on the application of the requirement of replacement, reduction and refinement and keep it informed of technical and scientific developments concerning the application of that requirement."

5.3.4 Synthesis of Evidence

The 3Rs are established in the EU directive. Each application for project authorisation is subject to a project evaluation by the competent authority. The application as well as the nontechnical summary must refer to the application of methods to replace, reduce, and refine the use of animals in procedures. In the Netherlands, special attention is paid for this purpose to synthesise evidence, any method providing full research evidence relevant to a specific question by identifying, selecting, appraising, and synthesising in order to enable evidenced-based decisions. Systematic review is one of these methods. Systematic reviews are standard practice in clinical studies but are not yet widely conducted in the field of laboratory animal science. Given that many studies using laboratory animals are aimed at improving human health (and health care), it seems reasonable that research using animals be reviewed in a similar way and adheres to the similar high-quality standards as in clinical research.

A systematic review can contain a meta-analysis. In a meta-analysis, the results of several independent studies are statistically combined. In other words, an average effect of two or more studies addressing the same question in more or less the same way is calculated (www.syrcle.nl). The quality of a review relies of course on the quality of the underlying scientific publications.

5.3.5 3Rs and Imaging Techniques

The availability of imaging techniques has opened a new area for reduction and refinement as has radiotelemetry. MRI, PET, SPECT, CT, IVIS, and others provide anatomical information, as well as measurements of physiology, metabolism, pathology, and pharmacology. In cancer research, neurological research, and transgenic research, among other research areas, one or several imaging techniques have been added to the toolbox. Imaging can be used to refine traditionally invasive procedures, so reducing the suffering of experimental animals, decreasing the number of animals required in each study, and permitting real-time measurements. In addition, imaging techniques enable that data of multiple timepoints are taken from each animal and that individual animals can act as their own controls, which greatly reduces variation, thus improving the quality of the scientific output and increasing the validity of the conclusions (Hudson 2006).

Where the imaging technique itself is subject to research, reduction is less evident. Nuclear medicine is auxiliary for many medical disciplines, and the development of tracers for new target organs, e.g. biochemical receptors, generates a wide range of research projects where animal experiments on mice, rats, or larger species are often involved. In the ethical review process, these distinct applications of imaging techniques require different approaches. Imaging used as a refinement technique is often performed at several time points in the same animal. For tracer development, establishing the value of a tracer may require comparison of images and measuring the amount of tracer in selected tissues and organs. After imaging, the animal is humanely killed, and analysis on separate organs is performed.

For these imaging directed projects where procedures on animals are involved, the general rules for reduction and refinement should be applied as for all projects.

5.4 Part III. The Use of Genetically Modified Animals in Nuclear Medicine Imaging

In the last 5–10 years, nuclear medicine imaging is increasingly used in animal research. Adapted equipment has been developed to make it possible to use this technique on small animals, such as rodents. It is not always possible to utilise the equipment within the building of an animal facility, and often the research is done under the auspices of a Nuclear Imaging Center which is also responsible for human diagnostics. This means that animals have to be transported from the animal facility to the imaging facility and, but not in all cases, back. The use of genetically modified animals in research, especially rodents, has become more common in the last decade, and as a consequence, these animals are also used more often for nuclear medicine imaging research. In this section, important issues are addressed that should be taken into account when planning research with genetically altered animals within the nuclear medicine imaging facility.

5.4.1 European Law

In Europe, working with genetically modified animals for research purposes is guided by Directive 2010/63/EU (http://eur-lex.europa.eu/LexUriServ/LexUriServ.do?uri=OJ:L:2010:276:0033:0079:en:PDF). In the Netherlands, the use of genetically modified animals is also regulated by law concerning the contained use of genetically modified organisms. The main purpose of this law is to prevent the escape of a modified animal into the environment, meaning that measures need to be taken in the construction of the room in which the animals are analyzed (see below). When blood and tissue need to be analyzed or stored for later research, the institute also needs to observe the Animal By-Products Regulation (Regulation (EC) No 1069/2009 (http://eur-lex.europa.eu/LexUriServ/LexUriServ.do?uri=OJ:L:2009:300:0001:0033:EN:PDF)). This regulation also dictates measures to be taken when the material is sent to another institute or company. When the modified animal has been created by the use of viral vectors or the animal serves as a host for (genetically modified) microorganisms, regulations concerning public health come into play. In European countries, viral vectors and other genetically modified microorganisms are regulated by law based on Directive 2009/41/EC (http://eur-lex.europa.eu/legal-content/en/ALL/?uri=CELEX:32009L0041) "on the contained use of genetically modified micro-organisms." The use of wild-type microorganisms is covered by Directive 2000/54/EC (http://eur-lex.europa.eu/legal-content/en/ALL/?uri=CELEX:32000L0054) "on the protection of workers from risks related to exposure to biological agents at work." The abovementioned European directives and regulations should be incorporated into national law. In many cases, permits are required before the start of experiments on animals in the nuclear medicine imaging facility. The institutional office responsible for health, safety, and environment is available for advice. In the next sections, we ignore the use of microorganism-associated animals and stick to the use of genetically modified animals created by non-viral techniques and free of microorganisms.

5.4.2 Construction of the Laboratories

Laboratories where animals are kept need to be constructed in a manner which prevents them from escaping. In case of an incident, in which the animal is released from the experimental setup, there should therefore be no cracks or holes. A window in the entrance door allows to check for released animals before opening the door. A warning sign outside the lab prevents unexpected opening of the door by colleagues when an experiment is in progress. When the animals are associated with microorganisms, more stringent demands for the construction of the lab are required. Information about the measures to be taken can be found in the section V of the Centers for Disease Control publication "Biosafety in Microbiological and Biomedical Laboratories"(Biosafety in Microbiological and Biomedical Laboratories (BMBL) 2009).

5.4.3 Infection Prevention

In order to prevent contamination, the research with laboratory animals should be performed by using SPF (specified pathogen free) laboratory animals. These animals should be obtained from approved vendors (commercial or noncommercial) breeding laboratory animals under FELASA (Federation of Laboratory Animals Science Associations) recommendations (FELASA working group on revision of guidelines for health monitoring of rodents and rabbits et al. 2014). The SPF laboratory animals have a health status report based on the FELASA recommendations and are documented free of specified pathogen microorganisms. The housing procedures for the SPF laboratory animals as well as the experimental procedures at the Nuclear Medicine Imaging Center should be performed under standardised operation procedures (SOPs) preventing microbiological contamination of the SPF animals. These SOPs must describe the experimental procedures as how many animals are imaged at the same time and what microbiological status the animals must have and disinfection of the adapted equipment by using specified sterilins. For more information and for the local SOPs, contact the local biosafety officer.

5.4.4 Housing Procedures

The housing of the genetically modified animals should be preferably in a permanent individually ventilated cage (IVC) unit. In this way, the microbiological status of the genetically altered animals can be guaranteed during the whole period of research. The risk of contamination of the genetically altered animals is low when following the IVC procedures. All manipulations should be performed in laminar flow cabinets (changing cabinets). All caging material must be sanitised, and food, bedding, and drinking water should be autoclaved. The transportation of the genetically altered animals toward the Nuclear Medicine Imaging Center is preferably in a mobile IVC System.

The Nuclear Medicine Imaging Center can be present in a separate department at the Laboratory Animal Facility where the genetically modified animals are originally housed or at another location outside the Laboratory Animal Facility. When the Nuclear Medicine Imaging Center is not able to provide the legally required housing conditions, it is obligatory to keep the animals only temporarily (not overnight) at the Nuclear Medicine Imaging Center. After imaging, the genetically altered animals are transported in the mobile IVC system back to their original housing in the permanent IVC housing system.

References

Art 47 in http://eur-lex.europa.eu/LexUriServ/LexUriServ.do?uri=OJ:L:2010:276:0033:0079:en:PDF. https://www.humane-endpoints.info/en

Balls M. Special anniversary volume — issue 1: reduction, preface. Atla. 2009;37:21.

Balls M. Replacement. Atla. 2013;41:512–53.

Biosafety in Microbiological and Biomedical Laboratories (BMBL). 5th ed. Antlanta: Centers for Disease Control and Prevention; 2009. http://www.cdc.gov/biosafety/publications/bmbl5/.

Council of Europe. European Convention for the Protection of Vertebrate Animals used for Experimental and Other Scientific Purposes. European Treaty Series 123. 1986.

Council of Europe. Appendix A of the European Convention for the protection of vertebrate animals used for experimental and other scientific purposes (ETS No. 123). Guidelines For Accommodation And Care Of Animals (Article 5 Of The Convention). Approved By The Multilateral Consultation. Cons 123 (2006) 3. 2006.

EC transposition score board updated on the 2nd of May 2014 still showed four countries that had not notified the EC of transposition 2010/63/EU into national legislation: Italy, The Netherlands, Poland and Romania. http://ec.europa.eu/environment/chemicals/lab_animals/transposition_en.htm.

FELASA working group on revision of guidelines for health monitoring of rodents and rabbits, Mähler Convenor M, Berard M, Feinstein R, Gallagher A, Illgen-Wilcke B, Pritchett-Corning K, Raspa M. FELASA recommendations for the health monitoring of mouse, rat, hamster, guinea pig and rabbit colonies in breeding and experimental units. Lab Anim. 2015;49(1):88.

Festing M. Editorial fifty years after Russell and Burch, toxicologists continue to ignore genetic variation in their test animals. Atla. 2009;37:1–5.

Guillén J, Editor. Laboratory animals: regulations and recommendations for global collaborative research. Amsterdam, etc.: Elsevier, Academic Press; 2013.

http://ec.europa.eu/environment/chemicals/lab_animals.

http://ec.europa.eu/environment/chemicals/lab_animals/pdf/Endorsed_E-T.pdf.

http://ec.europa.eu/environment/chemicals/lab_animals/pdf/qa.pdf.

http://eur-lex.europa.eu/legal-content/en/ALL/?uri=CELEX:32000L0054.

http://eur-lex.europa.eu/legal-content/en/ALL/?uri=CELEX:32009L0041.

http://eur-lex.europa.eu/LexUriServ/LexUriServ.do?uri=OJ:L:2009:300:0001:0033:EN:PDF.

http://eur-lex.europa.eu/LexUriServ/LexUriServ.do?uri=OJ:L:2010:276:0033:0079:en:PDF.

Hudson M. The EU Physical Agents (EMF) directive and its impact on MRI imaging in animal experiments: a submission by FRAME to the HSE. Atla. 2006;34:343–7.

Rose Gaines D, et al. Planning for *reduction*. Atla. 2009;37:27–32.

Russell WMS, Burch RL. 1959. (as reprinted 1992). The principles of humane experimental technique. Wheathampstead (UK): Universities Federation for Animal Welfare.

The European Parliament and the Council of the European Union. Directive 2010/63/EU of the European Parliament and of the Council of 22 September 2010 on the protection of animals used for scientific purposes. *Official Journal of the European Union* 2010; L 276/33–79.

Website humane-endpoints.info. Department of Animals in Science and Society.

Website Syrclc. www.syrcle.nl.

6 Contract Research and Investigator Driven Research

Wietse Russchen

6.1 Introduction

The discussion in this chapter is referring to a situation where clinical research has been performed by healthcare organizations in the Netherlands in the last decade.

Contract research by definition is assigned and financed by the pharmaceutical industry, while investigator-driven research is financed by nonprofit organizations. This is one of the reasons for the historically grown difference in having more means available and a higher level of knowledge of regulatory requirements in favor of contract research.

The Declaration of Helsinki, principles of conducting research noted down in a Research Code by the World Medical Association, and best practice applied to the execution have always been the backbone of performing clinical research in healthcare organizations.

Through a changed regulatory environment, it became mandatory for both types of research to comply with the same set of rules, directed by the law "Wet medisch-wetenschappelijk onderzoek met mensen (medical-scientific research with humans, WMO)."

6.2 Healthcare Organizations

The law means a challenge for the healthcare organizations to find the resources and to facilitate the requirements prescribed in the law. The global standard Good Clinical Practice (GCP) for the conduct of clinical research plays a key role in this. The basis of GCP is the well-being of the patient, consistent with the principles of the abovementioned Declaration of Helsinki and the credibility of trial data.

W. Russchen
Quality Solutions, Roderwolderweg 38, Foxwolde 9314 TB, The Netherlands
e-mail: info@qualitysolutions.nl

A.W.J.M. Glaudemans et al. (eds.), *Quality in Nuclear Medicine*,
DOI 10.1007/978-3-319-33531-5_6

Healthcare organizations have had and still have their own approach to strive for compliance with the regulatory requirements. A common model is the integration of clinical research in the daily operation of providing care to patients. Many healthcare organizations choose for this solution which of course resulted in as many different settings as outcomes. A newly established entity disconnected from the care for patients is also realized as an option.

For years the regulatory authorities did not seem to follow or show interest in the rules being applied to clinical research in healthcare organizations. The regulatory authorities could have used their power to support and guide the healthcare organizations in order to improve and harmonize the circumstances under which clinical research has to be performed. Generally spoken this supportive and guiding role is not preferred or taken up by the governmental inspectorate for the GxP regulations of which they monitor the compliance in the industry and healthcare organizations. They see themselves not as a consultancy. The inspectors keep to their inspection program to assess the level of compliance the moment they visit an organization. The inspectors review documents, records, facilities, and any other relevant resources.

This approach implies "learning by doing" for the inspected organization, including the healthcare organizations, in the process of reaching a level of compliance that is satisfactory in view of the governmental inspectorate.

6.3 Central Committee on Research Involving Human Subjects (CCMO)

The committee "Central Committee on Research involving Human Subjects (CCMO)" has issued a number of publications that can be of help for the investigator for both types of research. The committee was installed in 1999 based on the law WMO, effective from 1998. The primary task of the CCMO is to supervise the activities of the Medical Ethics Committees. The CCMO is also a(n) (inter)national center for questions and information with respect to clinical research. On their website, you can find guidelines and/or examples for, e.g., the following items:

- Clinical trial agreement
- Requesting for a EudraCT number
- Reporting SAEs and SUSARs
- Trial/study report
- Content of the trial master file

6.4 Good Clinical Practice (GCP)

GCP is addressing the different roles of those involved in conducting clinical research. The most important are the roles of the ethics committee, investigator, and sponsor. The ethics committee without doubt oversees the patient safety and ethical aspects of a clinical trial. The investigator, responsible for the conduct of the clinical trial, must have the scientific qualifications, be able to supply the accountable resources and potential participants, and foresees in an adequate facility to perform the clinical trial. The more difficult ones to a certain extent are the responsibilities of the sponsor. GCP describes the role of the sponsor as if it concerns an in-house clinical research, whereas in practice the investigator takes over some of these tasks and responsibilities of the sponsor.

A quality assurance system to assure and control clinical research of the trial execution, data registration, and reporting is one of the most striking examples. Other duties taken over and performed by the investigator are filing a request for approval to start the trial at the ethics committee, warehousing, and preparing and distributing the investigational medicinal product in compliance with the relevant rules of the standard good manufacturing practice (GMP) in cooperation with the pharmacy of the healthcare organization.

Probably these examples are the reason why the pharmaceutical industry, as a sponsor, has strongly supported and still is supporting their own clinical trials at the healthcare organization of the selected investigator. The support may include delivering the relevant documents needed for the trial like a protocol, informed consent, and case report forms. The sponsor also takes care of trial-specific training and monitoring. The monitoring of a trial is overseeing the progress and compliance with the protocol, standard operating procedures (SOPs), GCP, and other applicable regulatory requirements.

For investigator-driven research, the tasks and responsibilities of sponsor and investigator as a whole have to be encountered by the healthcare organization with a smaller budget and less support when compared to contract research.

6.5 Quality Assurance System

Healthcare organizations often have already a quality assurance system in place, e.g., ISO 9001 related. In this case, the choice to be made is either to include contract research and investigator-driven research according to GCP in the existing quality system or to set up a separate GCP quality system for clinical research. The distinction in contract research and investigator-driven research can be made in the quality system chosen for and does not require two separate quality systems.

If clinical research is integrated in the process of the daily operation of providing care to patients than for practical reasons, the existing quality system may be adapted to a GCP proof quality system also.

In order to establish the GCP level with respect to the role of the investigator in your current quality assurance system, you can use the checklist in the attachment. The results may serve as a quick reference and a first impression of what needs to be done to design a quality assurance system as described in the sections below.

A well-designed quality assurance system goes beyond the mandatory requirements in GCP.

The difficulty is how to design, by whom, and after implementing who becomes responsible for the system. Integrity, protection of patients (safety and confidentiality), registration of credible and reliable data (validation and safety of information management systems), traceability of critical materials, accountability of investigational products, and a potential reconstructing of a trial must be embedded.

Validation becomes more and more an issue in the last years, not only applied to equipment that is used but also to information technology and software, e.g., in use for statistical calculations with the registered data of a trial. The principle of validating is collecting evidence of suitability and reliability for a piece of equipment, a specific function, a process, calculation models, etc. Validating is often done with support of the supplier and consists at least of an installation qualification (IQ = received what is requested?) and an operational qualification (OQ = function complies with what is required?). The user is responsible for the performance qualification (PQ = compliance testing of the performance over a longer period of time).

The development of procedures with respect to safety of information management systems is recently of high interest. In this respect, the standards ISO 27001 and ISO 20000 are helpful to read.

One should be aware of the fact that implementing the applicable regulatory requirements is an ongoing process.

Reading GCP the quality assurance system for clinical trials should basically be built on the following two elements:

- Quality assurance (verification that quality control is working, performed on taken samples at random)
- Quality control (designed to achieve quality, performed on each output every time)

However, today many of us think that the quality assurance system should also inspire all involved in clinical research to improve continuously for the benefit of those who make an appeal to the (future) services offered by the healthcare organizations.

Techniques to be used for continuously improving are:

- Measuring key indicators that may have an influence on the quality of the trial
- Discussing the status and the problems encountered in a short daily meeting
- For analyzing a problem, use one of more of the following instruments:
  - Circle of Deming (based on plan, do, check, and act)
  - Pareto analysis (decision-making technique)
  - Ishikawa diagram (cause and effect diagram)

6.6 Plan-Do-Check-Act

The plan-do-check-act cycle (Website ASQ: The Global Voice of Quality) is a four-step model for carrying out changes. Just as a circle has no end, the PDCA cycle should be repeated again and again for continuous improvement.

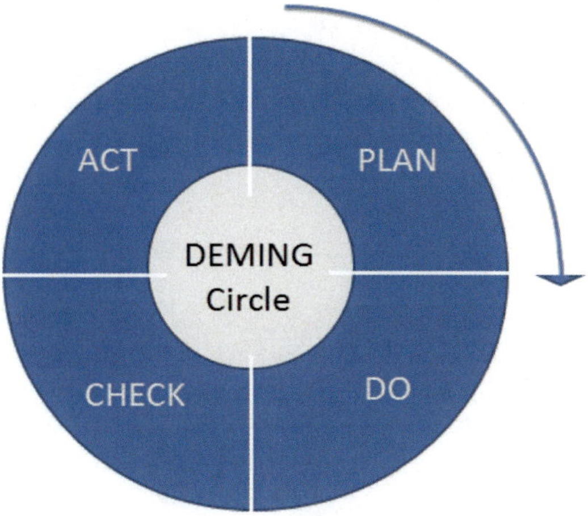

PDCA Procedure

Plan: recognize an opportunity and plan a change.
Do: test the change and carry out a small-scale study.
Check: review the test, analyze the results, and identify what you have learned.
Act: take action based on what you have learned in the study step; if the change did not work completely, go through the cycle again with a different plan.

6.7 Pareto Analysis

Pareto analysis uses the Pareto Principle, also known as the "80/20"rule, stating that 20% of causes generate roughly 80% of the effects that arise from the 20% of the causes.

Pareto Analysis is a simple technique for prioritizing possible changes by identifying the problems that will be resolve by making these changes. By using this approach, you can prioritize the individual changes that will most improve the situation (Source: website Mind Tools: Management training and leadership training online).

How to use the tool?

Step 1: identify and list the problems.
Write a list of all the problems that you need to resolve. Where possible, talk to team members and patients to get their input, and draw on surveys, helpdesk logs, and such like, where these are available.
Step 2: identify the root cause of each problem.
For each problem, identify its fundamental cause.

Step 3: score problems.

Now you need to score each problem. The scoring method you use depends on the sort of problem you are trying to solve.

For example, if you are trying to improve customer satisfaction, you might score them on the basis of the number of complaints eliminated by solving the problem.

Step 4: group problems together by root cause.

Group problems together by cause. For example, if three of your problems are caused by lack of staff, put these in the same group.

Step 5: add up the scores for each group.

The group with the top scores has the highest priority, and the group with the lowest scores has the lowest priority.

Step 6: take action.

Deal with the top-priority problem or groups of problems.

Cause and effect analysis helps to think through the causes of a problem thoroughly, including its possible causes. It is by identifying the main causes that permanently remove the problem. The inventor is Professor Kaoru Ishikawa of Tokyo University.

By going through the process of building the diagram with colleagues, everybody gains insights into the problem, alongside possible solutions. The people involved benefit from the shared contributions, leading to a common understanding of the problem.

The analysis enables a team to focus on the content of the problem rather than its history or the differing interests of team members. Indentify the problem, write it in a box, and draw an arrow pointing towards it. Draw four or more potential causes or categories off the large arrow. Categories could include equipment, environment, procedures, and people. Make sure that the categories used are relevant for the particular problem (Fig. 6.1).

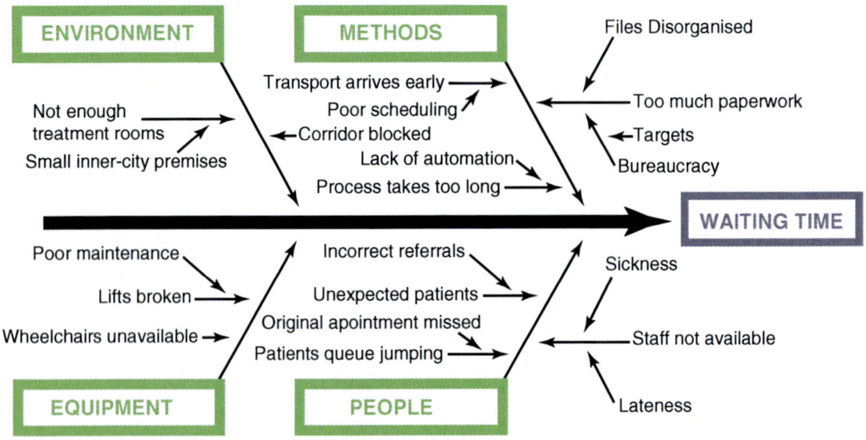

Fig. 6.1 Example of a cause and effect analysis (Source: website NHS Institute for Innovation and Improvement)

6.8 Attachment 1: Quality Assurance System

A written and documented Quality Assurance System for clinical research may consists of:

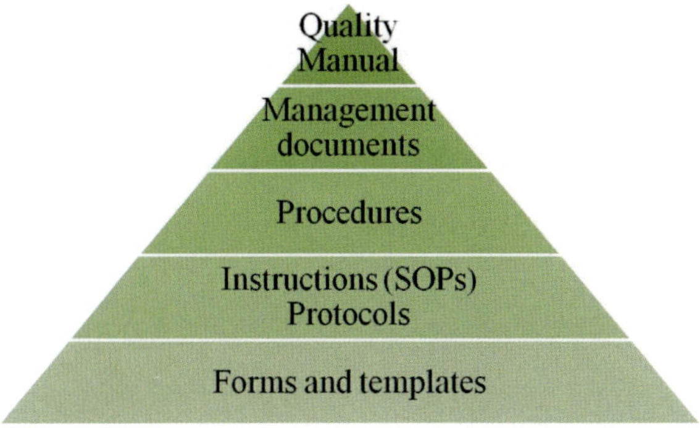

Having procedures and instructions is minimally required. Procedures and instructions are designed to achieve uniformity in the conduct of clinical research and important for the potential reconstruction.

A procedure is a summing up of activities to be followed. A procedure indicates who does what and who is responsible. An instruction describes in detail how an activity as mentioned in the procedure must be carried out and appoints to only one person. In writing procedures and instructions, you should avoid long sentences and difficult and vague words.

Some organizations combine the procedures and instructions in one document: standard operating procedure (SOP).

Essential documents to set up are:

- Change control
- Qualification and training of employees
- Accountability
- Data management
- Internal auditing of facilities, processes, and clinical trials
- Subcontracting (testing, analyzes)
- Archiving of the essentials documents
- Validation of equipment
- Investigational medicinal product (receipt, warehousing, and accountability)
- Monitoring study progress and study data registered

A quality assurance department should manage the documented system. For the reason of independency, the quality assurance department must report to the board of the healthcare organization.

The quality assurance department should focus on measuring compliance through an independent and systematic review (internal audit), initiate continuous improvement, implement a system for good document control (e.g., revision of documents every 2–3 years and archived for at least 10 years), and maintain the system in cooperation with the users.

6.9 Attachment 2: Checklist GCP Level Concerning Investigator Activities

		Ranking				
Number	Activities of the investigator (ICH GCP Sect. 6.4)	1	2	3	4	5
1	Is the investigator qualified to perform clinical research (education, CV, and experience)?					
2	Is the knowledge of the investigational products present and explained by the sponsor?					
3	Do the staff have knowledge of GCP and other relevant regulatory requirements?					
4	Is monitoring and auditing permitted by the investigator?					
5	The staff involved is competent and qualified for the job they have to perform					
6	Is there a list of names of the staff including the activities they are qualified for (site signature log)?					
7	Are the means to be used adequate (apparatus and facilities)?					
8	Does the investigator have the population to recruit participants for the trial?					
9	Is there a procedure to acquire informed consent?					
10	Is medical care for participants adequate?					
11	Is there a procedure for obtaining approval of the ethics committee?					
12	Is a signed protocol required before the start of the trial?					
13	Are deviations of the protocol registered and judged upon?					
14	Is randomization procedure available?					
15	Is there a procedure for subcontracting tests and/or analyzes?					
16	Is there a procedure on how to fill in case report forms and make corrections if needed?					
17	A progress report which is periodically sent to the ethical committee is part of the Quality System					
18	Is a procedure for AEs and SAEs available?					
19	Is document management described in a procedure?					
20	Documents are archived for a minimal time frame. The handling is confirmed in a procedure					
21	Is the reporting of study results by the investigator described in a procedure?					

1 = insufficient, 2 = poor, 3 = reasonable, 4 = sufficient, 5 = excellent

Part II

Radiation Safety

Personnel and Public People

7

Johan R. de Jong

Abstract

In most countries, legislation for working with ionizing radiation is based on the "recommendations of the ICRP" in which the ALARA principle for optimization of radiological work to minimize risk was introduced, dose limits for personnel and public people were defined, and the principle of justified use of ionizing radiation was introduced. Application of ionizing radiation is performed by radiological workers in radiological zones that have to meet certain safety requirements and facilities for dose monitoring and prevention of radioactive contamination. Furthermore, personal dosimetry of radiological workers is obligatory as well as risk analysis of the radiological work. Apart from the protection of workers themselves, legislation is in place to protect the general public as well, such as dose limits, expelling of radioactive substances in air, and water and exemption limits for open radioactive substances. The protection of the general public applies also to the unborn child such that in case of pregnancy, the dose limits for radiological workers no longer apply to the mother, but those of the public people have to be met instead.

7.1 Introduction

Most of current legislation for working with ionizing radiation is based on the "recommendations of the ICRP" of the International Commission on Radiologic Protection (ICRP 1950). The first version of the recommendations was published in

J.R. de Jong
Department of Nuclear Medicine and Molecular Imaging, University of Groningen, University Medical Center Groningen, Hanzeplein 1, Groningen 9700 RB, The Netherlands
e-mail: j.r.de.jong@umcg.nl

A.W.J.M. Glaudemans et al. (eds.), *Quality in Nuclear Medicine*,
DOI 10.1007/978-3-319-33531-5_7

1958 and introduced dose limits for radiological workers and for public people. The dose limits for workers were primarily based on genetic effects and external radiation. ICRP-2 (1959) added limits for internal contamination.

In 1965, ICRP-9 was published and the ALARA principle was introduced. The ICRP acknowledged the absence of a threshold for radiation dose below which no risk is involved. The ALARA principle involves optimization of radiological work to minimize risk. The acronym first stood for "As Low As Readily Achievable," but in ICRP-22 this was changed into "As Low As Reasonably Achievable."

In 1978, ICRP-26 was published and included for the first time explicitly the principles of justification, ALARA/optimization and individual dose limits.

In 1991, ICRP-60 was published. The dose limits for the general public and for radiological workers were decreased based on new data of the Hiroshima/Nagasaki survivors. For radiological workers the total body dose limit was reduced to 100 mSv in 5 years, with a yearly maximum of 50 mSv. For the public people, a dose limit of 1 mSv/year was introduced.

Legislation for working with ionizing radiation mostly follows the ICRP recommendation and involves the basic principles of justification, optimization and individual dose constraints. A list of justified use of ionizing radiation is present for which a permit may be requested. Often also a list is present of applications that cannot be justified and for which no permit is possible. For each justified use of ionizing radiation, a permit is obligatory except for devices or sources for which there is an exemption.

The optimization principle of ALARA is specifically stated in legislation obligating the holders of any permit to reduce the dose as the result of any work with ionizing radiation as much as reasonably achievable. In most countries the dose limits are as follows:

7.2 Personnel

7.2.1 Dose Limits

Dose limits for personnel are listed in Table 7.1. Often a distinction is made between A-workers and B-workers. For A-workers the effective dose limit is 20 mSv/year, whereas for B-workers the effective dose limit is 6 mSv/year. These limits are maximally tolerated doses and cannot be claimed as rights or as limits below which the dose is always justified. Always the ALARA principle has to be taken in consideration.

Table 7.1 Yearly dose limits for radiological workers and public people

Category	Effective dose (mSv)	Eye lens (mSv)	Skin/extremities (mSv)
Radiological workers	20	20	500
Non-radiological workers	1	15	50
Public people in location	1	15	50
Public people outside location	0.1	–	–

7.2.2 Laboratories and Radiological Zones

Applications of ionizing radiation for which a permit is required must be performed in a radiological zone. This radiological zone could be a laboratory where work on open radioactive sources is performed, an examination room in which a device emitting ionizing radiation is present, an examination room in which patients are present that have received radioactivity for diagnostic nuclear medicine examinations, a room in which radioactivity is administrated to patients, a waiting room in which patients (injected with radioactivity) are waiting for nuclear medicine diagnostic imaging, therapy rooms, etc.

The entrance of a radiological zone must be marked with a radioactivity sign, a warning for ionizing radiation and/or radioactive substances. Depending on the maximum dose that can be achieved by a person on a yearly basis, the radiological zone is often categorized as low-risk and high-risk. For example, often the distinction is made between a zone for which the dose is lower than 6 mSv (corresponding to the work of B- workers) and a zone for which the dose is higher than 6 mSv (corresponding to the work of A-workers).

For radionuclide laboratories various regulations exist. These include regulations about ventilation, underpressure, walls and floors (e.g. the presence of seams), taps and such. Laboratories are categorized in risk levels (such as a B-, C-, or D-lab). These categories have their own regulations (D is least strict). The differences in these regulations are usually:

- Classification of workers (A or B workers)
- Maximum allowed amount of radioactivity for work
- Obligation to wear a personal dosimeter or not
- Requirements on the radiation safety officer responsible for overseeing work and regulations

The maximum amount of radioactivity allowed for work at a radionuclide lab is coupled to the risk/radiation dose as a result of the unintentional spread of radioactive substances. The parameters that determine this limit are:

- The radiotoxicity of the radionuclide
- The risk category of the lab
- Ventilation (including flow cabinets, gloveboxes, etc.)

Since usually the work at a lab involves various processes with possibly different nuclides, amounts and duration of the work, the “load” of a laboratory must be monitored. One way of doing this is to sum for each nuclide and for each process the product of the fraction of the activity used in relation to the maximum allowed activity and the cumulative duration of the process in relation to a workweek.

7.2.3 Zone Monitoring

Usually, the monitoring of the radiation dose rate on a radiological zone is not obligatory. However, it is recommended for increasing the safety on a radionuclide laboratory. Instructions for workers on a lab should include using a dose rate monitor during work, especially when opening a flow cabinet, opening a shielded location and generally approaching an area where a radioactive source may be present. As an alternative or an additional measure, zone monitoring may be used in combination with an alarm dose rate level to warn radiological workers of high radiation dose rates. Especially when interlocks or other safety measures cannot be utilized to increase safety or when just not present, zone monitoring may be employed and even augmented by wearing an electronic personal dosimeter (EPD).

7.2.4 Contamination

In radionuclide laboratories where work is performed with open radioactive substances, there is always a risk of the spread of radioactivity. This spread may result in external contamination of objects and persons or in the internal contamination of persons (inhalation or ingestion). Moreover, it may result in spread of radioactivity and contamination outside the radiological zone. It is therefore important to monitor possible contamination on a radiological lab. Aside from working safely and using personal safety instruments such as gloves, lab coats and glasses, the following describes various methods to monitor and contain contamination and can be used in combination.

7.2.4.1 Contamination Check After Work

After completing work, the workplace should always be checked for contamination with a contamination monitor. If a contamination is found, it should be contained and cleaned up. Large contaminations of high amounts of radioactivity are not considered in this case but are rather incidents and discussed elsewhere.

7.2.4.2 Hand-Foot Monitors

A hand-foot contamination monitor may be placed at the entrance of a radionuclide lab. The device checks for contamination of the extremities and should be used whenever leaving the lab.

7.2.4.3 Wipe Tests

Wipe tests should be performed regularly (e.g. once a month) on a radionuclide lab where long-lived radionuclides are used. This way, build-up of contamination is detected, and it also monitors the (continued) safe and clean working of the radiological workers, especially after change of personnel or change of work. The wipe tests involve mapping locations at the lab at which accidental contamination is most likely or at which contamination is most likely to happen when work becomes "sloppy." These locations are wiped with a tissue and measured for radioactivity. Notorious are keyboards and mice (forgot to change gloves), pipettes and spots in hot cells or flow cabinets where radioactivity is extracted from closed systems.

7.2.5 Risk Assessments

All use of sources of ionizing radiation must be licensed, justified, and optimized. When applying for a license, risk assessment should be part of the application. In order to make a proper risk assessment, the processes that are part of the application need to be mapped and written down and divided into separate steps. Since SOPs (standard operational procedures) usually are already part of the operational management as well as the application for a license, these can be used to create an overview of all steps. For the risk assessment, the exposure (dose obtained by the worker) for all steps is determined. This includes the regular exposure due to the activities that are part of the work as well as foreseen unintentional events.

Anything else could be seen as an incident. For foreseen unintentional events, the risk may be evaluated by determining the product of the probability (frequency that the event may take place) and severity (in this case the dose obtained). In this way, each step is evaluated, and either deemed acceptable or judged unacceptable, such that additional measures need to be taken or procedural changes and improvements need to be put in place. One of the methods of risk assessment ideally suited in this case is the Fine-Kinney method.

When all steps have been evaluated, the total exposure due to steps in the application is summed to obtain the total exposure attributed to the application and its processes. In turn this total exposure is used to determine the classification of workers and of radiological areas. The classification of radiological workers into low-risk or high-risk is determined by the expected exposure obtained by summing up the doses that they receive according to the risk assessments of all processes and applications that they take part in. This depends, for example, on the size of the pool of workers that perform the job. In addition, the classification of a radiological area is determined by the sum of the expected exposures that follow from the risk assessment of all steps from all processes and applications that take place in the radiological area, in other words, the dose that would be obtained by a worker that is taking part in all work being done in the radiological area.

Calculation of the exposure due to the application of ionizing radiation is just one part of a proper risk analysis. Aside from the calculation of the dose, the risk assessment should also explain the basic assumptions and principles underlying the risk assessment as well as the proper context. Finally, the risk assessment should contain proper assessments of the calculated risks and exposures and evaluate whether these are acceptable and if the criteria of optimization are met. The calculated exposure of the workers can be used as a dose reference level of what is deemed "normal." Any significant elevation of the dose that workers obtain from the dose reference level may be a reason to look into the way the worker is performing his duties and to reevaluate whether the risk assessment is actual and realistic.

The risk assessment should be evaluated by performing actual measurements of the dose obtained by workers. Ideally, the real dose obtained by workers should be close to the expected dose from the risk assessment. Finally, the risk assessment should be re-evaluated periodically and checked for being actual. As this is usually also the case for the SOPs in operational management, the update of the SOPs and the re-evaluation of the risk assessment could be linked together.

7.2.6 Personnel Dosimetry and Dose Monitoring

Personal dose monitoring for radiological workers is mandatory. Often this is implemented by wearing a TLD badge that is exchanged on a monthly or 4-weekly basis. The badge is read-out by an external organization with government approval. The radiation safety officer overseeing the radiological work is responsible for monitoring the read-out data of the personal TLD badges in order to check for irregularities (sudden increase of dose per period) and checking that personal dose constraints are not exceeded. In addition, the badge read-outs can be used to check the effectiveness of measures that have been taken to increase radiation safety.

For laboratory personnel it may be necessary to monitor the extremity dose as well by wearing a TLD finger tip (ring). This is particularly the case when working with positron emitters as the contribution of the positrons on the dose on the fingers is much higher than the contribution of the gamma photons. Recently, recommendations have been published on this matter as the result of a European study of extremity dose in nuclear medicine: ORAMED.

In cases where a high amount of dose may be received in relatively short time, the timing resolution of monthly TLD badge read-outs is not sufficient. Such situations should be prevented by safety precautions such as interlocks on hot cells, but this is not always possible or present. As mentioned earlier, zone monitoring can play an important role here as well as wearing EPDs.

An additional advantage or use for an EPD is monitoring the dose of certain (new) processes or incidental work. This can be put in relation to prospective risk assessments.

It should be stressed that EPDs have no legal status. They cannot replace TLD badge read-outs for the legally mandatory and nationally central registration of personal dosimetry. In this central register, all badge read-outs are stored by all radiological workers during their radiological work in all organizations. This tracks the life dose of radiological workers even when changing organization.

7.2.7 Medical Inspection of Radiological Workers

Radiological workers should be medically monitored. Usually this is only performed for radiological A- workers and implemented as a yearly checkup. For this yearly checkup, the radiological worker is examined by a radiation physician, but this may also be done by filling in a survey after which the need for examination is judged by the radiation physician.

7.2.8 Pregnancy

Pregnant radiological workers are carrying, in the sense of the law, a member of the general public. Therefore, usually a dose limit of 1 mSv for the unborn is maintained from the moment the pregnancy is reported to the manager or radiation safety officer until the end of the pregnancy. In practice this means that the dose limit of 1 mSv is enforced for the mother as well. The tasks and activities of the pregnant worker have to be adapted to this dose restraint. In addition, the personal dose monitoring is continued if the work still involves radiological work. In nuclear medicine practices, ways to adapt the work involve doing administrative work or work that minimizes exposure to sources and patients as well as stopping work with (open) radioactive sources. Operating a medical imaging device may still be possible.

7.2.9 Breastfeeding

The risk for the infant in case of a breastfeeding radiological worker is internal contamination. In turn this can be the result of external contamination of the mother or internal contamination of the mother in which case the breast milk may be contaminated as well. This leads to restrictions on the amount of radioactivity the radiological worker is allowed to work with. In practice this could mean that working with open radioactive substances is ceased altogether.

7.2.10 Sealed Radioactive Sources

Sealed radioactive sources are sources that cannot leak radioactivity under normal circumstances. There are often requirements for these sources in terms of resistance to pressure, impact, temperature, etc. Nonetheless, sealed sources should be checked regularly for leakage by performing a wipe test to exclude the risk of contamination. When not in use, a sealed radioactive source should be placed in a depot. This depot should be used exclusively for radioactive sources and has to meet certain criteria regarding indication of radioactive sources, shielding requirements, lock, etc. An administration should be present listing all sealed sources present, their strength, nuclide and their use.

7.2.11 Quality Control of Dosimetric Devices

Dosimetric devices such as contamination monitors, dose monitors and area monitoring play a vital role in the radiation safety strategy. Therefore, these dosimetric devices should be subject to a quality control system. It may often be necessary to send the devices to an external agency for calibration with a yearly frequency. On the basis of a few dosimetric devices that are periodically calibrated externally, the remainder of the devices may be calibrated internally by qualified personnel.

Aside from calibration, the dosimetric devices should undergo quality control to check their proper function. Examples of this are the dose calibrators that are used to measure and prepare the amount of radioactivity that will be administered to a patient. Aside from the need to have quality control of the dose calibrator for the safety of the patient, the exposure of radiological workers also depends on the proper function of the dose calibrator: external exposure due to syringes or patients injected with radioactivity will be unjustifiably higher if the dose calibrator underestimates radioactivity amounts systematically.

7.2.12 Incidents

Any event that is both unintentional and unforeseen is an incident. It is important to have general protocols for handling incidents. These protocols should be targeted at minimizing the effect (exposure) for workers and helpers (e.g. fire department) and at decontamination of contaminated workers. Also, taking measurements to estimate the extent of the contamination should be performed. In case of internal contamination, taking urine samples at regular intervals may be considered to be able to estimate the severity of the contamination and to estimate the radiation dose.

Any quality management system should include a PDCA (Plan, Do, Check, Act) cycle to learn from incidents that do occur. Retrospective risk analysis and analysis of the incident (such as the PRISMA method) help finding the high risk factors that make it possible for the incident to occur. After performing the analysis, a plan is made to improve the security of the procedures, and the SOPs and risk analyses should be updated. After implementation of the plan, its effect should be evaluated in practice. To complete the cycle, the evaluation leads to action and a new plan for improvement.

7.3 Public People

7.3.1 Dose Limits

An organization that applies ionizing radiation is obligated to ensure that the licensed applications do not cause the radiation dose received by the public people to exceed legal limits (see Table 7.1). Note that the legal limits are exclusive of natural background. The sources of ionizing radiation in case of a nuclear medicine department that must be considered are outlined below.

7.3.1.1 Sealed Radioactive Sources

Sealed radioactive sources normally do not contribute significantly to the dose of public people as they are stored in a depot when not in use. In addition, when used, the radiological workers wielding them obtain by far the highest dose. Nonetheless, in a dosimetric analysis of the exposure to public people, the use of sealed radioactive sources should be analysed, and their contribution to the public people present in or traversing through public areas in the vicinity of the radiological area should be evaluated as well as their contribution to the dose at the terrain border (see Environment).

7.3.1.2 Open Radioactive Sources

In most regards, the contribution of open radioactive sources is similar to that of sealed radioactive sources regarding external irradiation of public people. However, in case of open radioactive sources, there is the additional risk of spread of radioactivity, contamination that may lead to external irradiation as well as external and internal contamination of public people. Usually, in the dosimetric analysis of the required shielding of rooms, only external radiation is considered. Contamination is dealt with through the safety measures present for radionuclide laboratories and the rooms for the administration of radiotracers. A check for contamination of the working area after a procedure, regular wipe tests, area monitoring and personal contamination checks using a hand-foot contamination monitors are all required tools to detect and prevent the spread of open radioactive sources beyond the radiological areas in which they are utilized.

In case of spread of open radioactivity in a hot cell or flow cabinet, the radioactivity is expelled in the open air. Depending on the type and amount of radioactivity, filters may need to be installed in the venting systems of a radionuclide lab. Evaluation of the risk to the public people in event of venting radioactivity in air must be part of the risk analysis that is part of the process of planning the facilities prior to building them. See also Environment.

7.3.1.3 Patients

Patients injected with radioactivity contribute to the exposure of the public people. In general, except for radionuclide therapy, patients leaving the hospital do not pose a risk for the public people as the exposure of individual members of the public to a radioactive patient is relatively rare, the duration of the exposure short, the dose rate at 1 m from the patient low, and the (biological) half-life of the radionuclide relatively short. This is true even for family members of the patient.

It is different in case that the concentration of radioactive patients is rather high and/or the probability of public people to be exposed to radioactive patients is high as well. These areas include the nuclear medicine department in general and more specifically the waiting areas for patients that have received radioactivity prior to scanning, the rooms in which radioactivity is administered and the rooms where (imaging) diagnostics are performed. These rooms generally require lead shielding in order to decrease the exposure to the public people.

In the dosimetric analysis in which the required shielding is determined, a distinction may be made between a nearby office (in which nonradiological workers that are considered to be public people may reside 100 % of the working hours) and, for example, corridors (in which a residence time of 50 % or even 10 % may be accounted for). Of course, the same may also be applied to the contribution to the exposure of public people from other sources of ionizing radiation.

Patients that have to remain in the hospital due to administration of high amounts of radioactivity as in the case of radionuclide therapy are a much larger source of ionizing radiation than diagnostic patients in general. Since in this case the exposure to family members and in some worst-case scenarios the exposure to members of the public may exceed legal limits, these patients remain in the hospital until the radiation dose rate has decreased sufficiently (in the case of 131-I therapy for ablation of thyroid tissue, a dose rate of 20 μSv/h at 1 m is the norm for dismissal). Even after the patient is allowed to leave, certain rules may have to be obeyed to limit the external exposure to family members and to limit the risk of contamination.

During their stay, radionuclide therapy patients remain a source of exposure for the public people both in the hospital and beyond the terrain border. A dosimetric analysis is part of the design of the suites in which the patients stay. Lead shielding of the walls may prove a requirement, but to increase hospitality windows are recommended. For shielding purposes these windows can include lead glass, but as an alternative or additional measure, the suites may be installed in the top level of the building rather than the ground level as to increase the distance to the terrain border.

7.3.1.4 Devices

Devices that emit ionizing radiation at a nuclear medicine department are usually limited to devices containing a roentgen tube and perhaps a cyclotron. One of the handy advantages of roentgen devices is that the exposure stops as soon as the tube is shut down enabling the use of interlocks to shut down the system when a door is opened. The main contribution of exposure to the public people is due to the scattered radiation from the patient during a radiological procedure. The lead shielding in the walls of the room due to the shielding of radiation from the patient is more than enough to effectively shield the much lower energy of the scattered x-rays provided that the lead shielding is installed from floor to floor covering the full wall.

In case of a cyclotron, it is the shielding of the neutrons that is the main concern. This topic is covered in Chap. 9.

7.4 Volunteers in Nuclear Medicine Research

As mentioned before, any use of ionizing radiation needs to be optimized and justified. In case of diagnosing or treating patients, the decision is made by the nuclear medicine physician whether the treatment or diagnostic procedure is justified. In case of research with volunteers, it is the medical ethics committee that makes judgement. There are however international guidelines that are taken from ICRP publication 62.

ICRP distinguishes four risk levels corresponding to four different ranges of exposure: (i) less than 0.1 mSv, (ii) 0.1–1 mSv, (iii) 1–10 mSv, and (iv) more than 10 mSv. Each risk level corresponds to a minimal societal benefit that the research should meet to justify the exposure, ranging from (i) the increase of knowledge to (iv) direct benefit (cure) for the volunteer. See ICRP 62 for more details and explanation of the societal benefit.

7.5 Environment

Another topic of concern regarding the public people is the environment as the risk of exposure to the public people is covered here as well and translated into legislation. Those points relevant to the public people for a nuclear medicine department are briefly covered in the following text.

7.5.1 Expelling in Air

Radioactive substances expelled in air contribute to the exposure of the public people through inhalation. Based on a risk analysis and dose limits for the general public, an institute is allowed to expel a certain amount of radioactivity in air. This amount is usually expressed in the license in terms of the amount of radiotoxic equivalents (RE). One RE is the amount of radioactive substance of a certain nuclide or radiofarmacon that would cause an effective dose upon inhalation of the substance equal to 1 Sv.

Causes of expelling of radioactive substances are mostly the unintentional spread of radioactivity that is vented from flow cabinets or hot cells. For radionuclide laboratories this is coupled to the equation for determining the maximum amount of radioactivity that may be regularly used in the lab as covered earlier in the chapter. The fraction of radioactivity that may unintentionally be vented is dependent on the type of procedure (spread parameter). This is covered for the application in the request for the license.

The distance to the terrain border and the half-life of the radionuclide are important factors in determining the risk for the public people. As the cloud of radioactive substances spreads towards the terrain border, the concentration decreases by dilution in air and by decay in time.

7.5.2 Expelling in Water

Expelling in water usually means sewage. The main contribution of expelling of radioactivity in sewage is excretion from patients. Just as in the case of expelling in air, the license usually includes a maximum amount of radioactivity in RE (RE ingestion in this case) that may be expelled in sewage. For the occasional toilet of diagnostic patients, there is usually a low risk as the amount of radioactivity is relatively low and the half-life of the radionuclide is relatively short. For therapy patients however, especially those for radioiodine treatment who stay at the hospitals for a number of days, the amount of radioactivity is often too high. Therefore, toilets in the suites for radioiodine patients are often connected to containers that collect the excretion for decay prior to expelling in sewage.

As is the case of expelling in air, dosimetric models exist to evaluate the risk to the public people from expelling radioactivity in sewage.

7.5.3 Dose at the Terrain Border

The dose at the terrain border due to the use of sources of ionizing radiation is calculated as the sum of all external radiation exposure of all applications of ionizing radiation in the hospital, including all departments that use sealed radioactive sources, open radioactive sources as well as devices that emit ionizing radiation. Often, legislation prescribes that the maximum dose at the terrain border, and thus the maximum expected dose to a member of the public people, is one tenth of the dose limit for a member of the public, i.e. 100 μSv per year. This is due to the assumption that the terrain border may be shared with a maximum of ten institutions that utilize ionizing radiation.

7.5.4 Exemption Limits for Radioactive Sources

Some applications of open radioactive substances are inherently very low risk due to the nature of the radioactive substance as well as the amount. Also, some users of open radioactive substances work with such low amounts that licensing the use of these may seem excessive. Also, especially in the case of natural sources of radioactivity, the total amount of radioactivity may be rather high, but due to the bulk of the materials the concentration may be as low as to be very low risk. For this reason exemption limits are defined. One of these is the total amount of radioactivity (summed and weighted by nuclide) that may be used on a yearly basis without the need of a license. The other is the maximum concentration for a radioactive substance that may be stored or used without a license. The exemption limits are defined separately for each radionuclide.

Usually the exemption limits for waste are equal to the exemption limits for usage. In other words, there is a total amount of (radionuclide weighted) radioactivity that may be thrown away as waste as well as a maximum concentration of radioactivity in waste. If either one of these criteria is met, a license is not required. Usually, a licensed removal of waste involves the transferral of waste to an institution that has a license to store radioactive waste.

Appendix A: The Fine-Kinney Method

The Fine-Kinney method of risk assessment comprises the calculation of a risk factor for each possible intentional or unintentional exposure of radiological workers, patients or members of the general public. The calculated risk factor is then evaluated, and depending on its value the risk can be acceptable, unacceptable, or acceptable once certain actions are taken or precautions are met.

The risk factor (*R*) is calculated as:

$$R = S \times E \times P$$

Here *S* denotes the severity, *E* the exposure, and *P* the probability of the exposure occurring. There is a certain freedom in choosing the values for each of these factors, but in radiation safety risk assessment a possible choice for the numerical values is listed in Tables 7.2, 7.3, and 7.4

The total risk factor of a task is calculated as the sum of all risk factors of the regular events and the foreseen unintentional events. Table 7.5 shows a possible assessment of the total risk factor depending on the class of radiological worker (in this case A worker = max 20 mSv/year and B worker = max 6 mSv/year).

Table 7.2 Severity as function of the radiation dose

S	Effective dose (mSv)
0	$E_{eff} \leq 0.001$
1	$0.001 < E_{eff} \leq 0.02$ mSv
3	$0.02 < E_{eff} \leq 0.1$ mSv
4	$0.1 < E_{eff} \leq 0.3$ mSv
5	$0.3 < E_{eff} \leq 0.5$ mSv
7	$0.5 < E_{eff} \leq 1$ mSv
10	$1 < E_{eff} \leq 2$ mSv
15	$2 < E_{eff} \leq 6$ mSv
40	$6 < E_{eff} \leq 20$ mSv
100	$E_{eff} > 20$ mSv

Table 7.3 Exposure as function of the frequency of occurrence of a task

E	Frequency
Regular work/events	
1	Independent of frequency
Foreseen unintentional events	
0.5	<1 time per year
1	Yearly
2	Monthly
3	Weekly
6	Daily
10	Continuously

Table 7.4 Probability as function of the probability of exposure happening during work

W	Description	Numerical probability
Regular work		
15	Certain	1 (100 %)
Foreseen, unintentional events		
10	To be expected	0.5–1
6	Quite possible	0.1–0.5
3	Unusual	10^{-2}
1	Unlikely	10^{-3}
0.5	Very unlikely	10^{-4}
0.2	Virtually impossible	10^{-5}
0.1	Virtually unthinkable	10^{-6}
0.01	Theoretically possible	$<10^{-6}$

Table 7.5 Risk factor vs required action

R_{total}	A-worker	B-worker
>1500	Measures required	Measures required
600–1500	Further analysis required	Measures required
150–600	No further analysis required	Further analysis required
<600	No further analysis required	No further analysis required

References

IAEA safety standards series No. GSR Part 3, Radiation protection and safety of radiation sources: International basic safety standards, International Atomic Energy Agency Vienna, 2014.

ICRP Publications. http://www.icrp.org/publications.

ORAMED. http://oramed-fp7.eu.

Sans Merce et al. Extremity exposure in nuclear medicine: preliminary results of a European study. Radiat Prot Dosimetry. 2011;144(1–4):515–20.

Radiation Safety in Patients

8

Marcel Greuter, Emmy Meijne, Johan R. de Jong, and Wim Tukker

Abstract

With the use of modern hybrid imaging techniques that use the advantages of radiologic and nuclear techniques, not only anatomical information of the patient can be obtained but instantly also functional information. Functional information from different nuclear tracers in positron emission tomography (PET) or single-photon emission computed tomography (SPECT) can be combined with anatomical information from computed tomography (CT) or magnetic resonance imaging (MRI) in novel hybrid imaging systems. However, the use of nuclear activity and ionizing radiation induces concerns about the radiation dose for the patient. What is the probability of inducing dose effects, what effects can be expected, and what will be the dose in the case of a pregnant patient to the fetus? What different dose reduction techniques are available, and how can the protocols on the hybrid systems be optimized so that the patient gets the optimal imaging with a dose as low as reasonably achievable? This chapter addresses these questions and gives insight in the risk of ionizing radiation in molecular imaging techniques.

M. Greuter (✉)
Department of Radiology, University of Groningen, University Medical Center Groningen, Hanzeplein 1, 9713 GZ Groningen, The Netherlands
e-mail: m.j.w.greuter@umcg.nl

E. Meijne
Department of Radiation Safety, University Medical Center Groningen, Groningen, The Netherlands

J.R. de Jong
Department of Nuclear Medicine and Molecular Imaging, University of Groningen, University Medical Center Groningen, Hanzeplein 1, Groningen 9700 RB, The Netherlands

W. Tukker
Department of Radiology, University Medical Center Groningen, Groningen, The Netherlands

A.W.J.M. Glaudemans et al. (eds.), *Quality in Nuclear Medicine*,
DOI 10.1007/978-3-319-33531-5_8

8.1 Imaging and Tracers

8.1.1 Imaging Modalities

In nuclear medicine, chemical compounds or pharmaceutical compounds are combined with radionuclides to form radiopharmaceuticals. These radiopharmaceuticals are administered to the patient and allow dedicated nuclear medicine imaging modalities to image the extent of a disease in the body. Whereas in conventional radiology imaging gives typical anatomical information, nuclear medicine imaging typically allows for the imaging of functional information and of physical changes in cellular functions in a disease. In addition, efficiency of treatment of diseased tissue can be followed in time. Because the radiopharmaceuticals emit radiation within the body, the uptake of these chemicals inside the diseased areas can be detected by dedicated detectors surrounding the patient. Therefore, nuclear medicine provides information in the field of molecular medicine. The use of dedicated radiopharmaceuticals allows for the visualization of biological processes on the cellular level and can provide quantitative information on the progression of the disease or efficiency of the treatment.

Traditional imaging techniques such as computed tomography (CT) and magnetic resonance imaging (MRI) typically provide anatomical information of the patient. With the use of nuclear imaging techniques, functional information can be added. Because the radiopharmaceuticals used in nuclear medicine are more disease or organ or tissue specific, the functional information on the diseased tissue can be superimposed on the anatomical information in the body. Typical applications are single-photon emission computed tomography (SPECT) and positron emission tomography (PET).

In SPECT, two-dimensional images are taken from the distribution of the radionuclide in the body. By taking these images over multiple angles, a three-dimensional reconstruction can be made just like in CT. This provides a three-dimensional data set from which thin slices can be reconstructed which show the uptake of the radionuclide in the diseased body area. Technetium 99 m is used for SPECT with a half-life of 6 h. Effective doses range up to 12.8 mSv for typical SPECT studies (Table 8.1) (Mettler et al. 2008).

In PET, the patient is injected with a radiopharmaceutical that emits positrons. The positron annihilates with an electron in the body under the emission of gamma rays. These gamma rays are detected by dedicated cameras around the patient and can produce a three-dimensional image of the uptake of the radiopharmaceutical in the patient. Generally, for PET, the radiopharmaceutical fluorodeoxyglucose (^{18}F-FDG) is used, which is a molecule similar to glucose and accumulates in the body where the metabolic activity in the body is high. Other tracers can also be used for oncology imaging, neuroimaging, and cardiology imaging. A typical application of FDG-PET is the diagnosis of cancer metastasis with an approximate effective dose of 14.1 mSv (Table 8.1). Recent developments in camera systems make it possible to provide high-resolution images with less amounts of administered radionuclides. When following the EANM guidelines correctly, the effective dose of FDG-PET is nowadays around 4 mSv in an adult person of approximately 70 kg.

Table 8.1 Effective doses for adults in radiology and diagnostic nuclear medicine (Mettler et al. 2008)

Examination[a]	Effective dose (mSv)	Administered activity (MBq)[b]	Effective dose (mSv/MBq)[c]
Brain (^{99m}Tc-HMPAO-exametazime)	6.9	740	0.0093
Brain (^{99m}Tc-ECD-Neurolite)	5.7	740	0.0077
Brain (^{18}F-FDG)	14.1	740	0.019
Thyroid scan (sodium iodine 123)	1.9	25	0.075 (15 % uptake)
Thyroid scan (^{99m}Tc-pertechnetate)	4.8	370	0.013
Parathyroid scan (^{99m}Tc-sestamibi)	6.7	740	0.009
Cardiac stress-rest test (thallium 201 chloride)	40.7	185	0.22
Cardiac rest-stress test (^{99m}Tc-sestamibi 1-day protocol)	9.4	1100	0.0085 (0.0079 stress, 0.0090 rest)
Cardiac rest-stress test (Tc-sestamibi 2-day protocol)	12.8	1500	0.0085 (0.0079 stress, 0.0090 rest)
Cardiac rest-stress test (Tc-tetrofosmin)	11.4	1500	0.0076
Cardiac ventriculography (^{99m}Tc-labeled red blood cells)	7.8	1110	0.007
Cardiac (^{18}F-FDG)	14.1	740	0.019
Lung perfusion (^{99m}Tc-MAA)	2.0	185	0.011
Lung ventilation (xenon 133)	0.5	740	0.00074
Lung ventilation (^{99m}Tc-DTPA)	0.2	1300 (40 actually inhaled)	0.0049
Liver-spleen (^{99m}Tc-sulfur colloid)	2.1	222	0.0094
Biliary tract (^{99m}Tc-disofenin)	3.1	185	0.017
Gastrointestinal bleeding (^{99m}To-labeled red blood cells)	7.8	1110	0.007
Gastrointestinal emptying (^{99m}Tc-labeled solids)	0.4	14.8	0.024
Renal (^{99m}Tc-DTPA)	1.8	370	0.0049
Renal (^{99m}Tc-MAG3)	2.6	370	0.007
Renal (^{99m}Tc-DMSA)	3.3	370	0.0088
Renal (^{99m}Tc-glucoheptonate)	2.0	370	0.0054
Bone (^{99m}Tc-MDP)	6.3	1110	0.0057
Gallium 67 citrate	15	150	0.100
Pentetreotide (^{111}In)	12	222	0.054
White blood cells (^{99m}Tc)	8.1	740	0.011
White blood cells (^{111}In)	6.7	18.5	0.360
Tumor (^{18}F-FDG)	14.1	740	0.019

[a]*DMSA* dimercaptosuccinic acid, *DTPA* diethylenetriaminepentaacetic acid, *ECD* ethyl cysteinate dimer, *18 F* fluorine 18, *FDG* fluorodeoxyglucose, *HMPAO* hexamethylpropyleneamine oxime, *111In* indium 111, *MAA* macroaggregated albumin, *MAG3* mercaptoacetyltriglycine, *MDP* methylene diphosphonate, *99 mTc* technetium 99 m

[b]Recommended ranges vary, although most laboratories tend to use the upper end of suggested ranges

[c]From radiation dose to patients from radiopharmaceuticals (addendum 2 to ICRP publication 53). *Ann ICRP* 1998;28(3):1–126

In multimodality imaging, the radiological anatomical information can be fused together with the nuclear functional information by acquisition of data at different times (asynchronous) or by simultaneous acquisition of data (synchronous). In asynchronous postprocessing, the data of SPECT or PET has to be fused with the CT data. This process has some various constraints, such as patient uncomfort, and different positioning of the patient in the two scans at different times in both scanners. Although dedicated software is available to semiautomatically merge these data sets, the best solution to overcome these constraints is to acquire both data sets at the same time and space by synchronous image acquisition. Therefore, system manufacturers offer multimodality solutions such as SPECT-CT and PET-CT. Recently, also the combination of PET with magnetic resonance imaging (PET-MRI) has appeared on the market. MRI has the advantage, that is, it provides excellent soft tissue contrast at a high spatial and temporal resolution. In addition, MRI does not use ionizing radiation and therefore can reduce dose to the patient with respect to CT.

8.1.2 Tracers

Nuclear medicine diagnostic imaging, i.e., PET and SPECT, works by virtue of generating two-dimensional or three-dimensional images of the radioactivity distribution in a subject's body. A radioactive nuclide is used to "trace" the whereabouts of chemical compounds in living subjects. Whether a series of short static images are produced to follow the kinetics of the compound or if a single static image is produced after the distribution of the compound reaches a steady state, the principle remains the same. Any single image shows the distribution of the compound at a certain time as long as the kinetics of the compound is slow compared to the timescale of the imaging process.

If the compound that is being traced interacts with physiological processes such that there is a time-dependent distribution that is mediated by functional properties of tissue or organs, the imaging becomes functional imaging. If, in addition, the amount or volume of the compound is small enough to not disturb the function itself (especially important in case of ligands in receptor studies), the tracer principle is satisfied allowing for unperturbed functional imaging.

Key to nuclear medicine imaging is the fact that the tracer has to be labeled with a radioactive nuclide. This radioactive nuclide has to meet certain criteria for the purpose of imaging. First, during decay, the emitted particles must include particles that can be detected outside of the body. In general, only those particles that are generated on the emission site and leave the body without interaction provide useful imaging information on detection. In practice, this means that only high-energy gamma photons are suitable. In order to get a precise spatial localization of the particle, required to generate good- or even high-resolution reconstructed images of the radioactivity distribution, the gamma photon should be detectable in a small volume of detector material (also to reduce cost). For this purpose, scintillation detectors with high densities are used. There is a certain tension between the need for high-energy photons on the one hand (since these have a larger probability of leaving the tissue without interaction) and the need for low-energy photons in order to detect them with good efficiency and good spatial resolution. In practice, the gamma energies of nuclides that are being used in the field are in the order of 0.1–0.5 MeV.

Unfortunately, the perfect nuclide does not exist: having a gamma energy that shows no interaction with tissue, but is detected with perfect efficiency by the external detectors. This has several disadvantages. One of those is the disadvantage for the imaging itself. Gamma photons that have interaction with tissue are either lost for detection, and hence imaging, or degrade image quality because of detection while the spatial correlation between origin and detector is lost. Two main effects of this that show up in images are attenuation effects and the effects of scatter. In modern PET/CT and SPECT/CT, these effects can be corrected quite well. A second disadvantage is the fact that interaction with tissue means that energy is deposited in the tissue in the form of ionizations; hence, a radiation dose to the tissue is caused.

The dose that a tissue receives is the amount of ionizing energy per unit of mass of tissue that is being deposited. This is dependent on: (i) the number of particles traversing the tissue, (ii) the probability of interaction taking place, and (iii) the amount of energy transferred to the tissue upon interaction. The latter two are a function of the nuclide that is being used for labeling and the density of the tissue. The first is dependent on the amount of radioactivity that is being administered and the distribution of the tracer.

The MIRD schema provides the most commonly used method for calculating dose from internal uptake of radioactivity. The program OLINDA/EXM incorporates the MIRD schema on an organ level base. The use of phantom models for humans of different gender and age and an internal database of radionuclides simplifies the calculation of doses to organs and effective dose for reference men (phantoms) to the point that only the number of disintegrations of radionuclides in organs needs to be measured or calculated (e.g., by quantitative imaging).

So the question becomes, how to reduce dose while maximizing image quality. One way of achieving this is by more efficient detection systems in order to reduce the required amount of injected radioactivity. Another way of reducing the number of disintegrations in tissue is by using radionuclides with a short half-life. The short limit on the radionuclide half-life is given by the requirement that sufficient radioactivity is available at and during the moment of imaging. The moment of imaging may vary a lot. In case of dynamic studies that acquire a time series for the purpose of kinetic modeling, the imaging starts directly after administration of tracer well into the range in which a steady state has established and, if applicable, washout of tracer has become the governing process. Thus, this is mainly dependent on tracer kinetics. Also, the production of tracer can be rather time-consuming, and at the end of the production process, there should still be sufficient radioactivity left.

In case of static studies, imaging usually takes place well into the range in which a steady state has established itself or when it can be considered to be so in good approximation. For some tracers, this could be a matter of minutes, but for proteins (such as in the case of antibody imaging), this could be days. The other extreme is the case of water PET studies during which blood perfusion through a tissue is being measured and in which the measurement is done from administration to a few minutes after. This brings about the need for radionuclides with a half-life of only 2 min up to radionuclides with a half-life of several days.

Excretion is another factor that plays a role in the final dose received. If a tracer binds on a longer timescale to a few tissues and the remainder is excreted on a short timescale, the dose is often considerably lower than in the case of negligible excretion. In case of urinary excretion, it is important to have a short interval between bladder voidings.

Ideally, the radionuclide that is being used only emits particles that are useful candidates for detection. Often, this is not the case. Aside from one of a few gamma emissions of useful energy, there may be other gamma emissions, X-rays, beta particles, Auger electrons, etc. Some of these may be the result of competing modes of decay such as electron capture is a competing mode for positron emission. In case of PET, the positron that is emitted prior to annihilation into gamma photons causes ionizations along its trail, resulting in dose to the tissue. Some longer-lived PET radionuclides have a plethora of other gamma emissions as well. All of these do contribute to dose but have no value for imaging.

Finally, there is the distribution itself. This plays a role in two ways. One is the capacity for an organ containing radioactivity at any time to irradiate another tissue or organ. This is highly dependent on the anatomical relationship of both organs. Different distributions of the same total amount of activity can result in significantly different doses. The other factor is the tissue weighting factors as defined by the ICRP to convert absorbed doses to the effective dose. Some tissues are much more sensitive to stochastic effects than others. In most cases, one cannot influence the distribution of the tracer into sensitive organs. In some cases, it may be possible to block certain tissues. Also, it is important to take into account abnormal biological behavior in patients that may well influence the distribution of tracer such as in the case of hyperthyroidism.

8.1.3 Radiochemical Impurities

Checking for radiochemical impurities is an important factor in quality control of the production of radiopharmaceuticals. The presence of impurities in the form of nonlabeled radionuclides, labeled by-products, or unwanted (long-lived) nuclides contributes to the dose, but not to image quality and should be avoided. One well-known quality control is in the case of elution of ^{99}mTc from a ^{99}Mo generator where a check on the breakthrough of ^{99}Mo is performed. Others are measuring the half-life of cyclotron-produced positron emitters to check for impurities with a different half-life. Also, in case of radionuclides produced in a reactor, a check on the radiochemical purity is performed.

8.2 Risks of Ionizing Radiation

8.2.1 Deterministic Effects

The biological effects of radiation can be grouped into two main categories: (a) deterministic effects (also called [harmful] tissue reactions) and (b) stochastic effects (cancer and heritable effects).

Deterministic means "causally determined by preceding events," and a deterministic effect is described as "an injury in a population of cells, characterized by a threshold dose and an increase in the severity of the reaction as the dose is increased further. In some cases, deterministic effects are modifiable by postirradiation procedures including biological response modifiers."

The induction of deterministic effect is generally characterized by a threshold dose, and deterministic effects are therefore only observed after high radiation doses. With deterministic effects, the absorbed dose is averaged over the volume of tissue irradiated (SI unit is Gy).

The reason for the existence of a threshold dose is that a critical population of cells needs to be damaged or killed before detectable tissue reactions or malfunction will occur. The magnitude of the threshold depends on the dose rate and linear energy transfer of the radiation, the organ or tissue irradiated, the volume of the irradiated part of the organ or tissue, and the clinical effect of interest. Below the threshold dose, detrimental effects are not observed; above the threshold dose, the severity of the injury, the impairment of tissue recovery, and the probability of occurrence steeply increase with dose up to 100 %. Depending on the type of tissue and the dose tissue reactions may occur early or late after irradiation.

Early tissue reactions occur within hours to a few weeks after irradiation. Examples are inflammatory-type reactions like erythema or mucositis. Late tissue reactions are observed after months to years after irradiation. A list of tissue reactions that can be observed after high doses of irradiation is given in Table 8.2 (ICRP 2012). The estimates for the threshold doses for cataract and cardiovascular disease have recently been decreased by the ICRP which had let to the proposal of much lower dose limits for the lens of the eye (20 mSv/year instead of 150 mSv/year).

The most severe deterministic effect is mortality (Table 8.3) (ICRP 2012). Mortality is generally the result of severe cell depletions in vital tissues or organs of the body. After whole-body X-irradiation, death occurs from one of several distinct syndromes which are characteristic for particular dose ranges. After partial body irradiation, the probability of mortality depends on the particular part of the body that is exposed, the volume that is exposed, and the dose.

The dose limits for workers and members of the public are set at such levels that they prevent the occurrence of deterministic effects. Only at doses above the dose limits used for radiation protection or with accidental exposures deterministic effects can occur.

8.2.2 Stochastic Effects and Tumor Induction

In recent years, the use of diagnostic radiology has shown a rapid growth (Brenner and Hall 2007; Fazel et al. 2009; Hricak et al. 2011). Especially, the use of computed tomography contributed to this growth (Brenner and Hall 2007; Einstein 2012; Hall and Brenner 2008). CT usage over the past quarter of a century has risen approximately 12-fold in the UK and 20-fold in the USA (Hall and Brenner 2008). It has been estimated that more than 70 million CT scans per year are obtained in the USA, including at least 5 million CT scans of children (Brenner and Hall 2007; Brenner 2010).

Table 8.2 Estimated threshold doses for 1 % incidence of morbidity in tissues and organs in adults exposed to acute, fractionated or protracted, and chronic irradiation (From ICRP 118)

Effect	Organ/tissue	Time to develop effect	Acute exposure (Gy)	Highly fractionated (2-Gy fractions) or equivalent protracted exposures (Gy)[a]	Annual (chronic) dose rate for many years (Gy/year)
Temporary sterility	Testes	3–9 weeks	~0.1	NA	0.4
Permanent sterility	Testes	3 weeks	~6	<6	2.0
Permanent sterility	Ovaries	<1 week	~3	6.0	>0.2
Depression of hematopoiesis	Bone marrow	3–7 days	~0.5	~10–14	>0.4
Xerostomia	Salivary glands	1 week	NA	<20	MA
Dysphagia, stricture	Esophagus	3–8 months	NA	55	NA
Dyspepsia, ulceration	Stomach	2 years	NA	50	NA
Stricture	Small intestine	1.5 years	NA	45	NA
Stricture	Colon	2 years	NA	45	NA
Anorectal dysfunction	Rectum	1 year	NA	60	NA
Hepatomegaly, ascites	Liver	2 weeks–3 months	NA	<30–32	NA
Main phase of skin reddening	Skin (large areas)	1–4 weeks	<3–6	30	NA
Skin burns	Skin (large areas)	2–3 weeks	5–10	35	NA
Temporary hair loss	Skin	2–3 weeks	~4	NA	NA
Late atrophy	Skin (large areas)	>l year	10	40	NA
Telangiectasia at 5 years	Skin (large areas)	>l year	10	40	NA
Cataract (visual impairment)	Eye	>20 years	~0.5	~0.5	~0.5 divided by years duration[b]

NA not available

Some of these diseases may not be fatal, if good medical care or biological response modifiers are used (see Section 3). In the cases of cardiovascular disease and cerebrovascular disease, from the evidence currently available, the values given here are also assumed to apply to morbidity from these diseases

[a]Most values rounded to nearest Gy: ranges indicate area dependence for skin and differing medical support for bone marrow

[b]Derived from fractionated radiotherapeutic exposures, generally using 2-Gy fractions. For other fraction sizes, the following formula can be used, where D is total dose (number of fractions multiplied by d), d is dose per fraction (2 Gy in the case of D_1, and new value of d the case of D_2), and the ratio α/β can be found in the appropriate section of this report: $D_1[1+2/(\alpha/\beta)]=D_2[1+d_2/(\alpha/\beta)]$. Protracted doses at a low dose rate of around 1 cGy/min are approximately iso-effective to doses delivered in 2-Gy fractions at high dose rate for some issues, but this equivalence is dependent on the repair half-time of the particular tissue. Further details can be found in Joiner and Bentzen (2009). Bentzen and Joiner (2009), and Van der Kogel (2009)

Table 8.3 Estimated threshold doses for mortality in adults exposed to acute, fractionated or protracted, and chronic irradiation (From ICRP 118)

Effect	Organ/tissue	Time to develop effect	Absorbed dose[a] resulting in approximately 1 % incidence		
Mortality			Acute exposure (Gy)	Highly fractionated (2-Gy fractions) or equivalent protracted exposures (Gy)[b]	Annual (chronic) dose rate for many years (Gy/year)
Bone marrow syndrome					
Without medical care	Bone marrow	30–60 days	~1	10	NA
With good medical care	Bone marrow	30–60 days	2–3	>10	NA
Gastrointestinal syndrome					
Without medical care	Small intestine	6–9 days	~6	NA	NA
With conventional medical care	Small intestine	6–9 days	>6	40	NA
Pneumonitis – mean lung dose	Lung	1–7 months	7–8	15	NA
Cardiovascular disease – whole-body exposure	Heart	>10–15 years	~0.5	~0.5	~0.5[c] divided by years duration
Cerebrovascular disease	Carotid artery	>10 years	~0.5	~0.5	~0.5[c] divided by years duration

NA not available

Some of these diseases may not be fatal, if good medical care or biological response modifiers are used (see Section 3). In the cases of cardiovascular disease and cerebrovascular disease, from the evidence currently available, the values given here are also assumed to apply to morbidity from these diseases

[a]Most values rounded to nearest Gy: ranges indicate area dependence for skin and differing medical support for bone marrow

[b]Derived from fractionated radiotherapeutic exposures, generally using 2-Gy fractions. For other fraction sizes, the following formula can be used, where D is total dose (number of fractions multiplied by d), d is dose per fraction (2 Gy in the case of D_1, and new value of d the case of D_2), and the ratio α/β can be found in the appropriate section of this report: $D_1[1+2/(\alpha/\beta)]=D_2[1+d_2/(\alpha/\beta)]$. Protracted doses at a low dose rate of around 1 cGy/min are approximately iso-effective to doses delivered in 2-Gy fractions at high dose rate for some issues, but this equivalence is dependent on the repair half-time of the particular tissue. Further details can be found in Joiner and Bentzen (2009). Bentzen and Joiner (2009), and Van der Kogel (2009)

[c]The values quoted for the circulatory system assume the same incidence of injury irrespective of the acute or chronic nature of the exposure, with >15 years follow-up. It is emphasized that great uncertainty is attached to these values

However, radiation-induced carcinogenesis is a potential risk of diagnostic radiology (Hall and Brenner 2012; Hendee and O'Connor 2012; Mathews et al. 2013; Pearce et al. 2012; Shah et al. 2012). The estimated attributable risk of diagnostic X-rays worldwide ranged from 0.6 % in the UK up to 3.2 % in Japan (Berrington de González and Darby 2004). Especially, the use of recurrent and relatively high-dose CT exposure leads to an increased tumor risk (Brenner and Hall 2007; Mayo 2008). It has been estimated that CT is responsible for 1.5 to 2.0 % of all cancers in the USA and that 29,000 future cancers could be related to CT scans performed in the USA in 2007 (Berrington de González et al. 2009; Brenner and Hall 2007).

Depending on the machine settings, the organ being studied typically receives a radiation dose in the range of 10 mSv to 30 mSv for a single CT scan, with an average of two to three CT scans per study (Brenner and Hall 2007). At these doses, the most likely (though small) risk is for radiation-induced carcinogenesis.

Radiation-induced carcinogenesis is a stochastic effect of ionizing radiation. The probability of the effect increases with dose, but the severity of the effect is independent of dose. Stochastic effects are assumed to have no threshold, and the risk of radiation-induced tumors is estimated at 5 % per Sv (ICRP 2007). The most important source for the estimate of the stochastic effects is the epidemiological data from the Life Span Study (LSS) of the atomic bomb survivors in Hiroshima and Nagasaki. A significant increase in the overall risk of cancer was observed in the survivors who received low doses from 5 to 150 mSv with a mean dose of approximately 40 mSv, which approximates the effective dose from two or three typical CT scans. Although most of the quantitative estimates of the radiation-induced cancer risk are derived from the LSS cohort, there are other supporting studies, including a recent large-scale study of 400,000 radiation workers in the nuclear industry who were exposed to an average dose of approximately 20 mSv. Also in this cohort, a significant increase in cancer risk was reported among the workers who received doses between 5 and 150 mSv. The risks were quantitatively consistent with those reported for atomic bomb survivors. Moreover, there has been growing awareness regarding the long-term effects from radiation in children undergoing CT, because children have more years of life during which a potential cancer can be expressed (Andreassi and Picano 2014; Meulepas et al. 2014; Miglioretti et al. 2013). Some patients are exposed to recurrent CT examinations from an early age due to chronic diseases or long-term follow-up of cancer. In the USA, it has been estimated that about 500 individuals will die from radiation-induced cancer because of annual CT exposure under the age of 15 years (Brenner 2001). In summary, there is direct evidence from epidemiologic studies that the organ doses corresponding to a common CT study result in an increased risk of cancer (Brenner 2007; Hall and Brenner 2012), Fig. 8.1.

8.2.3 Pregnancy

The developing fetus is more sensitive to ionizing radiation than adults (McCollough et al. 2007; Dauer et al. 2012). Therefore, special precautions have to be taken to protect the unborn child against radiation. For female workers, a dose limit of 1 mSv for

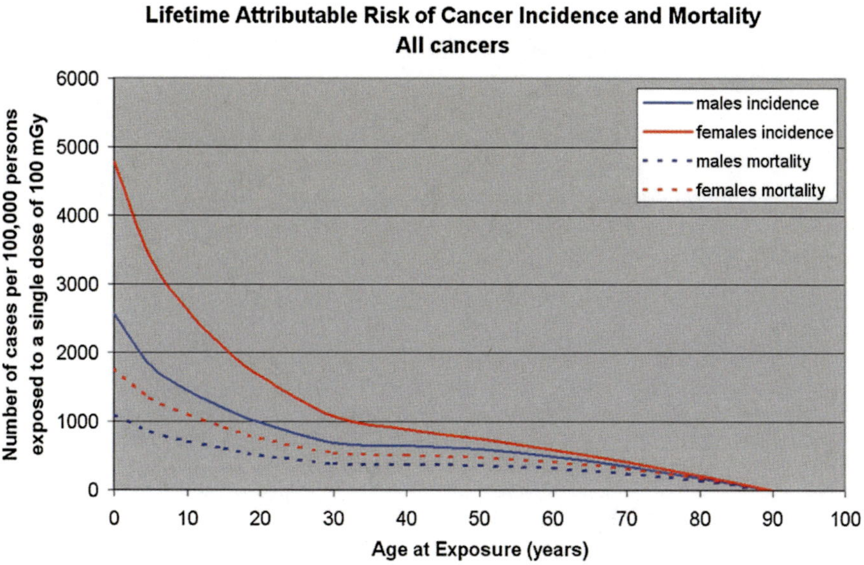

Fig. 8.1 Lifetime attributable risk of cancer incidence and mortality for all cancers for males and females

the fetus is applicable from the moment she declares that she is pregnant till the end of the pregnancy period. This dose limit is however not applicable to female patients.

Exposure of the developing fetus to irradiation leads to the same types of adverse health effects as exposure of adults: deterministic effects leading to tissue effects due to cell killing and stochastic effects due to unrepaired/misrepaired DNA damage.

The developing fetus is radiosensitive throughout the gestational period. The effect of radiation exposure is however not only dependent on the absorbed radiation dose but also on the stage of the pregnancy. High doses of ionizing radiation can cause embryonic death, congenital malformations, growth retardation, and neurologic detriment. There is however little evidence that very low doses lead to tissue effects and malformations in the developing fetus and adverse effects to the outcome of the pregnancy outcome. Much of the current knowledge of the harmful effects of ionizing radiation to the fetus is derived from the follow-up of atomic bomb survivors, from patients who received radiation therapy for nonmalignant conditions, and from animal studies.

8.2.3.1 Deterministic Effects Observed After Fetal Irradiation

There are radiation-related risks throughout pregnancy, which are related to the stage of pregnancy and the fetal absorbed dose. Radiation risks are most significant during organogenesis and the early fetal period, somewhat less in the second trimester, and least in the third trimester. There is no evidence that radiation doses below 100 mGy are associated with an increased incidence of congenital malformation, stillbirth, miscarriage, growth, or mental disability. Possible deterministic effects

Table 8.4 Deterministic radiation effects at different stages of gestation

Stage of gestation (wk)	Possible radiation effect	Dose characteristic	Estimated threshold dose (mGy)
3–4	Most sensitive period for the induction of embryonic death	Minimum lethal dose (from animal studies)	100–200
4–8	Embryo is also predisposed to the induction of major malformations and growth retardation	Minimum lethal dose (from animal studies)	250 (at 18 d), >500 (at >50 d)
		Minimum dose for growth retardation	200–500
8–15	Most sensitive period for irreversible whole-body growth retardation, microcephaly, and severe mental disability	Minimum dose for growth retardation	250–500
		Threshold tor severe mental disability	60–500
		Decrease in IQ can occur at lower doses	~100
		Microcephaly	≥20,000
16–Term	Higher exposures can produce growth retardation and decreased brain size and intellect, although the effects are not as severe as occurs from similar exposures during midgestation	Minimum lethal dose (from animal studies)	>1,500
		Minimum dose for severe mental disability	>1,500
		Decrease in IQ can occur at lower doses	>100

Dauer et al. (2012)
IQ intelligence quotient

that can be observed after fetal irradiation are listed in Table 8.4. These effects are associated with doses above a threshold dose of more than 100–200 mGy, with increasing risks at doses greater than 200 mGy. Since the fetal neural system is the most sensitive and has the longest period of development, radiation-induced abnormalities are rarely seen in humans without neuropathology.

Central Nervous System Effects

Development of the central nervous system occurs over a prolonged period during the first and second trimesters. The most sensitive prenatal period is between 8 and 15 weeks postconception and has a threshold dose of approximately 300 mGy or more. The associated data on mild retardation, as measured by decreases in intelligence quotient (IQ), suggest a loss of approximately 25–31 IQ points per Gy at a threshold dose greater than 100 mGy. Any effect on IQ following in utero doses of a few tens of mGy is of no practical significance since they will not have substantial influence on school achievements. Doses for typical diagnostic examinations are below these dose values. There is therefore no evidence that radiation exposure in typical diagnostic ranges is associated with a measurably increased incidence of congenital malformation, stillbirth, miscarriage, growth, or mental disability.

Prenatal Death, Congenital Malformations, and Growth Retardation

In the first weeks after conception, the only deterministic effect of radiation is prenatal death or induced abortion, with high doses of 1 Gy or more resulting in a high rate of lethality.

In most cases, these effects will not be noticed as the pregnancy is not yet known. The likelihood of inducing this effect at doses of less than 50 mGy is unlikely and undistinguishable from zero. After 4 weeks of gestation, there may be a risk of radiation-induced malformation of organs and growth retardation. The threshold for major effects during this period is approximately 100–200 mGy. Survivors of the atomic bombs on Hiroshima and Nagasaki that had received a fetal dose of more than 200 mGy were 2–3 cm shorter and 3 kg lighter than controls and had a 1 cm smaller head circumference.

8.2.3.2 Stochastic Fetal Effects Observed After Fetal Irradiation

Cancer

A number of studies have suggested an appreciable childhood cancer risk from in utero radiation. Other studies on cancer risk following irradiation of the fetus found a lifetime cancer risk from in utero exposure that is not greater than that from exposure in early childhood. The risk of cancer induction is at least as likely following exposure in the first trimester as in later trimesters. From a radiation protection perspective, it is prudent to assume that in utero radiation exposure confers a nontrivial risk to the fetus for future cancer induction and that this risk is, at most, a few times that of the population as a whole (5 % per Gy for lifetime risk of fatal cancer) with no dose threshold. Therefore, the risk of childhood fatal cancer is approximately 5 %–15 % per Gy, i.e., at most three times that of the general population as a whole.

8.2.3.3 Treatment of Pregnant Patients

Prenatal doses from most (properly) performed diagnostic procedures present no measurable increased risk of prenatal death, malformation, or impairment of mental development over the background incidence. Higher doses, such as those involved in therapeutic procedures, can however result in significant fetal harm and are essentially contraindicated in patients who are known to be pregnant.

There are no dose limits that are applicable to pregnant patients. Justification of the examination should however be carefully considered. With women of childbearing age, the possibility of pregnancy has to be considered and ascertained by questioning and information on advisatory posters. Women with an overdue menstrual period have to be treated as pregnant. Pregnant patients have the right to know the potential radiation effects that may result to in utero exposure of their unborn child.

If a diagnostic radiology examination is medically indicated, the risk to the mother of not performing the procedure is usually greater than the risk of potential harm to the fetus (Table 8.4). When a nuclear medicine examination is proposed for a pregnant woman, care has to be taken to ascertain that the examination is indeed indicated for a medical condition that requires prompt therapy. Also for these procedures, the risk to the mother of not performing the examination is usually greater

Table 8.5 Estimated absorbed fetal dose from common extra-abdominal radiologic procedures

Examination	Nominal fetal dose "Typical estimate" (mGy)	Reported range (mGy)
Dental	–	~0–0.001
Skull (radiographic)	~0	–
Head-cervical spine	—	<0.005–0.03
Cervical spine	<0.001	—
Extremities	—	<0.001–0.18
Shoulder	—	<0.005–0.03
Thoracic spine	0.07	<0.001–0.55
Chest	<0.01	0.0001–0.43
Mammography	<0.1	—
Femur (distal)	—	0.01–0.50
Foot	<0.0001	—
Pulmonary embolism scan	—	0.64–0.8
CT, head	<0.005	—
CT, chest	0.06	0.02–0.2
CT, pulmonary angiography	—	0.003–0.23
CT, lung	1.2	1.0–1.4
CT, angiography of coronary arteries	0.1	—
CT, pulmonary embolism	0.7	0.2–0.7

Dauer et al. (2012)

than the radiation risk to the fetus. The possibility of reducing the administered activity should however be considered.

Most diagnostic nuclear medicine procedures are done with short-lived radionuclides (such as technetium-99 m) that do not cause large fetal doses. For radionuclides that do not cross the placenta, fetal dose is derived from the radioactivity in maternal tissues. There are, however, some radiopharmaceuticals (such as iodine isotopes, P-32) that do cross the placenta and concentrate in a specific organ or tissue and which can therefore pose significant fetal risks.

8.2.3.4 Breast-Feeding

Females should also be asked to indicate if they are breast-feeding, since many radiopharmaceuticals can be transferred to a baby via breast milk. Cessation of breast-feeding for at least some period is recommended for most nuclear medicine examinations. Breast-feeding is usually stopped for 3 weeks after all I-131 and I-125 treatments except labeled hippurate. For other nuclides, shorter cessation periods can be considered. When therapeutic doses have to be given, breast-feeding should be stopped completely (Tables 8.5 and 8.6).

Diagnostic Reference Levels

Diagnostic reference levels are used in medical diagnosis to indicate whether, in routine conditions, the levels of patient dose or administered activity from a specified imaging procedure are unusually high or low for that procedure. The diagnostic reference level is an upper limit for the exposure of the patient that still can be

Table 8.6 Estimated fetal dose from common nuclear medicine examinations in early pregnancy and at term (doses include maternal and fetal self-dose contributions) ICRP 1988 en ICRP 1998

Radiopharmaceutical	Procedure	Administered activity (MBq)	Early (mGy)	9 months (mGy)
^{99m}Tc	Bone scan (phosphate)	750	4.6–4.7	1.8
^{99m}Tc	Lung perfusion (MAA)	200	0.4–0.6	0.8
^{99m}Tc	Lung ventilation (aerosol)	40	0.1–0.3	0.1
^{99m}Tc	Thyroid scan (pertechnetate)	400	3.2–4.4	3.7
^{99m}Tc	Red blood cell	930	3.6–6.0	2.5
^{99m}Tc	Liver colloid	300	0.5–0.6	1.1
^{99m}Tc	Renal DTPA	750	5.9–9.0	3.5
^{67}Ga	Abscess/tumor	190	14–18	25
^{123}I	Thyroid uptake[a]	30	0.4–0.6	0.3
^{131}I	Thyroid uptake[a]	0.55	0.03–0.04	0.15
^{131}I	Metastases imaging[a]	40	2.0–2.9	11.0

[a]Fetal thyroid doses are much higher than fetal whole body dose, namely, 5–15 Gy/MBq for ^{123}I and 0.5–1.1 Gy/MBq for ^{131}I

considered as "good medical practice." Diagnostic reference levels should not be exceeded in standard procedures associated to common clinical referrals and good diagnostic and technical performance. In the Netherlands, DRN values have been established for a number of radiology and cardiology procedures. The examinations for which diagnostic reference levels have been established are mammography, radiography, computed tomography, and diagnostic fluoroscopy. Because a much lower dose level compared to the diagnostic reference level is achievable when modern imaging equipment is used and acquisition protocols are optimized in addition to DRN values, achievable dose levels have been defined for certain practices. If diagnostic reference levels are exceeded, a local review should be initiated to determine whether protection has been adequately optimized or whether corrective action is required.

8.3 Dose Reduction Techniques

In order to avoid unnecessary radiation exposure to patients, the as low as reasonably achievable (ALARA) principle should always be applied [ICRP 2006]. A CT should only be ordered when the outcomes of the diagnostic test results are expected to affect patient care. Especially nonionizing alternatives as ultrasound and MRI should be considered. The European Commission issued guidelines for imaging referral for use by health professionals referring patients for medical imaging [RP 2008]. The guidelines aim to ensure that radiological imaging prescriptions are justified, in application of Articles 3.1 and 6.2 of Council Directive 97/43/EURATOM on health protection of individuals against the dangers of ionizing radiation in relation to medical exposure. Once the indication for a patient's CT is justified, several approaches are available to reduce the patient dose. The most important available options to reduce CT radiation doses include optimization of CT acquisition parameters (e.g., tube voltage, tube current, pitch, and collimation), application of dedicated patient protection methods (e.g., automatic tube current modulation), and recently available advanced reconstruction techniques (e.g., iterative reconstruction) (Costello et al. 2013).

8.3.1 Lower Tube Voltage

Lowering the tube voltage is particularly advantageous in slim patients with a relatively small body mass index (BMI), pediatric patients, and patients undergoing CT examinations with intravenous iodinated contrast medium. However, increased noise levels and variations in tissue contrast resulting from decreased tube voltages limit the widespread application of this technique (Kalra et al. 2004). Recently, (semi)automated tube voltage selection has become available on most state-of-the-art CT scanners, and it has been shown that the combined use of automated tube voltage selection and automated tube current modulation allows for a reduction of radiation exposure while maintaining good image quality (Lee et al. 2012).

8.3.2 Automatic Tube Current Modulation

Lowering the tubes' current is another method to reduce the patients' dose. This can be done by use of a low fixed tube current or by automatic tube current modulation, where the tube current is automatically adjusted on the basis of differences in tissue attenuation. Body regions that require fewer doses for an adequate data reconstruction are imaged with a reduced tube current. This results in an improved dose efficiency and lowers the effective dose of the patient while maintaining an acceptable level of quantum noise (Kalra et al. 2004). The automatic tube current modulation can be used with either angular (x-y axis) or z-axis modulation. In angular modulation, the tube current is adjusted as a function of the projection angle. For low-attenuation projection angles, the tube current is reduced, whereas for high-attenuation projection angles, the tube current is increased. In z-axis modulation, the tube current is adjusted so that in the z-direction of the patient, a predefined noise level is maintained. When differences in tissue density are detected, the tube current is altered to achieve the desired noise level. The aim of z-axis modulation is to generate CT images with similar noise levels, irrespective of patients' size and anatomy.

8.3.3 Iterative Reconstruction

A new dose reduction strategy has recently become commercially available from all major CT vendors with focus on the optimization of the CT image reconstruction

Table 8.7 Currently available IR techniques from the major vendors

Vendor	IR technique	Theoretical maximal dose reduction according to vendor (%)	Reported dose reduction[a]
Philips Healthcare	iDose[4]	80	50–76 %
Siemens Medical Solutions	IRIS	60	20–60 %
	SAFIRE	60	50 %
Toshiba Medical Systems	AIDR 3D	75	52 %
GE Healthcare	ASIR	40	23–76 %
	MBIR	75	NA

IRIS Iterative Reconstruction in Image Space, Siemens Medical Solutions; *AIDR ID* Adaptive Iterative Dose Reduction 3D, Toshiba Medical Systems; *ASIR* Adaptive Statistical Iterative Reconstruction, GE Healthcare; iDose[4], Philips Healthcare; *SAFIRE* Sinogram-Affirmed Iterative Reconstruction, Siemens Medical Solutions; *MBIR* Model-Based Iterative Reconstruction, GE Healthcare; *NA* not available

[a]Dose reduction strongly depends on the applied anatomic region and calculation method ($CTDI_{vol}$, DLP, effective dose, tube current)

(Table 8.7). During the last decades, CT data was commonly reconstructed with a filtered back-projection algorithm, which has been shown to be fast and robust (Fleischmann and Boas 2011). Iterative reconstruction is an alternative image reconstruction method that allows for imaging at lower radiation doses with similar noise levels and image quality compared to routine-dose filtered back projection (Willemink et al. 2013). Therefore, with iterative reconstruction, a dose reduction can be achieved without compromising on image quality.

8.4 CT Protocols in Molecular Imaging

A low-dose attenuation CT is sufficient to generate a fusion image for PET and SPECT. However, a modern PET-CT or SPECT-CT is also able to generate images of diagnostic CT quality. For patients, this provides the benefit that they do not have to schedule two appointments on the nuclear and radiology department for the PET or SPECT and CT scan, respectively, but they can schedule one appointment for the combined scan. In order to obtain sufficient diagnostic image quality, at least a four-row CT scanner is needed for regular diagnostic imaging with sufficient spatial resolution in an acceptable imaging time. Cardiac imaging is feasible with at least a 64-row CT scanner, where beta blockers are used at heart rates above 60 bpm. Because the rotation time of the CT scanner is crucial for sufficient temporal resolution in cardiac scanning imaging, one might wish to refer the patient to the radiology department if a dedicated scanner is available there with a higher temporal resolution than the multimodality scanner on the nuclear department.

How does one organize sufficient knowledge of the scanning personnel in the startup phase using CT in a nuclear medicine department? The option is to train nuclear workers in CT scanning or to train radiology workers in nuclear imaging. In most departments, the first option is preferred because it is more cost-effective and more efficient. Because most of the Dutch nuclear workers already have a radiology education or background, the additional knowledge of CT is obtained in a relatively shorter time. In any case, a training of the radiology department is advised to learn the specific nuclear protocols in oncology and to be able to respond quickly at complications in contrast administration. If the required knowledge is obtained, a certificate can be issued by the responsible educator to the nuclear worker. After the first scan is started, the principle of teach the teacher can be used to spread the knowledge of CT in the nuclear department. In addition, it is necessary to provide a special training of about two weeks on a radiology oncology scanner in case of new employees. This training combined with a positive judgment and enough scanning hours can also result in a certification.

Training is not the only reason to have a close contact between the two departments. Because patients can have a CT scan on the radiology department and, e.g., a combined PET-CT in the nuclear medicine department, the CT scan protocols of both departments have to be equal to ensure a reliable comparison of both examinations. Usually, the first CT scan is made on the radiology department to confirm diagnosis. The CT scan protocol on the nuclear department has to be the same in order to ensure proper follow-up.

Not only the CT acquisition and reconstruction protocols but also the protocols for preparation, protocols for contrast administration, and patient safety have to be harmonized. In general standard, neck, chest, and abdomen CT protocols are sufficient in most of the patients. Specific multiphase CT protocols can be useful in follow-up or for the detection and determination of new lesions or abnormalities. If also a brain scan with contrast is requested, this scan can be made at the end of the examination.

In the protocol for oral preparation, the patient has to start drinking one hour before scanning in order to fill the stomach and small intestine. This can be combined with the administration of radiopharmaceuticals needed for molecular imaging. Just before the actual diagnostic scan, the patient has to drink another glass of water mixed with iodine contrast. Rectal contrast is not recommended because of the additional radiation exposure to the technicians. Close contact with the patient has to be avoided and has to be kept as short as possible. Protocols for allergic patients can be provided by the radiology department. It is also important that the nuclear workers react adequately during calamities in the administration of iodine contrast. This is an important aspect of the practical training during the traineeship on radiology.

References

Andreassi MG, Picano E. Reduction of radiation to children : our responsibility to change. Circulation. 2014. pii: CIRCULATIONAHA.114.010699. [Epub ahead]. doi:10.1161/CIRCULATIONAHA.114.010699.

Berrington de González A, Darby S. Risk of cancer from diagnostic X-rays: estimates for the UK and 14 other countries. Lancet. 2004;363:345–51.

Berrington De Gonzalez A, Mahesh M, Kim KP, Bhargavan M, Lewis R, Mettler F, Land C. Projected cancer risks from computed tomographic scans performed in the United States in 2007. Arch Intern Med. 2009;169(22):2071–7.

Brenner DJ. Should we be concerned about the rapid increase in CT usage? Rev Environ Health. 2010;25(1):63–8.

Brenner D1, Elliston C, Hall E, Berdon W. Estimated risks of radiation-induced fatal cancer from pediatric CT. AJR Am J Roentgenol. 2001 Feb;176(2):289–96.

Brenner DJ, Hall EJ. Computed tomography – an increasing source of radiation exposure. N Engl J Med. 2007;357(22):2277–84. doi:10.1056/NEJMra072149.

Costello JE, Cecava ND, Tucker JE, Bau JL. CT radiation dose: current controversies and dose reduction strategies. Am J Roentgenol. 2013;201:1283–90. doi:10.2214/AJR.12.9720.

Dauer LT, Thornton RH, Miller DL, Damilakis J, Dixon RG, Marx MV, Schueler BA, Vano E, Venkatesan A, Bartal G, Tsetis D, Cardella JJ. Radiation management for interventions using fluoroscopic or computed tomographic guidance during pregnancy: a joint guideline of the society of interventional radiology and the cardiovascular and interventional radiological society of Europe with endorsement by the Canadian interventional radiology association. JVIR. 2012;23:19–32.

Einstein AJ. Effects of radiation exposure from cardiac imaging: how good are the data? J Am Coll Cardiol. 2012;59(6):553–65. doi:10.1016/j.jacc.2011.08.079.

Fazel R, Krumholz HM, Wang Y, Ross JS, Chen J, Ting HH, Shah ND, Nasir K, Einstein AJ, Nallamothu BK. Exposure to low-dose ionizing radiation from medical imaging procedures. New Engl J Med. 2009;361(9):849–57.

Fleischmann D, Boas FE. Computed tomography—old ideas and new technology. Eur Radiol. 2011;21:510–7. doi:10.1007/s00330-011-2056-z.

Hall EJ, Brenner DJ. Cancer risks from diagnostic radiology. Br J Radiol. 2008;81(May):362–78. doi:10.1259/bjr/01948454.

Hall EJ, Brenner DJ. Cancer risks from diagnostic radiology: the impact of new epidemiological data. Br J Radiol. 2012;85(December):e1316–7. doi:10.1259/bjr/13739950.

Hendee WR, O'Connor MK. Radiation risks of medical imaging: separating fact from fantasy. Radiology. 2012;264(2):312–21. doi:10.1148/radiol.12112678.

Hricak H, Brenner DJ, Adelstein SJ, Frush DP, Hall EJ, Howell RW, Mccollough CH, Mettler FA, Pearce MS, Suleiman OH, Thrall JH, Wagner LK. Managing radiation use in medical imaging: a multifaceted. Radiology. 2011;258(3):889–905.

ICRP. The optimisation of radiological protection – broadening the process. ICRP Publication 101b. Ann ICRP 36; 2006. p. 3.

ICRP. The 2007 recommendations of the International Commission on Radiological Protection. ICRP Publication 103. Ann ICRP 37; 2007. p. 2–4.

ICRP. ICRP statement on tissue reactions/early and late effects of radiation in normal. Tissues and organs – threshold doses for tissue reactions in a radiation protection context. ICRP Publication 118. Ann ICRP 41(1/2); 2012.

Kalra MK, Maher MM, Toth TL, Hamberg LM, Blake MA, Rcsi FFR, Shepard J. Radiology strategies for CT radiation. Radiology. 2004;230(9):619–28.

Lee KH, Lee JM, Park JH, Flohr TG, Kim KW, Kim SJ. Attenuation-based automatic tube voltage selection and tube current modulation for dose reduction at contrast-enhanced. Radiology. 2012;265(2):437–47. doi:10.1148/radiol.12112434/-/DC1.

Mathews JD, Forsythe AV, Brady Z, Butler MW, Goergen SK, Byrnes GB, Giles GG, Wallace AB, Anderson PR , Guiver TA , McGale P, Cain TM, James G, Bickerstaffe AC, Darby SC. Cancer risk in 680 000 people exposed to computed tomography scans in childhood or adolescence : data linkage study of 11 million Australians. 2013;2360(May):1–18. doi:10.1136/bmj.f2360.

Mayo JR. Radiation dose issues in longitudinal studies involving computed tomography. Proc Am Thorac Soc. 2008;5:934–9. doi:10.1513/pats.200808-079QC.

McCollough CH, Schueler BA, Atwell TD, Braun NN, Regner DM, Brown DL, LeRoy AJ. Radiation exposure and pregnancy: When should we be concerned? Radiographics. 2007;27:909–18.

Mettler Jr FA, Huda W, Yoshizumi TT, Mahesh M. Effective doses in radiology and diagnostic nuclear medicine: a catalog. Radiology. 2008;248(1):254–63.

Meulepas JM, Ronckers CM, Smets AMJB, Nievelstein RAJ, Jahnen A, Lee C, Kieft M, Laméris JS, van Herk M, Greuter MJ, Jeukens CR, van Straten M, Visser O, van Leeuwen FE, Hauptmann M. Leukemia and brain tumors among children after radiation exposure from CT scans : design and methodological opportunities of the Dutch Pediatric CT Study. Eur J Epidemiol. 2014;29:293–301. doi:10.1007/s10654-014-9900-9.

Miglioretti DL, Johnson E, Williams A, Greenlee RT, Weinmann S, Solberg LI, Feigelson HS, Roblin D, Flynn MJ, Vanneman N, Smith-Bindman R. The use of computed tomography in pediatrics and the associated radiation exposure and estimated cancer risk. JAMA Pediatr. 2013;167(8):700–7. doi:10.1001/jamapediatrics.2013.311.

Nederlandse commissie voor stralingsdosimetrie, Diagnostische referentieniveaus in Nederland, Rapport 21, juni 2012.

Pearce MS, Salotti JA, Little MP, McHugh K, Lee C, Kim KP, Howe NL, Ronckers CM, Rajaraman P, Sir Craft AW, Parker L, Berrington de González A. Radiation exposure from CT scans in childhood and subsequent risk of leukaemia and brain tumours: a retrospective cohort study. Lancet. 2012;380(9840):499–505. doi:10.1016/S0140-6736(12)60815-0.

Radiation Protection 118, 2008. Referral Guidelines For Imaging, Guidelines for Healthcare Professionals who prescribe Imaging Investigations involving Ionising Radiation, Final Report to the European Commission for Grant Agreement SUBV99/134996

Shah DJ, Sachs RK, Wilson DJ. Radiation-induced cancer: a modern view. Br J Radiol. 2012;85(1020):e1166–73. doi:10.1259/bjr/25026140.

Willemink MJ, de Jong P a, Leiner T, de Heer LM, Nievelstein R a J, Budde RPJ, Schilham AMR. Iterative reconstruction techniques for computed tomography Part 1: technical principles. Eur Radiol. 2013. doi:10.1007/s00330-012-2765-y.

The Decommissioning of Cyclotron Facilities for the Production of Radionuclides in Nuclear Medicine

9

Anne M.J. Paans and Johan R. de Jong

Abstract

The problem of decommissioning nuclear facilities has become more prominent in the last 10–15 years when accelerators have been put out of operation since better cyclotrons are available. A second-hand market for these machines is not obvious and for each machine a solution has to be found. Decommissioning a cyclotron facility involves the decommissioning and dismantling of the cyclotron itself and possibly the dismantling of the concrete vault. In this chapter, the process of decommissioning a cyclotron facility will be explained.

9.1 Introduction

Many types of accelerators (for electrons and charged particles) have been installed in the past mainly at universities for nuclear research and teaching. Since the interaction of electrons with matter is principally different from the interaction of nuclei with matter (weak and strong interaction), preferably charged particles are used for the production of radionuclides. For this reason only charged particle accelerators are considered in this chapter. Of the many Van de Graaff generators installed at universities in the second half of the twentieth century, virtually all have been dismantled because no new research areas could be defined. For the same reason most of the cyclotrons at universities also already have been removed. Sometimes they are still in use for unique topics within the energy range of the accelerator. Around 1980, the positron emission tomography (PET) technique became available, and the use of

A.M.J. Paans (✉) • J.R. de Jong
Department of Nuclear Medicine and Molecular Imaging, University of Groningen, University Medical Center Groningen, Hanzeplein 1, Groningen 9700 RB, The Netherlands
e-mail: a.m.j.paans@umcg.nl

A.W.J.M. Glaudemans et al. (eds.), *Quality in Nuclear Medicine*,
DOI 10.1007/978-3-319-33531-5_9

cyclotron facilities soon extended from university research facilities to the larger community hospitals in the developed countries. Around the world new cyclotrons were installed in the hospitals. Most of the cyclotrons installed for the production of the four most commonly used PET radionuclides (^{11}C, $T_{1/2}$=20 min; ^{13}N, $T_{1/2}$=10 min; ^{15}O, $T_{1/2}$=2 min; and ^{18}F, $T_{1/2}$=110 min) were accelerating protons to energies between 10 MeV and 50 MeV. Often also deuterons could be accelerated and in some cases also ^{4}He particles in order to have a versatile general radionuclide production machine. With the progress in radiochemistry, especially the ^{18}F chemistry, nowadays often only protons are used for radionuclide production. Moreover, more recently installed cyclotrons are accelerating H^- ions instead of the traditional protons. These H^- ions are extracted by stripper foils (100% efficient) and stripped of the electrons, converting them to protons. Prior to H^- acceleration, deflectors were used with often a much lower efficiency. The preference for protons is due to the often larger nuclear cross section for the desired radionuclide and the longer range (higher thick target yield) compared to heavier particles (deuterons, ^{4}He, etc.). With PET getting more and more common as a diagnostic tool, also the cyclotron facilities are spreading to the larger hospitals that want to have their own access to the shorter-lived radionuclides (^{18}F, ^{13}N, ^{11}C and ^{15}O). Nowadays, the newly installed cyclotrons are almost all H^- machines with proton end energy between 10 MeV and 20 MeV. Also older cyclotrons are being replaced by these new machines. At the moment ^{18}F-FDG is still the only widely used commercial PET radiopharmaceutical. The replacement of older cyclotrons by newer models brings about the need for decommissioning the obsoleted cyclotrons. In contrast to the tendency for a growing number of cyclotrons, sometimes the large costs involved due to mandatory GMP production facilities for radiopharmaceuticals are instead a reason for decommissioning a cyclotron as well.

The problem of decommissioning nuclear facilities has become more prominent in the last 10–15 years when accelerators have been put out of operation. A second-hand market for these machines is not obvious and for each machine a solution has to be found. Industry prefers to sell new accelerators, and transport is often not easy due to regulations on radioactive materials that are present due to activation of cyclotron parts. The amount of radioactivity induced inside the cyclotron or accelerator is luckily limited due to the relatively short half-life of the radionuclides involved. Over the course of years during the use of the cyclotron, an equilibrium between production and decay of induced radioactivity is reached, leading to saturation values for these radionuclides. For the concrete of the vaults, often a landscape filling is thought of but depends on the radioactivity level and the local regulations. To minimise the total amount of radioactivity induced in the materials of the cyclotron vault, the construction nowadays consists of a thick outer shell of concrete with enforcement steel and a thinner inner shell without any enforcement steel. Another problem in describing the decommissioning process is the individual variation of the different cyclotron facilities. Although sometimes the cyclotron may be the same, the construction of the vault and the building can be quite different. Probably the only exception on this is the Siemens 11 MeV cyclotron with its shielding (concrete and lead) wrapped around the machine, by Siemens sold as a self-shielding cyclotron.

In the decommissioning of cyclotron facilities in nuclear medicine, there are two major components to be discussed: (1) the cyclotron itself and (2) the vault in which it is positioned.

9.2 Induced Radioactivity into the Cyclotron

Inside the cyclotron positively or negatively charged particles are accelerated. These particles are extracted and guided to a target where desired radionuclides are produced. Next to the desired radionuclides also other radionuclides can be produced depending on the energy of the beam and the target material. In Table 9.1 the most commonly used nuclear reactions are given with the Q-value of the reaction (the difference between the masses before and after the reaction in MeV) and the energy threshold, the Q-value translated into the minimum energy. A correction for the Coulomb barriers has also to be applied; see Keller et al. (1974). For the production of radionuclides, the proton-induced reactions are often the preferred reaction because of the cross section of the reaction and because of the fact that the range of the protons is the longest. This makes it possible to use longer targets such that radioactivity can be produced along the full maximum range of the protons. Therefore, the thick target yield is at maximum for the proton-induced reaction. The maximum in cross section is 5–10 MeV above the threshold energy (usually about 5 MeV) which explains the preference for maximum cyclotron energies between 15 and 20 MeV. At higher energies more reaction channels open up and different (contaminating) radionuclides are produced. Indeed, from Table 9.1, the most used reactions are the proton-induced reaction and especially the (p,n) reaction is quite prominent. These neutrons, maximum energy often around 6 MeV, are leaving the target. Other products like α-particles do not have sufficient range to leave the target material. The thickness of the target material is optimised for the maximum yield or the lowest contamination, and if possible the beam should be stopped inside the target material. If not, the back side of the target should stop the beam.

The vast majority of the incoming charged particles will lose their energy due to the interaction between these particles and the electrons around the target nuclei. This is the limiting factor for the range of the protons, but does not produce

Table 9.1 Nuclear reactions for the four important PET radionuclides and some promising reactions on solid-state targets

Nuclear reaction	Q-value (MeV)	Ethr (MeV)
$^{18}O(p,n)^{18}F$	−2.4	2.5
$^{20}Ne(d,\alpha)^{18}F$	+2.8	0.0
$^{14}N(p,\alpha)^{11}C$	−2.9	3.1
$^{16}O(p,\alpha)^{13}N$	−5.2	5.5
$^{14}N(d,n)^{15}O$	+5.1	0.0
$^{15}N(p,n)^{15}O$	−3.5	3.7
$^{64}Ni(p,n)^{64}Cu$	−0.8	0.8
$^{89}Y(p,n)^{89}Zr$	−3.6	3.6
$^{100}Mo(p,2n)^{99m}Tc$	−7.7	7.8
$^{124}Te(p,n)^{124}I$	−5.5	5.5

radioactivity. Some of the charged particles will penetrate into the nucleus of an atom. At that moment a nucleus of another element is created. The surplus of energy will be shared by the other protons and neutrons in the nucleus. The nucleus has to get rid of this surplus energy, and what will happen is determined by the amount of energy and the structure of the nucleus. In most cases, a neutron or an α-particle will be emitted. Often this process is called "evaporation" or "pre-equilibrium decay" (Blann 1975). The computer code ALICE is able to calculate the cross sections according to this evaporation or pre-equilibrium model of all competing nuclear reactions. Due to the thickness of the target and its mounting, no charged particles will escape into the air, only in target generated neutrons will they be able to do that and of course the γ-rays generated in the decay of excited nuclei.

So in the ideal cyclotron, no beam loss will occur: all induced radionuclides are inside the target, the target foil in front of the target and the foil at the exit of the cyclotron. Since often alloys (Havar, Fe, Ti) are used for thin and strong foils, quite different radioactive products will be found in these foils (Sunderland 2012). These targets and foils can easily be removed and are not part of the discussion. In cyclotrons accelerating positively charged particles, the beam is deflected to the external target by an electrostatic deflector or extractor. In this deflection process, particles are always lost and stopped in the deflector material (copper, aluminium). In the old days, all kinds of metals with high melting points and good electrical properties were used, e.g. molybdenum. So where beam loss occurs, nuclear reactions will occur with direct production of radionuclides and the production of neutrons which will also activate the materials inside the cyclotron.

In Table 9.2, the longer-lived radionuclides that have been observed after closing down a 17 MeV Scanditronix MC-17 are given (Sunderland 2012). The Scanditronix MC-17 can also be seen as the prototype for the GE PETtrace with 16 MeV protons. In the MC-17 machine, after 20 years of operation and 300.000 μAh of beam, the amounts of induced radioactivity inside the cyclotron components have reached their saturation value.

Table 9.2 Long-lived radionuclides in the cyclotron components produced during operations of the cyclotron

Nuclide	Half-Life	Reaction channel
^{7}Be	53 days	^{10}B(p,α)^{7}Be (Havar)
^{22}Na	2.6 years	^{27}Mg(p,α)^{22}Na (Havar)
^{52}Mn	5.6 days	^{52}Cr(p,n)^{52}Mn (Havar)
^{54}Mn	312 days	^{54}Cr(p,n)^{54}Mn (Havar)
^{56}Co	77 days	^{56}Fe(p,n)^{56}Co (Havar)
^{51}Cr	27 days	^{54}Fe(n,α)^{51}Cr, ^{50}Cr(n,g)^{51}Cr, ^{52}Cr(n,^{2}n)^{51}Cr (Havar and other)
^{57}Co	272 days	^{57}Fe(p,n)^{57}Co (Havar and other)
^{58}Co	71 days	^{58}Fe(p,n)^{58}Co (Havar and other)
^{60}Co	5.3 years	^{63}Cu(n,α)^{60}Co
^{59}Fe	44 days	^{59}Co(n,p)^{59}Fe, ^{58}Fe(n,p)^{59}Fe
^{65}Zn	244 days	^{65}Cu(p,n)^{65}Zn

Table 9.2 is split into two parts. In the upper part, the longer-lived activities originating from foils, etc., are listed. In the lower part, the longer-lived activities induced in the cyclotron itself (magnet, dees, coils, etc.) are listed. In practice for the decommissioning process, the highly active parts like foils, etc., can easily be separated and dealt with separately. What remains are the lower five radionuclides of which the longest-living radionuclide is ^{60}Co (half-life 5.3 year) with a total amount of roughly 200 GBq (5 mCi) in this case.

9.3 Induced Radioactivity into Construction Material of the Vault

The external shielding for a cyclotron is needed for the absorption of the generated neutrons and gamma-radiation. Free neutrons are chargeless particles with a half-life of 10.6 min. The energy loss mechanism for neutrons is quite different from the mechanism for charged particles as there is no interaction with electrons. There are two processes possible: first the kinetic energy loss due to elastic collisions (as with billiard balls), most effective if the collision is not against a nucleus with high mass (a wall) but with nuclei of the same weight, preferably protons. This is most effective at higher energies. The neutron energy spectrum generated in the nuclear reactions in the target is rather broad, depends on the energy of the incoming particles and often has its maximum intensity around 4–6 MeV. The second mechanism is neutron capture and this is most effective at low energies. There are elements with very large cross sections for neutron capture, e.g. cadmium, which can be used selectively. So the most effective shielding will be hydrogen. And indeed some cyclotrons have a complete water shielding with boron added for the neutron capture process. Also polyethylene (PE) is sometimes used for more local shielding, e.g. to catch the neutrons from the ^{18}F target, as being the most prominent source in the neutron production, immediately behind the target. The most economic material to shield both neutrons and gammas is ordinary concrete (2.35 g/cm^3) which always contains a low percentage of water which is very effective for the neutrons. Next to neutron emission, the compound nucleus can also lose energy by gamma-ray emission with energies usually about 6 MeV, and as rule of thumb one can calculate thickness of the concrete assuming the emission of three 2 MeV gamma rays for each event (Landolt-Bornstein).

The concrete will be reinforced with steel rods. This iron can be the source of long-lived radioactive nuclei. In the past all vaults were built from reinforced concrete with steel rods throughout the concrete. Due to the radioactivity in the steel nowadays, most vaults are built with the 20–40 cm most inward layer of pure concrete to avoid the induction of long-lived radioactivity in steel. Depending on the exact energy of the cyclotron, the local regulations and its geometrical position inside the building, the wall thickness of the vault can vary, but in general it will be around 2 m of concrete.

Most neutrons (80–90 %) will leave the target in a cone with top half angle of 30°. So, induced radioactivity in the vault will not be homogeneous, but depending on the location of the targets and the distance to the wall, areas of higher activity will be created EUR (1999), IAEA (2003), Philips et al. (1986).

The Siemens 11 MeV cyclotron is called a "self-shielding" cyclotron which means in this case that concrete with lead at the target positions is wrapped around the machine. Since neutrons are the source of the induced radioactivity, the only difference will be in the size and shape of the generated neutron spectrum. The most prominent generated radionuclides will be same as for cyclotrons with higher energies Calandrino et al. (2006).

The Scanditronix MC-17 cyclotrons often have a target ladder at the exit of the cyclotron, and the neutrons generated inside targets will all go in the same direction implying that the radionuclide production by fast neutrons will be concentrated to the vault area just opposite the target. The IBA Cyclone cyclotrons have their targets in the median plane of course but spread over the 360° circle. Also local neutron shielding of the ^{18}F targets is offered to reduce the neutron flux to the wall. So the distribution of the fast neutrons on the walls of the vault will be inhomogeneous and completely dependent on the type of the cyclotron, the geometry of the vault and whether local target shielding is employed. The neutron capture of the thermalised neutrons will be much more homogeneous, due to the randomisation of direction and the resulting spreading by multiple collisions.

Next to the so-called ordinary concrete, also "heavy" and "extra-heavy" concrete are sometimes used. The properties of all three different kinds of concrete are not well defined. Variations in the local composition of the concrete are common, so general quantitative statements on radioactivity and the specific activity are not possible. Also the definition of heavy (3.6 g/cm^3) and extra-heavy (4.8 g/cm^3) concrete is not well defined and may vary from site to site. So for specific cases, an individual sampling may be the appropriate procedure. In Table 9.3, the longer-lived radionuclides in concrete are listed. One has to realise that in concrete most of the elements needed for the production of these radionuclides are only available in ppm amounts. If the activity in the reinforcement steel of the concrete is analysed, much higher specific activities of ^{54}Mn and especially ^{60}Co can be found.

Before decommissioning, vault samples should be taken to measure the amount, specific activity and species. The activity level will go down with depth of course but only few data is available. To reduce the radioactivity induced in the vault, it is

Table 9.3 Long-lived radionuclides induced by neutrons in the concrete of the vault

Nuclide	Half-life	Reaction channel
^{40}K	1.28 × 109 year	Natural
^{55}Fe	0.27 × 10 year	$^{54}Fe(n,g)^{55}Fe$
^{59}Fe	4.46 × 10 year	$^{58}Fe(n,g)^{59}Fe$
^{152}Eu	1.36 × 10 year	$^{151}Eu(n,g)^{152}Eu$
^{154}Eu	0.88 × 10 year	$^{153}Eu(n,g)^{154}Eu$
^{60}Co	0.53 × 10 year	$^{59}Co(n,g)^{60}Co$
^{134}Cs	0.207 × 10 year	$^{133}Cs(n,g)^{134}Cs$
^{54}Mn	312 days	$^{54}Fe(n,p)^{54}Mn$

preferable that during the construction of the vault, no reinforcement steel is applied in the first 20–40 cm of concrete on the inside.

9.4 Disposal of Materials from the Cyclotron and Vault

In the previous sections, the activation of cyclotron parts and of the concrete in the vault has been discussed. In this section the disposal of radioactivity is discussed. In case of the concrete walls, samples should be taken for analysis. This could, for example, be done by drilling. However, before analysis it is unclear if the concrete contains radioactivity levels beyond the local exemption levels; this possibly involves working with, and possibly spreading of, radioactive materials. Therefore, precautions should be made and work should be done under guidance of a radiation safety officer. Prior to start of the operations, work instructions (SOPs) should be defined and well communicated, and a risk assessment should be completed. If analysis shows the radioactivity concentrations to be below the exemption levels, the concrete may be treated as non-radioactive. In principle the vault could be reused for non-radiological purposes or dismantled just as a conventional vault would be.

In case that the radioactivity concentrations are above the exemption levels, dismantling the vault becomes more complicated. It is not expected that the radiation levels from the concrete are such that a level significantly above background can be measured. As such, it is possible to reuse the vault either as a radiological area or a non-radiological area. If the vault is to be dismantled, the concrete must be transferred to an organisation that is licensed to store radioactive waste. During the work on dismantling the vault, precautions must be taken to prevent the spread of radioactive waste and dust. A dismantling plan covering the precautions as well as the risks must be defined. It is not expected that layers of concrete beyond the first 20 cm or so will have radioactivity concentration levels that exceed the exemption limits. Based on the order of magnitude of the concentration of radioactivity in the concrete, the radiation levels will most likely be low enough to package and transport the material as an excepted package (UN2910).

In case of the cyclotron itself, a distinction must be made between bulk materials that usually contain low concentrations of radioactivity and highly activated parts such as foils, targets, deflectors and such. After a cooling down period of several weeks or months, the shorter-lived nuclides will have decayed, and the longer-lived nuclides will remain (see Table 9.2). Longer-lived nuclides have reached their saturation values after years of use of the cyclotron and will not significantly decay on a timescale of months. Moreover, legislation often requires that the radioactive materials are removed as soon as is reasonable, but at least in two years time. After removal of the hottest parts, the bulk of the cyclotron may be placed in a crate or container and transported as an excepted package if the radiation levels on the outside of the container as well as the total amount of radioactivity inside do not exceed the local limits. The hot parts will have to be transported under conditions suitable and required according to local legislation. All parts must be transported to an organisation that is licensed to store and transport radioactive waste materials.

Conclusions

Decommissioning a cyclotron facility involves the decommissioning and dismantling of the cyclotron itself and possibly the dismantling of the concrete vault. In both cases one has to deal with activated materials. In case of the concrete vault, the concrete may, after analysis, prove to contain radioactivity concentrations below the exemption limits. In this case, the vault may be dismantled or reused according to wish or requirement. In case the concrete contains radioactivity concentrations that exceed exemption levels, the vault may be reused if the radiation dose levels permit. If (part of) the vault is dismantled, the concrete should be treated as a radioactive material, requiring safety precautions during work and transport.

The cyclotron will have hot parts and bulk parts that contain relatively low concentrations of long-lived nuclides. After a cooling down period, most short-lived nuclides will have decayed. The hot parts of the cyclotron should be removed and treated separately. The bulk of the cyclotron (e.g. the yoke) may be transported as an excepted package (UN2910) if the total amount of radioactivity as well as the radiation dose levels on the outside of the package allow this. Otherwise, the materials will have to be transported according to the requirements of local legislation. All materials that are removed and exceed the exemption levels should be transported to an organisation that is licensed to receive and store radioactive waste materials.

References

Blann M. Preequilibrium decay. Annu Rev Nucl Sci. 1975;25:123–66.

Calandrino R, del Vecchio A, Savi A, Todde S, Griffoni V, Brambilla S, Parisi R, Simone G, Fazio F. Decommissioning procedures for an 11 MeV self-shielded medical cyclotron after 16 years of working time. Health Phys. 2006;90:588–96.

European Commission on Nuclear Safety and the Environment. Evaluation of the radiological and economic consequences of decommissioning particle accelerators. Report EUR 19151, March 1999.

IAEA. Decommissioning of small medical, industrial and research facilities, IAEA Technical report series no. 414. Vienna: IAEA: 2003

Keller KA, Lange J, Münzel H. Numerical data and functional relationships in science and technology, 1. Q-values for nuclear reactions, Vol 5. Landolt-Bornstein, Springer (Heidelberg); 1974. p. 1–5.

Phillips AB, Prull DE, Ristinen RA et al. Residual radioactivity in a cyclotron and its surroundings. Health Phys. 1986;337–42.

Sunderland JJ, Erdahl CE, Bender BR, Sensoy L, Watkins GL. Considerations, measurements and logistics associated with low-energy cyclotron decommissioning. AIP Conf Proc. 2012;1509: 16–20.

The Role of a Nuclear Medicine Department in Nuclear Accidents

10

Anne M.J. Paans and Johan R. de Jong

Abstract

The term "nuclear accident" covers a wide variety of accidents from a simple radioactive contamination to the detonation of an atomic bomb and everything in between. A department of nuclear medicine should be prepared for accidents which can happen in the patient service area of the hospital. So a proper inventory of nuclear facilities in the area should be available or should be made.

In this chapter an overview will be given on the possible accidents which can be encountered in large general hospitals or university hospitals.

10.1 Introduction

In general, hospitals are not or not well prepared for patients from nuclear accidents with exception of hospitals in the near vicinity of nuclear installation, e.g., nuclear power plants or large nuclear research installations that have a special contract with these installations. The possible accidents can be split in five categories depending on the severity:

1. Nuclear detonation of an atomic bomb
2. Accidents in large nuclear installations, e.g., in nuclear power plants, uranium enrichment factories, and nuclear research facilities
3. Nuclear public health threats: dispersion of nuclear material in public by accident or terrorism

A.M.J. Paans (✉) • J.R. de Jong
Department of Nuclear Medicine and Molecular Imaging, University Medical Center Groningen, University of Groningen, Hanzeplein 1, Groningen 9700 RB, The Netherlands
e-mail: a.m.j.paans@umcg.nl

A.W.J.M. Glaudemans et al. (eds.), *Quality in Nuclear Medicine*,
DOI 10.1007/978-3-319-33531-5_10

4. Accidents during the transport of radioactive materials
5. Accidents in industrial and/or research laboratories or during medical diagnostic or therapeutic procedures

A department of nuclear medicine should be prepared for accidents which can happen in the patient service area of the hospital. So a proper inventory of nuclear facilities in the area should be available or should be made.

In this chapter an overview will be given on the possible accidents which can be encountered in large general hospitals or university hospitals.

10.2 Detonation of an Atomic Bomb

The detonation of an atomic bomb can only happen in a war zone. A normal department of nuclear medicine cannot be prepared for such an emergency event. This type of emergency situation should be handled by government-installed emergency systems which work countrywide. Organizations for a "national emergency" should take over and instruct lower governmental organizations how to work according to already prepared plans for this type of emergencies.

The individual countries will have taken their precautions already many years ago and put a nationwide plan in position having a special organization take over and instruct also the hospitals. The exact form of the organization will differ for each country and should be checked by the individual departments and be incorporated in the hospital-wide plans for emergencies.

Nationwide plans will incorporate measures to be taken on different levels. One such level consists of measures that should be taken to treat the wounded and the contaminated. Another will be on the level of damage control, containment, and prevention of follow-up damage. Hospitals in general and nuclear medicine departments in particular will, in case of calamities on a scale such as this, mostly focus on individual patient care under relatively safe conditions and will not have the capacity to decontaminate large groups of people. This will only be possible for patients from the outer rim of the detonation zone where radiation levels will be relatively low, survivors exist, and the infrastructure is not completely destroyed.

10.3 Accidents in Large Nuclear Installation

With large nuclear installations, one should not only think of nuclear power plants but also, e.g., of uranium enrichment facilities or the larger nuclear research facilities. In the planning process of such installations or facilities, all kinds of safety procedures have been taken in order to get the necessary licenses to operate the facility in a safe way. This includes also the cooperation with a hospital in case of incidents and/or accidents. Of course the facility itself has its own infrastructure and services to act on accidents and incidents, but especially specialized medical help has to be found in a hospital in the close vicinity. In the hospital the department of nuclear medicine has a special role in establishing the level of (possible) radioactive contamination and in the process of decontamination. In practice, the first aid department and the department of nuclear medicine together with the nuclear facility involved should make standard operating procedures (SOPs) based on an analysis of the possible accidents/incidents and how to act in case of emergency. Also, based on this analysis, the knowledge and equipment in the hospital should be adapted to the possible situations. The possible emergency situations should also be practiced by regular training sessions of the nuclear facility, the first aid department, and the department of nuclear medicine. Depending on the scale of the damage caused by the accident or terroristic attack, the number of people wounded or exposed may be limited to the amount of workers of the facility or include inhabitants from the surrounding area. In the first case, the hospital(s) in the area will probably have sufficient capacity to treat and decontaminate/contain the wounded. In the latter case, a nationwide approach will be required involving containment or isolation of the area and damage control.

10.4 Nuclear Public Health Threats: Dispersion of Nuclear Material in Public by Accident or Terrorism

Large amounts of nuclear material can enter by accident into the public environment because in hospitals often large quantities of nuclear material are available for therapeutic and/or diagnostic purposes. The nuclear source has to be replaced after a certain time. "Famous" are the stories of the loss of radium needles during illegal transport to the hospital by the individual medical specialist. Under the present regulations, the disposal of the old sources should be according to the rules and should not be sold as scrap metal as happened once, e.g., in Brazil where the new owner of the scrap distributed the ^{137}Cs source among relatives, friends, and children contaminating nearly 250 people and causing four deaths.

The development of nuclear weapons started around 1940 (Manhattan Project) and resulted in the world's first radiologic public health emergency: the first test of an atomic bomb near Alamogordo (New Mexico) in July 1945 followed by the bombs on Japan in Hiroshima and Nagasaki. see at Office of History https://www.osti.gov/opennet/manhattan-project-history.

After World War II, the USA, the Soviet Union, the UK, France, and China started testing nuclear weapons under atmospheric conditions. This resulted in a worldwide elevation of the radiation level in the atmosphere due to the long-lived radionuclides produced in the detonation of the atomic bombs, both fission and fusion bombs. Since the Non-Proliferation Treaty of Nuclear Weapons in 1968, the radiation level in the atmosphere has gone down according to decay laws and the atmospheric conditions.

Another well-known public health threat was the Chernobyl accident in April 1986. The accident was not reported immediately to the public right after the accident, but after some weeks the accident was detected due to an elevated atmospheric radiation level in Western Europe and Sweden. In the struggle against the continuation of the nuclear contamination in the first days and weeks after the accident, reactor employees and firemen received a lethal dose. The emergency workers, the so-called liquidators, have been highly exposed, and this is the part of the population that received (too) large radiation doses. Death by an acute radiation syndrome (ARS) occurred in these cases. Large quantities of radioactive ^{131}I (half-life 8 days) were released from the reactor contaminating the nearby farmland with large quantities. No measures were taken to reduce the consumption of fresh milk and vegetables, and also no stable iodine was provided to the population to suppress the accumulation of ^{131}I in the thyroid. This resulted in a large amount of thyroid cancers, especially in children in the near vicinity of Chernobyl. The contaminated area moved up into Sweden where the long-lived ^{137}Cs (30 years) was found and also detected in the meat of animals (e.g., deer). The effect on the population in general was, as UNSCEAR concluded: "there is no evidence of a major public health impact attributable to radiation exposure (Cardis et al. 2006; Steinhausler 2005) 14 years after the accident. There is no scientific evidence of increases in overall cancer incidence or mortality or in non-malignant disorders that could be related to radiation exposure."

The last example of a public health threat is the Fukushima accident on March 11, 2011. Due to an earthquake in the sea near Japan, a tsunami was created which seriously damaged, and partly destroyed, the nuclear power plant complex Daiichi in Fukushima. Large areas of land with villages were and are contaminated, and people were evacuated and still remain evacuated. A time path for eventual return is not established yet. The spill of contaminated water is still not under control, and large quantities of contaminated water are being released into the sea.

Next to these disasters due to nature or to human failure, there is a fear for terrorism using a radiological dispersal device, a RDD, or better known as "dirty bomb." A RDD consists of two parts: (1) conventional (Barnen et al. 2006) explosives and (2) long-lived radioactive material. The goal is to contaminate by the conventional explosion not only a large area (in the order of hundreds of thousands of square meters) but also all people in this area. The explosion will take place in, for example, a downtown area or shopping area in order to contaminate as much people as possible.

Of all possible longer-lived radioactive, there are four isotopes which are very frequently used in medicine or industry. ^{60}Co (half-life 5 years) is used in radiotherapy, industrial radiography, and food irradiations. The amount of activity used in these sources is in the order of 10 PBq. ^{137}Cs (half-life 30 years) is used in medicine for diagnostic and therapeutic procedures, blood irradiation, industrial radiography, and food irradiation. Source strength is in the order of 1 PBq. ^{192}Ir (half-life 74 days) is used for medical therapeutics and industrial radiography, source strength 10 TBq. ^{241}Am (half-life 432 years) is used for industrial radiography, source strength in the order of 1 TBq. Especially in radiotherapy and in sterilization procedures, the replacement of radioactive sources by electron accelerators has priority in minimizing the possible accidents with long-lived radioactive sources. For the use as a RDD, the half-life of ^{192}Ir is rather short but the other three are certainly candidates.

Next to the four abovementioned radionuclides, one can also think of ^{235}U (half-life 7×10^8 years) or ^{239}Pu (half-life 24,400 years). Especially, the use of uranium worries the governments because basically it is a natural element and enriched; it is used worldwide, e.g., in nuclear power plants. The enrichment grade can vary from a few percent to over 95 % ^{235}U as weapons-grade uranium for use in a nuclear explosive device. Highly enriched uranium is also used in nuclear reactors for special use like research reactors with high neutron fluxes. Worldwide nowadays one tries to limit the use of highly enriched uranium. Enriched uranium is now divided into two classes: (1) highly enriched uranium or HEU (>20 %) and (2) low-enriched uranium or LEU (<20 %). Worldwide, a program is initiated to replace all HEU in nuclear reactors by LEU in order to minimize the amount of HEU worldwide available. The Nuclear Security Summit 2014, the third in a row, in The Hague (Netherlands) is a platform where these problems are discussed worldwide. Plutonium is of course another radionuclide which can be used by terrorists but is available in much lesser degree than uranium. Plutonium is also used as an admixture in uranium for use in nuclear power plants. This so-called mixed oxide fuel (MOX) uses the plutonium generated in the reactors of nuclear power plants in order to reduce the amounts of Pu. The whereabout of this plutonium should be strictly controlled. For the production of ^{99}Mo, the mother radionuclide of ^{99m}Tc, up till now HEU was used but is in the process of being replaced by LEU. The production of ^{99}Mo as the mother nuclide of ^{99m}Tc is rather critical because all the production nuclear reactors are rather specific, e.g., the high flux reactor in Petten (Netherlands), because of the requirements on the neutron flux for the production of ^{99}Mo. ^{99m}Tc is the most frequently used radionuclide in nuclear medicine diagnostic procedures. In the Netherlands alone, this amounts to about 500,000 procedures yearly.

The health effects of a RDD can be split in two parts, the conventional part and the nuclear part. The conventional part is due to the explosives used in the RDD. Estimates are that it can cause several deaths and a series of wounded depending on the strength of the explosion and these victims will be localized to the place of the explosion. Due to the explosion, nuclear material will be dispersed in the surrounding. Depending on the specific area, this can be rather limited, but if the RDD is used in open air in a windy environment, the radioactivity can cover some hundreds of thousands of square meters. Depending on the source and the strength of radioactive material, the contamination of the people can differ. Ingestion or inhalation is not considered at this moment. In the worst case the strength is so high that deterministic effects can be expected. Deterministic effects have a threshold of about 0.7 Gy which is rather high and are expected not to be reached, and thus, no ARS, as was the case with the liquidators, will occur. Contamination of a much lower level is expected so only stochastic effects are to be expected. At present it is assumed that stochastic effects do not have a threshold and that the increased probability of developing lethal cancer is 5 % per Sievert. As noted before, such high doses are not to be expected. All people in the contaminated area should be decontaminated. This means that all clothes should be collected and all people should wash with water and soap on the areas where radioactivity is expected. Since not only the cloth but also the water will be contaminated, the water has to be collected also. By this simple decontamination procedure, it is expected that >90 % of the radioactivity can be removed.

What will the public do after a "dirty bomb"? The expectation is that there will be some panic because of the explosion and soon police and fire and rescue services will be at the place of accident to control the situation. The fire fighters are able to measure the radiation level (standard procedure with available equipment), and as soon as the word "radioactivity" spreads, real panic will cause a run on the nearby medical help posts and more specifically the hospitals, also by not contaminated people. A well-educated guess is that only one out of every five at the reception desk of the hospital will really be contaminated. The local authorities will have an emergency plan to handle the calamity of a RDD, but nevertheless, a large crowd can be expected at the emergency entrance of the hospital. The hospital should also have a calamity plan to handle the situation of a RDD including separation of the "RDD" stream from the "regular" emergency patient into a special stream where first a triage can be done (<10 μSv/h, not contaminated; 10–100 μSv/h, cleaning by standard personnel; >100 μSv/h, cleaning under supervision of radiation expert). Medical emergencies have priority and can be supported by radiation experts. Contaminated people should be separated, cleaned, and checked again. Also a sample of the radioactivity should be obtained for further analysis so the radionuclide involved can be identified. This is especially important since the half-life and the nature of the emission of ionizing radiation of the radionuclide determine the final radiation dose and the duration of elevated radiation levels and continued risk. The pathway for these calamity patients should be predefined within the hospital organization as well as the personnel involved, so next to the normal calamity personnel are also personnel from the nuclear medicine department (radiation experts). Equipment, e.g., radiation monitoring, clothing, etc. should be predefined and available on the shelf.

There is also the possibility of internal contamination due to ingestion or inhalation. In case of ingestion or inhalation, it is important to know the radionuclide involved and also the chemical form in order to take appropriate measures. One can think of the induction of vomiting, administration of stable iodine to block the thyroid, increase diuresis and try to purge. One could collect urine and feces for identification for radionuclide and chemical analysis.

Not all departments of nuclear medicine and also not all hospitals will have a trained calamity organization available because the estimated urgency will be low in most organizations, but, e.g., the Dutch Society of Nuclear Medicine has the so-called recommendations (aanbevelingen in Dutch) in which also nuclear accidents are covered.

10.5 Accidents During Transport of Radioactive Materials

Many radioactive materials are transported every day in each country. One can think of relative small sources for vitro diagnostic procedures and for research. Special regulations for these transports are part of the nuclear legislation. In most countries these transports are only allowed from license holder to license holder. The packing of the radioactive materials is prescribed and is depending on the kind of radioactive material and the amount. Transports like the transport of nuclear fuel or nuclear waste in the so-called castor containers are well known because of the protest demonstrations against it in some countries, but most radioactive transports are very small and fit in a normal transport van. This van has to meet special conditions and should be equipped with warning signs and transportation forms which show all details of the transport. In case of accidents, these warning signs will alarm the police and fire and rescue services immediately, and they will take the necessary precautions. In case of injured people with open wounds, the hospital involved will also be warned for possible radioactive contamination, and the department of nuclear medicine should be warned to take care of the matter. For these events, a standard operating procedure or SOP should be available at the emergency entrance.

10.6 Accidents in Industrial and/or Research Laboratories or During Medical Diagnostic or Therapeutic Procedures

The fire and rescue services is the organization which has an overview of all industrial and laboratory dangers in their service area. The local industry and laboratories will have their own emergency plans, and within these plans, they will have made contact with nearby hospitals, and in cooperation between industry and hospital, SOPs should have been defined for emergency situations.

Conclusions

The nuclear accidents as described above can be split into three categories:

- Local size overstepping events (categories one and two)
- Local accidents which are covered by SOPs
- A RDD for which it is difficult to be fully prepared

In order to be prepared as a department of nuclear medicine, one should have available SOPs in cooperation with the emergency department. All materials required in the SOPs should be available on the shelf.

To be prepared for a RDD, not only the hospital organization should be prepared but also SOPs should be prepared together with the local authorities including the police and fire and rescue department.

The most important in all these preparation is to keep the knowledge updated for all people involved by a regular training scheme.

References

Barnen DJ, Parker CL, Blodgett DW, Wierzba RK, Links JM. Understanding radiological and nuclear terrorism as public health threats: preparedness and response perspectives. J Nucl Med. 2006;47:1653–61.

Cardis E, Howe G, Ron E, Behesko V, Bogdanova T, Bouville A, Carr Z, Chumak V, Davis S, Demidchik Y, Drozdovitch V, Gentner N, Gudzenko N, Hatch M, Ivanov V, Jacob P, Kapitonova E, Kenigsberg Y, Kesminiene A, Kopecky KJ, Kryuchkov V, Loos A, Pinchera A, Reiners C, Repacholi M, Shibata Y, Shore RE, Thomas G, Tirmarche M, Yamashita S, Zvonova I. Cancer consequences of the Chernobyl accident: 20 years on. J Radiol Prot. 2006;26:127–40.

Office of History and Heritage Resources, U.S. Department of Energy. The Manhattan Project: an interactive history. Available at: https://www.osti.gov/opennet/manhattan-project-history/. Accessed 11 Mar 2014.

Office of the Assistant Secretary for Public Affairs. Terrorism and other public health emergencies: a reference guide for media. Washington, DC: U.S. Department of Health and Human Services; 2005.

Steinhausler F. Chernobyl and Goiania: lessons for responding to radiological terrorism. Health Phys. 2005;89:566–74.

United Nations Scientific Committee on the effects of Atomic Radiation. Sources and Effects of Ionizing Radiation, UNSCEAR 2000 Report to the General Assembly, with Scientific Annexes: 451–566 Annex J: Exposures and effects of the Chernobyl accident. 2000. United Nations, New York.

Part III

Equipment

Medical Devices

11

R.M. (Marcel) Löhr, J.A.W. (Koos) van Ringelenstein, and G.E. (Gert) Drewes

Abstract

Since the number of medical equipment is growing and equipment becomes more diverse, specialized people are necessary for the technical management of these medical devices. In the UMCG, the Department of Medical Technology provides technical support in the application of medical technology and makes an important contribution to the continuity and safety of care, education, and research. In this chapter, it is explained how a tender for a new camera park at a nuclear medicine department was performed and how the Department of Medical Technology is embedded in all medical departments of a hospital.

11.1 General

The University Medical Center Groningen and University of Groningen are pioneers in the application of radioisotopes in medicine. This aspect of their history started in 1952 when the first in vivo and in vitro measurements were performed.

For in vivo measurements, external detectors were initially employed; later, a scanning detector system was used. Radioimmunoassays were developed. The first gamma camera was installed in 1965, and with the availability of the ^{99m}Tc generator, new in vivo diagnostic procedures were set up. Positron emission tomography (PET) became possible in 1972 after installation of a large cyclotron at the Kernfysisch Versneller Insituut (KVI), a university institution. Pioneering PET

R.M. (Marcel) Löhr (✉) • J.A.W. (Koos) van Ringelenstein • G.E. (Gert) Drewes
Department of Medical Technology, University Medical Center Groningen, Hanzeplein 1, Groningen 9700 RB, The Netherlands
e-mail: r.m.lohr@umcg.nl

A.W.J.M. Glaudemans et al. (eds.), *Quality in Nuclear Medicine*,
DOI 10.1007/978-3-319-33531-5_11

studies were performed in close cooperation between nuclear medicine, the KVI, and the University Laboratory of Organic Chemistry.

This led to financing by the Dutch government of a fully equipped PET-Center on hospital grounds in 1988. Nuclear medicine (headed by Dr. D.A. Piers) and PET-Center (headed by Prof. W. Vaalburg) developed via separate lines during the 1990s. Because of the clinical potential of nuclear imaging in diagnostics and radionuclide therapy, nuclear medicine and PET-Center were reunited in 2005.

The Department of Nuclear Medicine and Molecular Imaging was formed as a novel discipline group of the UMCG, headed by Prof. Dr. R.A. Dierckx (Nuclear Medicine and Molecular Imaging, History 2012).

11.2 History

Until 2008, the facilities in the Department of Nuclear Medicine and Molecular Imaging consisted of four gamma cameras, two PET scanners, and one bone density measurement system for clinical use and one microCT, one microCAT, and one microSPECT for preclinical use and furthermore one cyclotron.

- Siemens Orbiter, single head
- Siemens Diacam, single head
- Siemens MultiSpect2, dual head
- Siemens Ecam, dual head
- Siemens Ecat HR+
- Hologic Discover A bone density
- Siemens microPET Focus 220
- Siemens Imtek microCAT II
- Milabs microSPECT II
- Scanditronix cyclotron MC-17

The two dual-headed and the two single-headed gamma cameras were in use for clinical and research studies in humans. Three of the four systems showed errors on a regular basis and required more than occasional maintenance until 2006.

The complete single photon machine park and the computer platform of the present gamma cameras, the Siemens Icon, were outdated. Since the older PET scanner has been already acquired, in 1996 it was decided that this machine should be replaced by an up-to-date PET/CT system. The latest PET scanner, a Siemens Ecat Exact HR+, acquired in 2004, was decided to be replaced shortly after the replacement of the whole machine park.

11.3 European Tender

In 2006, the head of the Department of Nuclear Medicine and Molecular Imaging took the initiative to set up a program to replace the four gamma cameras, one PET camera, and the IT-infrastructure for processing and storage purposes. The reason was that these systems needed more attention than the regular services.

During 2008, a European Tender for four new gamma cameras and one new PET/CT with the complementary computer platform was evaluated.

European tendering is purchasing by government agencies (or government-funded organizations) with the EU guidelines followed (Information About European tender 2014). The guidelines apply above certain thresholds (€ 207,000 for supplies and services and € 5,186,000 for works, price level 2014). The guidelines are based on procurement, but there are other procedures for specific purchasing situations. The directives must be transposed into national laws. In the Netherlands this is called the Public Procurement Act. The guidelines consist of general principles that have to be followed during procurement processes.

The objectives of the EU directives are:

- Promotion of free trade in the European Union
- Providing equal opportunities to providers of works, supplies, and services to compete for public contracts
- Promoting the efficiency of public spending

The general principles of the directives are:

- Transparency, the process must be clear and unambiguous. It should be clear to suppliers in advance what you want to buy and how you will evaluate the offers.
- Equality, all bidders are equally treated.

European tendering begins with the preparation of a set of requirements (PVE). In the PVE must be described what the job is and what the demands and requirements are to which the tenderers and tenders will be assessed. If the PVE is completed, the contract notice may be sent to TenderNed, the Dutch publishing site for public contracts.

Interested industrial suppliers can take notice of the assignment and possibly enroll. Bids that are received are assessed after the closing of the tender. The best tender wins the round. A European tender will last between 3 and 4 months; in practice this may also be longer. The preparations, particularly the drafting of the PVE, usually takes about 3 months, but a complex tendering can easily take longer. An average time to complete a tender will run for 6–9 months.

The contract may be awarded on the basis of best value for money. In terms of law, this means "the most economically advantageous tender" or EMVI (Dutch abbreviation).

All tenders based on EMVI price and quality are taken into account. In fact, an entrepreneur can compensate a higher price by a higher quality.

The requirements (PVE) for the new gamma cameras, new PET/CT, and new IT platform was based on the following items:

- Functional and operational requirements, such as hardware, data handling, and specifications
- Operations
- Maintenance, based on high performance with respect to low total costs of ownership (TCO)

- Extensive cooperation in the field of research
- Training of staff, regarding technicians, doctors, and physicists
- Time of installation and delivery
- References

11.4 Current Medical Devices

Due to the outcome of the European tender, the Board of Directors of the UMCG was advised to replace all cameras and computers by a Siemens platform. This recommendation was adopted and results in the following configuration, which was installed in 2009.

- 2 Siemens Symbia S, gamma camera (both dual head gamma camera, Fig. 11.1)
- Siemens Symbia T2, SPECT/CT (dual head gamma camera with a dual slice CT)
- Siemens Symbia T16, SPECT.CT (dual head gamma camera with a 16 slice CT)
- Siemens Biograph mCT, PET-CT (PET/CT system with a 64 slice CT, Fig. 11.2)
- Pukka-J, PACS system
- Siemens MI workstations, incl. several processing applications

11.5 Department of Medical Technology

The Department of Medical Technology provides technical support in the application of medical technology in the UMCG and makes an important contribution to the continuity and safety of care, education, and research. This is done by instruction, testing, maintenance, and advising on medical devices and systems. This support is offered in all phases of the life cycle: acquisition, introduction, use, and rejection.

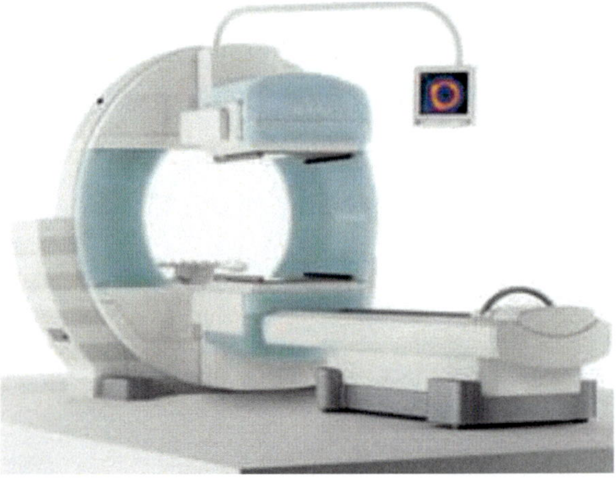

Fig. 11.1 Symbia S gamma camera

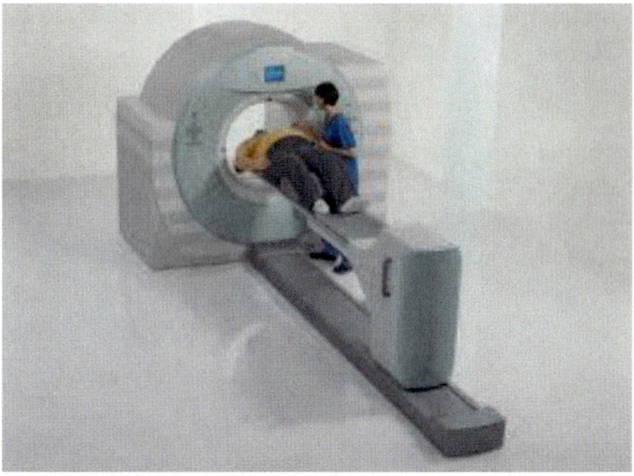

Fig. 11.2 Biograph mCT PET-CT

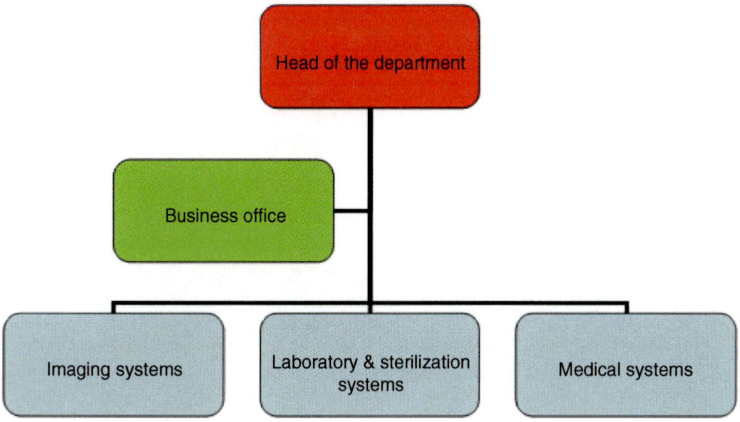

Fig. 11.3 Organization model medical technology

All medical departments, clinical laboratories, medical support departments, and research departments are increasingly using the services of the Department of Medical Technology. There are also a number of external companies and institutions within the UMCG who purchase our services. With all of our customers, we have a service level agreement (SLA).

The Department of Medical Technology is divided into three teams, each with its own focus, and a business office, in total 45 FTE (2014); see Fig. 11.3.

The head of the department is a general manager, and each team is led by a team leader. Each team consists of medical instrumentation technicians, medical instrumentation engineers, and technical specialists. The department has also a general clinical physicist. The business office consists of administrative staff, IT staff, and staff advisors. The Department of Medical Technology is ISO 9001 certified since 2002.

The total amount of equipment managed by the Department of Medical Technology includes more than 23,000 units with a total investment value of approximately € 190 million (2014) and has an enormous diversity.

- Imaging systems such as MRI, CT, PET/CT, gamma cameras, X-ray equipment, and PACS used at the Department of Radiology, Cardiology, Nuclear Medicine and Molecular Imaging, and Dentistry.
- Medical equipment such as patient monitors, infusion equipment, anesthesia and respiratory equipment, surgical instruments, electro surgery equipment, defibrillators, ophthalmic equipment, incubators, ultrasound equipment, pulmonary function equipment, dental treatment units, endoscopic equipment, and patient beds.
- Laboratory and sterilization equipment such as laboratory analyzers, mass spectrometers, microscopes, weighing equipment, centrifuges, incubators, DNA/PCR equipment, HPLC equipment, tissue processing machines, vacuum pumps, laboratory robots, samplers, sterilization equipment, instrument cleaners, bedpan washers, and pharmaceutical production units.

A few more figures: the annual number of work orders for periodical maintenance is about 9000, and the annual number of failures is 6000 (excluding the decentralized fault messages).

For the technical management of the medical systems, the Department of Medical technology uses Ultimo. Ultimo is a very wide software package for object and maintenance management. The Department of Finance and Control uses the objects module of Ultimo for the registration of all equipment (capital goods). Each device gets in the purchasing process a unique object-code. This object-code is recorded in the year-end database and applied physically on any device. The object-code contains data about equipment type, manufacturer, model, serial number, vendor, installation date, purchase price, department, etc.

As said earlier, the Department of Medical Technology has with all its customers a SLA, and there are now more than 50 active SLAs. Within in a SLA, there are agreements made about mutual responsibilities, response times to breakdowns, availability service, delivery, billing information, costs, etc. An important part of a SLA is the equipment list which comes from the maintenance management system (Ultimo). In the equipment list, it is indicated by device if maintenance should be carried out and how often it should be done, whether it is done by the Department of Medical Technology or external party, and who supervised the execution of maintenance.

A SLA evaluation is annually held with all the customers based on a checklist and some specific reports from Ultimo. These reports provide a detailed picture of carried out repairs, periodic maintenance, etc. In the evaluation, interviews are also agreements on service and maintenance of recently purchased equipment. An evaluation report is made of all the evaluation findings and actions (PDCA cycle). On the basis of all evaluation reports, there is a clear picture of how customers experience our services and if improvements have to be made.

In the maintenance, module of Ultimo data is recorded about maintenance such as period, frequency, protocol, performer, supervisor, etc. All the work that is performed on a device is recorded at object level in Ultimo, including things like maintenance costs (costs for parts, labor, contracts, etc.).

This means that we are capable to get a good and complete picture of all the maintenance work carried out at both object level and by equipment type, by department, and so on.

11.6 Service and Maintenance

In the UMCG, the maintenance of complex imaging systems are mainly based on shared service contracts with different suppliers. This is reflected at the departments of radiology, cardiology, nuclear medicine and molecular imaging, and dentistry. All activities such as preventive and corrective maintenance are carried out by both the Department of Medical Technology and the suppliers and recorded in Ultimo.

The shared service contracts for the imaging systems at the Department of Nuclear Medicine and Molecular Imaging are based on different participations levels, namely, 1st, 2nd, and 3rd level. A prerequisite for 2nd and 3rd level is that the engineers and technical specialists of the Department of Medical Technology are trained and certified. Training of the engineers and technical specialists for the several imaging systems of Siemens are taking place at the Siemens training facilities in Erlangen (Germany) or Gary (NC, USA). Regarding to the training, there is no distinction between training for engineers from Siemens or engineers, technical specialists from the Department of Medical Technology.

In 2009, a setup for a growth model was made, in consultation with Siemens and the Department of Nuclear Medicine and Molecular Imaging, on how to implement the different shared service levels and the training of the engineers and technical specialists of the Department of Medical Technology.

An overview of the different kinds of service levels is mentioned below.

- 1st level participation means that all activities regarding the preventive and corrective maintenance and upgrades/updates of hardware and software are performed by Siemens engineers. Only 1st level activities regarding corrective maintenance are done by engineers and technical specialists from the Department of Medical Technology.
- 2nd level participation means that all activities regarding the preventive and corrective maintenance and upgrades/updates of hardware and software are performed jointly by engineers from Siemens and engineers and technical specialists from the Department of Medical Technology. Prerequisite is that the engineers and technical specialists of the Department of Medical Technology are fully trained and certified for the regarding systems.
- 3rd level participation means that all activities regarding the preventive and corrective maintenance and upgrades/updates of hardware and software are performed by engineers and technical specialists of the Department of Medical

Technology. Prerequisite is that the engineers and technical specialists of the Department of Medical Technology are fully trained and certified for the regarding systems.

Before starting the work, such as application, repair, preventive maintenance, and validation, the system is transferred by the technicians, by means of a special transfer form, to engineers, technical specialists of the Department of Medical Technology, or engineers of the supplier.

After completion of the work, the system is transferred back to nuclear medicine and molecular imaging department by means of the same form. The engineers and technical specialists of the Department of Medical Technology or engineers of the supplier stated on the transfer form the description of the work performed and whether the system meets specifications and can be used again.

The temporary release for clinical use is done by the technician of the department. The ultimate responsibility for the final release lies with the medical physicist.

11.7 Current Developments

The Dutch hospitals, represented in the NVZ and NFU, and Rehabilitation Netherlands have covenants drafting the safe use of medical technology. This agreement is formally ratified in November 2011. The agreement gives substance to the risk management and safe use of medical technology in patient care. The Healthcare Inspectorate also uses the covenant as a framework for the inspections of hospitals.

The agreement covers the entire life cycle of medical technology, introduction, use, and disposal and states that the reliability of the applied medical technology is determined by various measures to be taken during the entire life cycle. A plan prior to the implementation of a new medical device/medical technology must be prepared. This plan should cover the need for the proposed acquisition, risk analysis, competence and training plan for users and technicians, and a maintenance and periodic evaluation. A procurement file must be created for each purchase in which all information mentioned must be stored. Risk management and competence of users of equipment is central to the covenant.

Against this background, the Department of Medical Technology has carried out a risk classification, done by an external company in early 2013. Included in the used model are a risk score and risk class assigned per equipment type, manufacturer, and model. This model distinguishes four risk categories: low, medium low, medium high, and high.

The function, application risk, disruption of the care process, use, environmental factors, as well as the necessary maintenance are taken into account. This risk classification is an integral part of medical technology module in Ultimo release 10. Ultimo release 10 is currently being implemented in the UMCG, and all departments are able to update the online risk class and risk scores of their medical equipment when the release is ready.

The UMCG is responsible for the requirements regarding education and training of users, the ability required, and assessments linked to the risk category. The Medical Technology department wants to use the risk classification in the securing of the periodic maintenance.

Equipment from a higher risk class will have a tighter maintenance regime than equipment from the middle risk class.

References

Information about European tender. Opgehaald van website of universiteit Leiden. 4 maart 2014. http://www.organisatie.leidenuniv.nl/inkoop/medewerkers/vragen/veelgestelde-vragen.html#wat-is-europees-aanbesteden.

Nuclear medicine and molecular imaging, history. Opgehaald van website university of Groningen. 2012. http://www.rug.nl/research/radiation-science/ngmb/history.

SPECT/CT and Image Quality

12

Yves D'Asseler

Abstract

In this chapter, we will look into image quality aspects of SPECT/CT technology. We will place the focus on the SPECT part of the technology, starting from the point of view that a SPECT/CT camera is used primarily as a SPECT camera that also acquires a CT image, registered to this SPECT image. Consequently, we will discuss SPECT image quality and show how the CT part of the technology can be used to improve the quality and readability of the SPECT images. Less attention will be given to the quality of CT images, although it is clear that this is also a very important issue.

In the first part of this chapter, the technology behind a SPECT/CT camera will be briefly discussed, as this is background information necessary in order to understand the issues arising in SPECT/CT imaging.

Next, a short introduction about general medical image quality will be given, which will serve as the reference framework for the further discussion about SPECT/CT image quality.

The subsequent part will handle the technological image quality in SPECT/CT, and the issues that may arise concerning this technological image quality.

We will dedicate some paragraphs to quantification in SPECT, since it is still widely assumed that SPECT, in contrast to PET, is a non-quantitative imaging modality. However, many advances have been made towards reaching the goal of quantitative SPECT in clinical practice.

Next, we will discuss image quality in SPECT/CT from a task-based perspective. As we will explain, the task-based point of view is of utmost importance in medical image quality assessment, and the optimisation of purely

Y. D'Asseler, PhD
Department of Nuclear Medicine, Ghent University Hospital,
De Pintelaan 185, Gent 9000, Belgium
e-mail: Yves.DAsseler@ugent.be

A.W.J.M. Glaudemans et al. (eds.), *Quality in Nuclear Medicine*,
DOI 10.1007/978-3-319-33531-5_12

technological image quality parameters, not taking into account the task at hand for a specific application, will often not be sufficient to guarantee optimal image quality.

Finally, some general conclusions are made and future prospects are discussed.

12.1 SPECT/CT Technology

SPECT/CT is an imaging technology that combines functional with anatomical information to obtain high diagnostic accuracy. This technology uses a gamma camera integrated with a CT scanner.

The gamma camera is used to produce single photon emission computed tomography (SPECT) images, using the tracer principle and the tomographic technique. Tomography consists in acquiring projection images of a three-dimensional object from many angles and using these projections to obtain a three-dimensional image of this object. The calculation of the 3D image from the projections is known as tomographic reconstruction.

The tracer principle refers to the use of a small quantity of a substance (a tracer) of which one desires to study the distribution in the body of a patient. This tracer is labelled with a marker in order to be able to measure its distribution after the administration to the patient. In the case of SPECT imaging, the marker is a radioactive substance known as a single photon emitter (Runge et al. 2015), which produces a high-energy gamma photon when it decays to its stable form. Typically and frequently used single photon emitters include ^{99m}Tc, ^{123}I, ^{111}In, ^{67}Ga and ^{201}Tl.

Computed tomography (CT) uses the same tomographic technique as mentioned above, but in this case, the quantity imaged is the attenuation of an X-ray beam as it traverses the patient body. In this way, anatomical images are obtained.

Combining these two diagnostic techniques in one device has a number of advantages compared to having the imaging modalities available separately (Buck et al. 2008; Jacene et al. 2008). Firstly, the reconstruction of the SPECT images requires accurate attenuation correction in order to be able to provide quantitatively correct information. The CT image can be used as the basis for an attenuation map that can be used for this correction.

Secondly, the combination of perfectly registered anatomical and functional information provides an important advantage in the interpretation of the images and the subsequent diagnosis, since SPECT images often lack anatomical landmarks necessary to pinpoint the specific organ or tissue type in which an important feature in the image was detected. An anatomical image such as CT can give this information.

SPECT images are acquired by a gamma camera. The gamma camera consists of a patient bed, one or more detector heads and a gantry which enables the positioning and movement of these detector heads relative to the patient (Cherry et al. 2012). In Fig. 12.1, the detector head of a gamma camera is shown schematically with its main components.

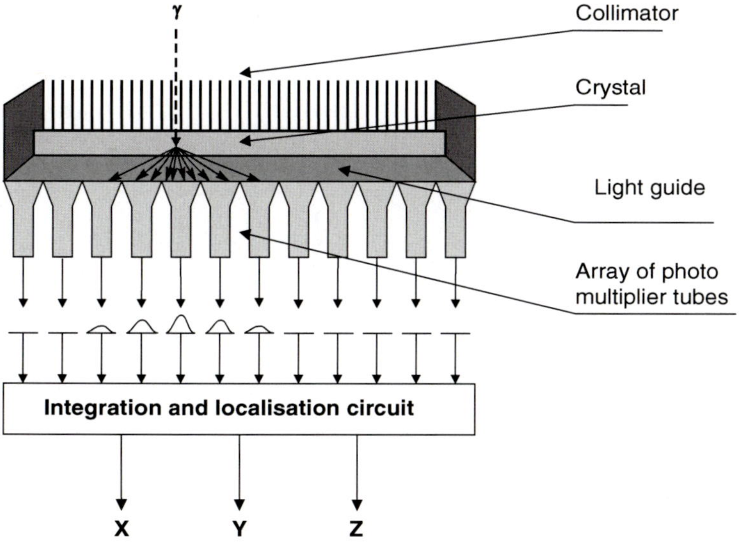

Fig. 12.1 Gamma camera detector head

As a gamma photon impinges upon the detector, it must first get through the collimator for a detection to be possible. A collimator is basically a block of highly attenuating material (e.g. lead or tungsten) with many holes. Only photons travelling approximately parallel to these holes can get through the collimator; other photons will be stopped by the attenuating material in between the holes known as the septa. In this way, projections of the activity distribution in the field of view of the detector are obtained. The most often used collimator is a parallel hole collimator, yielding projections perpendicular to the detector surface. However, other types such as fan beam or cone beam collimators exist.

Once the gamma photon makes it through the collimator, it falls upon a scintillation crystal. In the case of a gamma camera, the crystal used is typically a large NaI(Tl) monocrystal. This crystal produces a scintillation, a flash of visible light, when a high-energy photon interacts with it. This flash spreads within the crystal and reaches the photomultiplier tubes (PMTs) that are optically coupled to the crystal through a light guide. A PMT is a device that converts light into an electrical signal. It consists of a photocathode, which emits electrons as it gets hit by photons, and a cascade of anodes to which the electrons are accelerated by an electric potential, giving rise to more electrons as they collide with the anode. Thus, the small number of electrons originally released at the photocathode is amplified to a measurable signal.

In modern gamma cameras, the signal of each of the PMTs is converted into a digital signal by an analogue-to-digital converter (ADC). These digitised signals are then used as inputs to calculate the position and the energy of the impinging gamma photon using so-called Anger logic (after Hal Anger, inventor of the gamma camera). In this way, a projection of the activity distribution is obtained from an angle perpendicular to the detector surface. If the detector head is rotated around the patient, resulting in projections from many angles, a three-dimensional image can be computed by tomographic reconstruction.

12.2 Image Quality in Medical Imaging

When discussing image quality in medical imaging, one needs to keep in mind that these images are taken for a specific purpose. Image quality in this context does not imply "visually appealing" images but should be defined in terms of the aptness with which the task at hand can be successfully fulfilled using these images (Barrett et al. 2015; Barrett and Myers 2004).

Fryback et al. (1991) distinguish six levels of diagnostic efficacy. The first level is technical quality which refers to the parameters which are typically studied and optimised when designing and using an imaging system, such as resolution, sensitivity (in terms of number of recorded counts in the image), the absence of artefacts, quantitative accuracy, etc. The second level is diagnostic accuracy, often measured as the sensitivity and specificity of a diagnostic procedure. It is this level that describes how well the obtained images can be used for a certain task, such as differentiating between two possible diseases or detecting a malignancy. The third level is diagnostic impact and describes, for a certain disease or population, how the test changes diagnostic thinking about the patient. The fourth level, therapeutic impact, describes how the test changes therapeutic decisions for the patient undergoing the test. The fifth and sixth levels, patient outcome and societal outcome, describe the impact of the procedure on the patient in terms of, for instance, survival or improvement of quality of life and the impact on the society as a whole, such as expressed in global cost-benefit studies.

We will be discussing image quality mainly concerning the first level, i.e. technical quality, but, from a task-based perspective, improvements at this level are only relevant if they add a benefit to performance at higher levels. For example, in collimator design, there is a compromise to be made between resolution and sensitivity. To make an educated decision about which of the two parameters should be preferentially improved, one should take into account the specific application for which the collimators will be used, in other terms, which task is to be performed with the images (Fryback and Thornbury 1991).

The possible tasks for which an image can be used can be roughly subdivided into two categories, classification and estimation. In a classification task, the patient needs to be classified into two or more disjoint classes based on the image. Examples include benign or malignant tumour, lesion present or not present (binary classification), or type of tumour. The special case of determining whether a certain feature (e.g. a tumour) is present or not in the image is referred to as a detection task. Evaluating performance for a classification task is typically performed using receiver operating characteristic (ROC) studies. In this methodology, sensitivity and specificity of the classification are plotted against a threshold, generating a curve as shown in Fig. 12.2. The area under this curve is then used as a metric to evaluate

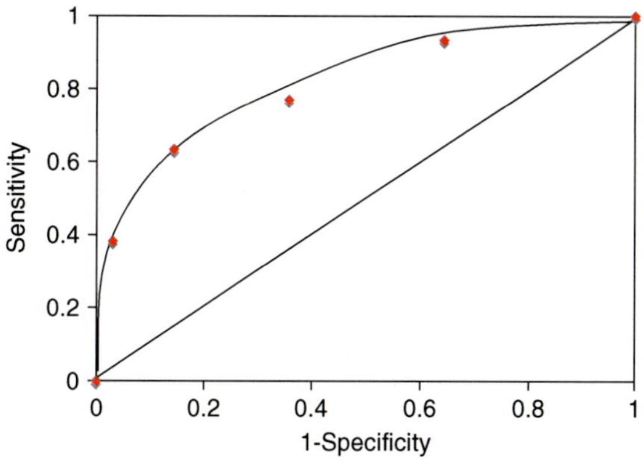

Fig. 12.2 Example of a ROC curve

classification and thus image quality. The classification itself can be performed by a trained observer (such as an experienced nuclear medicine physician) or by a numerical algorithm (a model observer). Results from this kind of studies allow predictions about the second level of diagnostic efficacy as defined above.

For an estimation task, the goal is to extract one or more numerical values from the image, for example, tumour uptake, volume, location of a lesion, etc. Typical metrics to assess the correctness of an estimation are bias and variance, which can be combined into a single parameter: the mean squared error (MSE). Typically, optimising these metrics relies on the first level of diagnostic efficacy, the technical image quality.

In image modalities that use ionising radiation, such as is the case with SPECT and CT, another aspect of image quality is that the ALARA principle should be adhered: the dose given to the patient should be as low as reasonably achievable (ALARA) while still keeping adequate image quality. Since image quality is directly linked with dose, the improvement in image quality by using higher doses should be weighed against the detrimental effects of the increased radiation burden to the patient and his surroundings (Moore et al. 2005). Optimising this trade-off is a typical example of enhancing level 5 and 6 in diagnostic efficacy.

12.3 Technical Image Quality in SPECT/CT

The technical image quality obtained by a SPECT/CT system is described by a number of parameters. In a first stage, the quality of the planar projections needs to be investigated. These planar images are used as a basis to calculate the reconstructed images, so it is evident that a decrease in image quality in the planar images will propagate to the reconstructions. In a second stage, there are a number of parameters that specifically define tomographic quality.

A first important system parameter is spatial image resolution. The resolution of the camera is governed by the intrinsic resolution and the collimator resolution. Of these two factors, collimator resolution is by far the dominant one. Intrinsic resolution is the resolution measured by the camera when using a perfectly collimated point source. A limited spatial resolution is due to the fact that the number of scintillation photons in the crystal is governed by statistical noise. The same is true for the number of photons reaching each PMT and the number of electrons in the amplifying process within the PMTs. All this noise leads to fluctuations in the position calculation for each gamma photon, thus leading to a blurry point spread function rather than a single unique position in the image.

The second term to take into account is the collimator resolution. This resolution is limited due to the finite width and height of the collimator holes, as can be seen in Fig. 12.3. As the holes of the collimator become higher and narrower, the angle under which the photons can reach the detector becomes smaller, thus increasing the resolution. However, this comes at the cost of a reduced sensitivity, since fewer photons will reach the detector. Since the collimator resolution is governed by the angle under which photons can reach the detector, resolution degrades linearly with the distance to the collimator. Thus, in order to improve resolution in the images, it is important that the detector head is positioned as closely as possible to the patient. For this reason, many vendors nowadays offer the possibility of automatic body contouring. If this option is not present, the user should define a scanning orbit that stays as close to the patient as possible during acquisition.

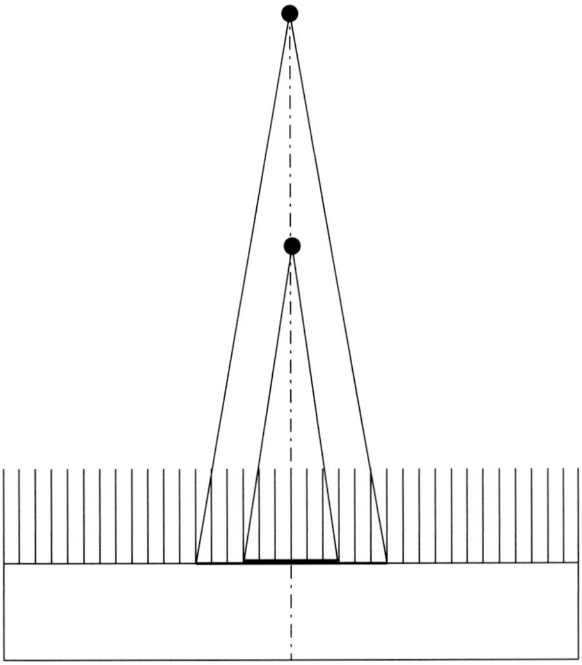

Fig. 12.3 The influence of the collimator on resolution

A second parameter of major importance in SPECT is sensitivity. Sensitivity is expressed as the fraction of emitted photons that are detected by the camera and thus contribute to the image. This sensitivity is limited by the thickness and material of the crystal used. Depending on the energy of the gamma photons used for imaging, only a part of the photons impinging on the crystal will interact with it and give rise to scintillation. A thicker crystal thus increases sensitivity, but, on the other hand, will lead to a certain loss in intrinsic resolution. The other main factor governing the sensitivity is the collimator. As was pointed out above, a high-resolution collimator will inevitably lead to low sensitivity. The thickness of the septa is also an important factor. As the energy of the gamma photons increases, thicker septa are needed to stop them from penetrating through the collimator. The thicker the septa are, the less surface is covered by the holes, leading to a decrease in sensitivity. Sensitivity is an important factor since the images are governed by noise. The noise in a planar projection is Poisson-distributed, meaning that the noise is proportional to the square root of the number of counts, and thus, the signal to noise ratio (SNR) is inversely proportional to the square root of the number of counts. An increase in SNR can either be obtained by increasing sensitivity, increasing the activity administered to the patient or increasing the acquisition time. However, increasing activity will lead to a higher radiation burden for the patient and his surroundings, whereas the acquisition time is limited by the time a patient can comfortably hold still during acquisition and by throughput considerations.

Since gamma photons can scatter within the patient, in the process losing energy and changing direction, it is important only to select primary photons that did not undergo any scatter and thus contain correct position information. To this end, the energy of each detected photon is measured, and only the events falling into the correct energy window are taken into account. However, measurement of the photon energy suffers from the same noise effects as described in the description of the spatial resolution. Therefore, energy resolution is finite, as can be seen from Fig. 12.4, showing a typical energy spectrum as measured by a gamma camera, along with a typical energy window as used in a SPECT acquisition. As a consequence, elimination of scattered events is imperfect. The better the energy

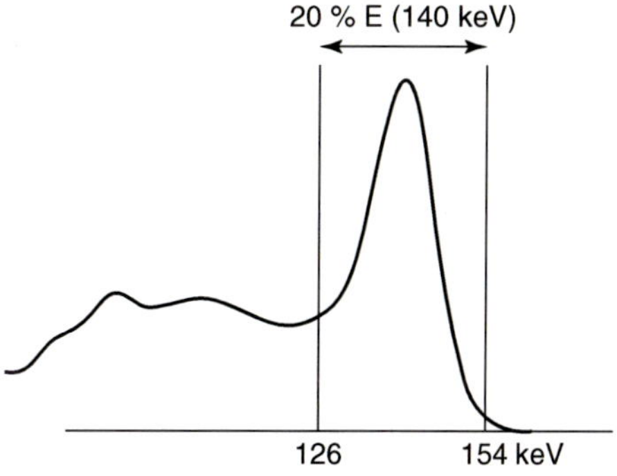

Fig. 12.4 The energy spectrum for Tc-99m gamma photons. The vertical lines indicate a typical energy window used for a SPECT acquisition

resolution is, the less scatter is detected in the energy window. Energy resolution depends on the scintillation crystal and the PMTs used. It should be noted that a next generation of gamma cameras, using solid state detectors such as cadmium zinc telluride (CZT) instead of the classical NaI(Tl) scintillation crystal, shows a marked improvement in energy resolution (Zaman et al. 2010).

Another aspect of the energy measurement is that for each acquisition with a certain isotope, the positioning of the energy window should be checked. An incorrectly positioned window will give rise to a decrease of counts and to artefacts in the image.

Finally, one last factor to take into account to evaluate planar image quality is uniformity and linearity of the image. The uniformity of the camera describes the property of the camera to produce a uniform image when imaging a uniform source. Uniformity is typically expressed as the uniformity index, calculated as the percentage of maximum number of counts minus minimum number of counts divided by the sum of maximum and minimum counts over a uniformly irradiated field of view (Tenhunen et al. 1996). Typically, uniformity is calculated in a useful field of view (UFOV) and a central field of view (CFOV). For integral uniformity, the maximum and minimum is taken over the whole field; for differential uniformity, the maximum difference between five consecutive pixels in the x- or y-direction is taken. Linearity expresses how good the image of a straight line is again a straight line. This is typically assessed by imaging a lead or tungsten bar phantom with straight slits in the x- and y-direction, irradiated by a uniform flood source or a point source at a large distance.

Apart from the previously mentioned planar image quality parameters, there are several additional aspects that are important for the image quality in a reconstructed tomographic image.

First of all, there is the centre of rotation (COR). In the reconstruction process, a certain image pixel is assumed to be positioned on the axis around which the detector heads rotate. This position should correspond to the physical axis of rotation. If this is not the case, this can result in image blurring and annular artefacts.

A major factor in tomographic image quality is the reconstruction algorithm used. Nowadays, analytical reconstruction algorithms such as filtered back projection (FBP) have been mostly replaced by iterative reconstruction algorithms. Iterative reconstruction algorithms, such as ML-EM (Shepp and Vardi 1982) and its faster variant OS-EM (Hudson and Larkin 1994), have better noise properties than FBP, and moreover, they make it possible to include corrections for various image degrading effects into the reconstruction. Examples of these effects include attenuation, scatter and detector response. In the following subsection concerning quantitative SPECT/CT, we will further discuss these effects and their corrections.

Finally, image quality can be seriously affected by artefacts in the image. We already briefly discussed the artefacts that an improper value of the COR can produce. Faulty or poorly calibrated PMTs or improper photo peak selection can also lead to artefacts. From the patient side, possible artefact sources are patient motion, contamination, metallic prostheses or metallic objects which were not removed during acquisition. Specifically for SPECT/CT cameras, there are a number of additional possible causes of artefacts that one should keep in mind (Gnanasegaran et al. 2009). Misregistration between the CT attenuation map and the SPECT image, either due to misalignment of the CT and the gamma cameras part of the scanner or to the movement of the patient in between the two scans can lead to local over- and under-corrections of the SPECT image. If breath hold is applied during the CT scan, while the patient is breathing normally during SPECT, this can lead to respiration artefacts. Metal streak artefacts in the CT images can propagate to the SPECT image through the attenuation map.

In order to assess the technical quality of the SPECT/CT camera after installation, acceptance testing of the device is needed (1993). On the one hand, this permits the user to check whether the camera achieves the quality parameters claimed by the vendor; on the other hand, it provides a baseline benchmark to compare later quality controls to. To ensure correct functioning of the camera over time, various instances have published protocols for periodic quality controls (Hines et al. 2000; Graham et al. 1995).

12.4 Quantitative SPECT/CT

We have already mentioned above that a possible task to be performed based on images is quantification: calculation of a certain physical quantity from the image. This might consist of a semi-quantification task, e.g. assessing left-right ratios in a certain volume of interest, or compare the counts in a volume, normalised to the counts in a certain region, to the counts observed from a database of "normal" subjects. On the other hand, the task at hand may be truly quantitative to evaluate the tracer uptake (in MBq/ml) in a certain area or at a certain location.

Until recently, SPECT was generally said to be a non-quantitative imaging modality, in sharp contrast with PET/CT, which has since long been regarded as quantitative. However, several groups have worked towards obtaining quantitative SPECT images (Willowson et al. 2008; Zeintl et al. 2008; Seret et al. 2012). With the advent of the integrated SPECT/CT camera, in combination with the now widespread iterative reconstruction methods including various corrections, the time seems there to introduce quantitative SPECT into clinical practice, and close the gap with PET/CT.

Quantitative SPECT requires a quantitative iterative reconstruction algorithm. Iterative reconstruction starts with a first "guess" of the image and forward projects this guess to the measurement space. This forward projection predicts what the measurement would be given a certain image using a model of the imaging process. The forward projection is then compared to the actual measurement, and the image guess is updated according to this comparison. These steps are then repeated (hence iterative reconstruction) until an adequate image is obtained.

The imaging model used in the forward projection is the key feature in incorporating corrections for image degrading effects needed for quantitative imaging.

Attenuation correction is the most important correction to perform for quantification. For this correction, an attenuation map is needed which contains the photon attenuation coefficient at each location of the image for the energy of the single photon emitter used. Before the advent of SPECT/CT, these attenuation maps were often acquired using transmission imaging with a long lived isotope (O'Connor et al. 2002). However, in a SPECT/CT scanner, the CT is used to compute the attenuation map (Zaidi and Hasegawa 2006). This has the advantage that the CT is much less noisy than transmission images, and moreover, CT acquisition is generally faster than transmission imaging. However, the fact that the X-ray spectrum in CT imaging is fundamentally different from the (usually) monoenergetic spectrum of the gamma photons in SPECT requires a translation of the measured CT map to an attenuation map for the correct energy. This is typically done with a bilinear transformation.

Scatter correction is a second very important factor to correct for. Some of the emitted photons undergo scatter within the body of the patient, thus losing energy and changing direction. Since, as we have discussed before, the energy resolution of a gamma camera is limited, many of these photons will be detected within the energy window, giving rise to counts that are incorrectly located. This leads to a decrease in image contrast and to errors in the quantitative accuracy of the image. In fact, correcting for attenuation without taking into account scatter will lead to overcompensation and thus incorrect results. Various scatter correction methods have been proposed, such as energy-based correction (of which the triple energy window method is the most well known), model-based methods such as effective-source scatter estimate (ESSE), and Monte Carlo based methods (Zaidi and Koral 2006).

Another image degrading factor is the finite (and relatively poor) spatial resolution of the camera, due to the intrinsic resolution and the distance dependent collimator resolution and septal penetration. These effects can lead to a serious underestimation of activities in small structures which is known as the partial volume effect. These effects can be compensated for by modelling the distance dependent detector response function within the forward projection of the reconstruction algorithm (Frey and Tsui 2006).

Whereas dead time corrections are important in PET, the presence of collimators in gamma cameras often insures that dead time is a negligible effect. However, for some applications, such as for post therapy imaging, the activity within the field of view can be such that correction for this effect is needed in order to obtain quantitative results (Hobbs et al. 2010).

Apart from all aforementioned corrections, absolute quantification requires that a calibration factor is known to convert numbers of counts per pixel to tracer uptake in MBq/ml. This factor can either be obtained from acquisition of planar images with known activities or from the acquisition of a uniform phantom with known activity, as has since long been customary in PET.

The previous paragraphs show that obtaining quantitative SPECT results is non-trivial and requires a lot of effort. A further complication is that all corrections depend highly on the isotope used, so each isotope requires a separate effort to obtain quantitative results (Elschot et al. 2013a, b). However, lately, with the advent of SPECT/CT and of sophisticated iterative reconstruction algorithms, quantitative SPECT seems to move from research to routine clinical application.

Achieving quantitatively correct SPECT images would enable the use of SPECT/CT in therapy monitoring, making it possible to measure an absolute decrease or increase of uptake in lesions after therapy. One of the major applications of quantitative SPECT would be in 3D dosimetry for radionuclide therapy, in which SPECT could be used to predict doses to tumours and normal organs using a test dose or to check doses after delivering the activity to the patient, bringing personalised medicine one step closer (Dewaraja et al. 2012).

12.5 Task-Based Image Quality in SPECT/CT

As mentioned before, technical image quality is a first prerequisite for the real goal of the images: the task for which the images are used. This task can be an estimation task, in which case proper quantification such as discussed above is important, or it can be a classification or detection task. In the past, improvements in image quality were often evaluated either on the level of technical image quality (e.g. improvement in SNR in the images) or on a subjective basis (e.g. by letting experienced observers score the perceived quality of images reconstructed with different algorithms) (Soderberg et al. 2012; Aldridge et al. 2006). However, more and more nowadays, image quality evaluation is done within a task-based framework (Barrett and Myers 2004).

In a classification or detection task, an observer is given the task to classify a number of cases based on images. The observer can consist in a mathematical calculation, such as absolute or relative uptake in a region of interest (ROI), or left/right asymmetry in a certain area. On the other hand, the classification may be performed by a human observer, such as an experienced nuclear medicine physician, who is asked to score images based on how likely he estimates the image to belong to a certain class. The classification task can also be combined with a localisation task, in which case the observer would have to point to the most likely location of, for example, a malignancy and then score the probability that there is in fact a malignancy present in the image.

Human observer studies are very labour-intensive and thus expensive. For this reason, model observers have been developed. These are mathematical algorithms that mimic the performance of a human observer. For reconstruction algorithm optimisation, for example, the parameter search space can be too large to be searched by a human observer study. In this case, model observers are used to narrow down the search space, this can be followed by a human observer study to further optimise the parameters within the reduced parameter space.

Another class of model observers are ideal observers. These are algorithms that extract as much relevant information from the image as possible to perform the task. These observers are typically used in system design and optimisation.

Observer studies have, for example, been used for optimising collimators for SPECT in various specific detection and quantification tasks and for specific isotopes (El Fakhri et al. 2006; Moore et al. 2005; Kijewski et al. 2001). The optimisation of reconstruction algorithms and spatial filtering has also been performed by observer studies (Lehovich et al. 2007; Nichols et al. 2007). Another study investigated the effect of CT-based attenuation correction on lesion evaluation using numerical and human observers (Shiraishi et al. 2006).

Finally, numerous authors have studied the advantages of SPECT/CT over SPECT or planar imaging using human observers for specific clinical applications and for specific isotopes (Franson et al. 2008; Perri et al. 2008; Luk et al. 2010; Barwick et al. 2010; Morrison et al. 2011; Wakabayashi et al. 2011; Sharma et al. 2012a, b, 2013).

12.6 Conclusion and Future Prospects

In this paper, we have discussed image quality aspects of SPECT/CT. Image quality is governed by various technical parameters which have to be taken into account when designing a system and choosing acquisition parameters. Evaluating and optimising image quality should take into account what the images will be used for, in a so-called task-based approach. This approach gains popularity in the SPECT research community, as can be observed from the many papers evaluating the gain SPECT/CT brings compared to regular SPECT or planar imaging in various clinical applications.

SPECT has long been regarded as a non-quantitative technique, in contrast to PET. However, many groups have worked towards quantitative SPECT in different applications and for various isotopes. In clinical practice, quantitative SPECT has been made more practically feasible with the advent of SPECT/CT. It seems that quantitative SPECT is now ready to move from a research environment to a clinical tool. This would be especially useful in therapy monitoring and in SPECT/CT-based dosimetry.

Future prospects in SPECT/CT may include, as mentioned, the further development of quantitative imaging and the use in 3D dosimetry. Advances in hardware and software, such as innovative collimator design and resolution recovery, may enable shorter scan times, thus making whole body SPECT/CT imaging feasible. Implementation of breathing correction methods may diminish the impact of attenuation correction artefacts and improve resolution in areas most affected by breathing. The use of solid state detectors such as CZT detectors can increase energy resolution, opening up possibilities in simultaneous multi-isotope imaging (DePuey 2012).

Although the gamma camera is a technology that has been remarkably stable over the decades, lately many technological advances have been achieved, most notably with the advent of SPECT/CT, and more developments can be expected in the near future.

References

Aldridge MD, Waddington WW, Dickson JC, Prakash V, Ell PJ, Bomanji JB. Clinical evaluation of reducing acquisition time on single-photon emission computed tomography image quality using proprietary resolution recovery software. Nucl Med Commun. 2006;34(11):1116–23.

Barrett HH, Myers KJ. Foundations of image science. Hoboken: Wiley; 2004.

Barrett HH, Myers KJ, Hoeschen C, Kupinski MA, Little MP. Task-based measures of image quality and their relation to radiation dose and patient risk. Phys Med Biol. 2015;60(2):R1–75.

Barwick T, Murray I, Megadmi H, Drake WM, Plowman PN, Akker SA, Chew SL, Grossman AB, Avril N. Single photon emission computed tomography (SPECT)/computed tomography using

Iodine-123 in patients with differentiated thyroid cancer: additional value over whole body planar imaging and SPECT. Eur J Endocrinol. 2010;162(6):1131–9.
Buck AK, Nekolla S, Ziegler S, Beer A, Krause BJ, Herrmann K, Scheidhauer K, Wester H-J, Rummeny EJ, Schwaiger M, Drzezga A. SPECT/CT. J Nucl Med. 2008;49:1305–19.
Cherry SR, Sorenson JA, Phelps ME. Physics in nuclear medicine. 4th ed. Philadelphia: Elsevier; 2012.
DePuey EG. Advances in SPECT camera software and hardware: currently available and new on the horizon. J Nucl Cardiol. 2012;19(5):551–81.
Dewaraja YK, Frey EC, Sgouros G, Brill AB, Roberson P, Zanzonico PB, Ljungberg M. MIRD pamphlet no. 23: quantitative SPECT for patient-specific 3-dimensional dosimetry in internal radionuclide therapy. J Nucl Med. 2012;53(8):1310–25.
El Fakhri G, Ouyang J, Zimmerman RE, Fischman AJ, Kijewski MF. Performance of a novel collimator for high-sensitivity brain SPECT. Med Phys. 2006;33(1):209–15.
Elschot M, Smits MLJ, Nijsen JFW, Lam MGEH, Zonnenberg BA, van den Bosch MAAJ, Viergever MA, de Jong HWAM. Quantitative Monte Carlo-based holmium-166 SPECT reconstruction. Med Phys. 2013a;40:112502.
Elschot M, Lam MGEH, van den Bosch MAAJ, Viergever MA, de Jong HWAM. Quantitative Monte Carlo–based 90Y SPECT reconstruction. J Nucl Med. 2013b;54:1557–63.
Franson T, Bardet S, Loiseau C, Switsers O, Allouache D, Allouache N, Gunzer K, Aide N. SPECT/spiral CT and bone scintigraphy in cancer patients: impact of a low dose CT acquisitions in indeterminate or suspicious solitary focus. Medecine Nucleaire-Imagerie Fonctionelle et Metabolique. 2008;32(5):273–80.
Frey E, Tsui B. Collimator-detector response compensation in SPECT. In: Zaidi H, editor. Quantitative analysis in nuclear medicine imaging. New York: Springer; 2006. p. 141–66.
Fryback D, Thornbury J. The efficacy of diagnostic imaging. Med Decis Making. 1991;11:88–94.
Gnanasegaran G, Cook G, Adamson K, Fogelman I. Patterns, variants, artifacts, and pitfalls in conventional radionuclide bone imaging and SPECT/CT. Semin Nucl Med. 2009;39(6):380–95.
Graham LS, Fahey FH, Madsen MT, van Aswegen A, Yester MV. Quantitation of SPECT performance: report of task group 4, nuclear medicine committee. Med Phys. 1995;22:401–9.
Hines H, Kayayan R, Colsher J, et al. National electrical manufacturers association recommendations for implementing SPECT instrumentation quality control. J Nucl Med. 2000;41:383–9.
Hobbs RF, Baechler S, Senthamizhchelvan S, Prideaux AR, Esaias CE, Reinhardt M, Frey EC, Loeb DM, Sgouros G. A gamma camera count rate saturation correction method for whole-body planar imaging. Phys Med Biol. 2010;55:817–31.
Hudson HM, Larkin RS. Accelerated image reconstruction using ordered subsets of projection data. IEEE Trans Med Imaging. 1994;13(4):601–9.
Jacene HA, Goetze S, Patel H, Wahl RL, Ziessman HA. Advantages of hybrid SPECT/CT vs SPECT alone. Open Med Imaging J. 2008;2:67–79.
Kijewski MF, Moore SC, Jadvar H, Zimmerman RE, Muller SP. Effects of SPECT collimation and system geometry on classification tasks related to parkinson's disease. IEEE Trans Nucl Sci. 2001;48(3):734–8 Part: 2.
Lehovich A, Gifford HC, Schneider PB, King MA. Choosing anatomical-prior strength for MAP SPECT reconstruction to maximize lesion detectability. In: IEEE nuclear science symposium conference record. 2007, Vol 1–11 IEEE nuclear science symposium – conference record, p. 4222–5.
Luk WH, Au-Yeung AWS, Yang MKW. Diagnostic value of SPECT versus SPECT/CT in femoral avascular necrosis: preliminary results. Nucl Med Commun. 2010;31(11):958–61.
Moore SC, Kijewski MF, El Fakhri G. Collimator optimization for detection and quantitation tasks: application to gallium-67 imaging. IEEE Trans Med Imaging. 2005;24(10):1347–56.
Morrison A, Brennan PC, Reed W, Pietrzyk M, Schembri G, Bailey E, Roach P, Evanoff M, Kench PL, Impact of hybrid SPECT/CT imaging on the detection of single parathyroid adenoma. Proceedings of SPIE 7966, Medical Imaging 2011: Image Perception Observer Performance, and Technology Assessment. 2011;7966:79661J.

Nichols KJ, Tronco GG, Tomas MB, Kunjummen BD, Siripun L, Rini JN, Palestro CJ. Phantom experiments to improve parathyroid lesion detection. Med Phys. 2007;34(12):4792–7.

O'Connor MK, Kemp B, Anstett F, Christian P, Ficaro EP, Frey E, Jacobs M, Kritzman JN, Pooley RA, Wilk M. A multicenter evaluation of commercial attenuation compensation techniques in cardiac SPECT using phantom models. J Nucl Cardiol. 2002;9(4):361–76.

Perri M, Erba P, Volterrani D, Lazzeri E, Boni G, Grosso M, Mariani G. Octreo-SPECT/CT imaging for accurate detection and localization of suspected neuroendocrine tumors. Q J Nucl Med Mol Imaging. 2008;52(4):323–33.

Runge VM, Marquez H, Andreisek G, Valavanis A, Alkadhi H. Recent technological advances in computed tomography and the clinical impact therein. Invest Radiol. 2015;50(2):119–27.

Seret A, Nguyen D, Bernard C. Quantitative capabilities of four state-of-the-art SPECT-CT cameras. EJNMMI Res. 2012;2:45.

Sharma P, Kumar R, Singh H, Bal C, Julka PK, Thulkar S, Malhotra A. Indeterminate lesions on planar bone scintigraphy in lung cancer patients: SPECT, CT or SPECT-CT? Skeletal Radiol. 2012a;41(7):843–50.

Sharma P, Kumar R, Das KJ, Singh H, Pal S, Parshad R, Bal C, Bandopadhyaya GP, Malhotra A. Detection and localization of post-operative and post-traumatic bile leak: hybrid SPECT-CT with 99mTc-Mebrofenin. Abdom Imaging. 2012b;37(5):803–11.

Sharma P, Dhull VS, Jeph S, Reddy RM, Singh H, Naswa N, Bal C, Kumar R. Can Hybrid SPECT-CT overcome the limitations associated with poor imaging properties of I-131-MIBG? Comparison with planar scintigraphy and SPECT in pheochromocytoma. Clin Nucl Med. 2013;38(9):E346–53.

Shepp LA, Vardi Y. Maximum likelihood reconstruction for emission tomography. IEEE Trans Med Imaging. 1982;1(2):113–22.

Shiraishi S, Tomiguchi S, Utsunomiya D, Kawanaka K, Awai K, Morishita S, Okuda T, Yokotsuka K, Yamashita Y. Quantitative analysis and effect of attenuation correction on lymph node staging of non-small cell lung cancer on SPECT and CT. AJR Am J Roentgenol. 2006;186(5):1450–7.

Soderberg M, Mattsson S, Oddstig J, Uusijarvi-Lizana H, Valind S, Thorsson O, Garpered S, Prautzsch T, Tischenko O, Leide-Svegborn S. Evaluation of image reconstruction methods for I-123-MIBG-SPECT: a rank-order study. Acta Radiol. 2012;53(7):778–84.

Specification and acceptance of computed tomography scanners (AAPM Report No. 39). 1993. College Park: American Association of Physicists in Medicine.

Tenhunen M, Pyykkönen J, Tenhunen-Eskelinen M, Jaatinen K, Kuikka JT. Components op the flood-field uniformity index in a gamma camera. Phys Med Biol. 1996;41(7):1209–16.

Wakabayashi H, Nakajima K, Fukuoka M, Inaki A, Nakamura A, Kayano D, Kinuya S. Double-phase I-131 whole body scan and I-131 SPECT-CT images in patients with differentiated thyroid cancer: their effectiveness for accurate identification. Ann Nucl Med. 2011;25(9):609–15.

Willowson K, Bailey DL, Baldock C. Quantitative SPECT reconstruction using CT-derived corrections. Phys Med Biol. 2008;53:3099–112.

Zaidi H, Hasegawa B. Attenuation correction strategies in emission tomography. In: Zaidi H, editor. Quantitative analysis in nuclear medicine imaging. New York: Springer; 2006. p. 167–204.

Zaidi H, Koral K. Scatter correction strategies in emission tomography. In: Zaidi H, editor. Quantitative analysis in nuclear medicine imaging. New York: Springer; 2006. p. 205–35.

Zaman MU, Hashmi I, Fatima N. Recent developments and future prospects of SPECT myocardial perfusion imaging. Ann Nucl Med. 2010;24(8):565–9.

Zeintl J, Vija AH, Yahil A, Ding X, Hornegger J, Towards quantitative SPECT: error estimation of SPECT OSEM with 3D resolution recovery, attenuation correction and scatter correction. In: IEEE nuclear science symposium conference record. IEEE; Dresden, Germany. 2008, 4106–10.

Technical Aspects of PET/CT Image Quality

13

Antoon T.M. Willemsen

13.1 Introduction

Nuclear imaging is based on the measurement of the radioactivity distribution of a tracer which was administered to a patient. This distribution is determined by the characteristics of the tracer as well as the tissue under investigation. By selecting an appropriate tracer, many different characteristics can be studied. As such it can be used for both diagnosis and therapy evaluation. This selection of the optimal tracer is an essential step to optimize both sensitivity and specificity. However, here we will focus on optimizing image quality.

Image quality is determined by many factors: from the amount of activity given to a patient to the uptake in the organ and the sensitivity of the PET system and finally the optimized image reconstruction and the quality of the imaging system used to display the data (Boellaard et al. 2015). In this chapter we will focus on the quality of the PET/CT system itself with some excursions into the other aspects. Readers interested in different example of image artifacts and their underlying causes are referred to the international atomic energy agency (IAEA) PET/CT atlas on quality control and image artifacts (International Atomic Energy Agency 2014).

Generally speaking, the quality of the CT scan is much higher than the quality of a PET scan. This is true both in resolution and in signal-to-noise ratio. Although both systems use ionizing radiation, the amount of signal in both systems is totally different. Whereas CT measures a current at the different detector elements, PET measures individual photons. As a consequence the signal-to-noise ratio of PET systems is still characterized by Poisson statistics. Considering this large difference in image quality, we will ignore image quality aspects of clinical CT. However,

A.T.M. Willemsen
Department of Nuclear Medicine and Molecular Imaging,
University Medical Center Groningen, University of Groningen, Groningen, The Netherlands
e-mail: a.t.m.willemsen@umcg.nl

A.W.J.M. Glaudemans et al. (eds.), *Quality in Nuclear Medicine*,
DOI 10.1007/978-3-319-33531-5_13

since CT is also used for attenuation correction of the PET data, we will look at the image quality of low-dose CT and its impact on the final image quality of PET.

So which are the main ingredients which determined the image quality of PET? As was already mentioned, the dose administered to a patient has a direct impact on the image quality. Although there is a limit to the count rate capability of PET systems, the maximum dose is limited by the radiation exposure of the tracer to the patient. Another obvious solution would be to increase the length of the scan, thereby increasing the total number of counts obtained and thus increasing the signal-to-noise ratio. However this approach is limited by the demands on throughput, the comfort of the patients, and the increased risk of motion artifacts. Consequently, both dose and scan duration are usually fixed within small boundaries. The only aspect which is generally taken into account is the weight-dependent distribution of the tracer. Often the dose administered is linearly related to the weight of the patients. However, for FDG whole-body studies, it has recently been shown (de Groot et al. 2013) that a quadratic relationship between dose and weight is optimal. For many other traces, the optimal relationship is currently unknown. It is conceivable that in many cases, a linear relationship would result in lower image quality for heavyweight patients. Please note that the optimal relationship between body weight and dose does not indicate that the image quality is optimal but rather that the image quality becomes independent of body weight.

Considering a specific patient, the next step in the imaging process is the PET/CT system. A PET/CT scan consists of several steps. First, a scout scan is made to determine the optimal area to be scanned. Once this has been done, a low-dose CT is made which can later be used for attenuation correction. The low-dose CT scan can also be used for anatomical correlation but should not be used for diagnosis. Then the actual PET scan is made. In most applications, the activity will be measured at different bed positions to construct a so-called whole-body scan. Particularly in research studies or cardiac studies, a so-called dynamic scan can also be made which measures the radioactivity distribution in an organ over time. If requested a diagnostic CT can be made at the end. The data is then reconstructed to give the 3-D radioactivity distribution.

Obviously the final image quality is directly related to the quality of the PET system. Therefore we will look at the construction of PET systems to obtain an understanding of the different processes that are involved and their potential impact on image quality. A description of the principles behind PET is beyond the scope of this chapter. The reader which is not familiar with PET is referred to other textbooks (Cherry et al. 2012; Powsner and Powsner 2006).

13.2 Construction of a PET/CT

PET systems measure coincidence radiation resulting from positron decay. For each individual photon, the energy must be measured as well as the position where it is detected. Since the energy of the photon is too high to be measured directly, a scintillation crystal is used which absorbs the photon and then gives a characteristic scintillation pulse which can be measured by a photosensitive device such as a photomultiplier. The scintillation pulse is always measured by multiple detectors. The total signal detected is related to the energy of the absorbed photon. If the measured energy is within the allowed energy window, the data will be processed further. If not, the data usually represents a scattered photon, and it will be omitted from further processing. The distribution of the signal over the photosensitive detectors gives information about the exact position where the photon interacted with the crystal. The signal from the many thousands of detectors in a PET system is then processed further to determine whether two signals were detected within a coincidence time window. If so, the two events are said to be in coincidence, and the corresponding line of response is stored.

Since the energy of the photon needs to be measured, the sensitivity of the photosensitive detectors needs to be known. This sensitivity can easily be determined by performing a measurement with a known source. Obviously it needs to be insured that this sensitivity is constant. Since the data of different detectors is combined both to determine the total energy and to determine the exact position of the incident photon, it is advantageous if all detectors have a similar sensitivity. Therefore all PET systems have the ability to determine and optimize the gain of the different detectors, thereby ensuring similar sensitivities. In the past, this optimization was often performed in a separate so-called normalization procedure. Nowadays, this optimization is often performed on the fly during the daily QC procedure. Even if the sensitivity of the different detectors is similar, small differences will remain which result in a nonlinear relationship between the detector signals, the calculated *X* and *Y* position, and the actual *X* and *Y* position; see Fig. 13.1. These differences in the position calculation are further influenced by the nonlinear response of the detectors particularly at the edges. Therefore, to determine the actual *X* and *Y*

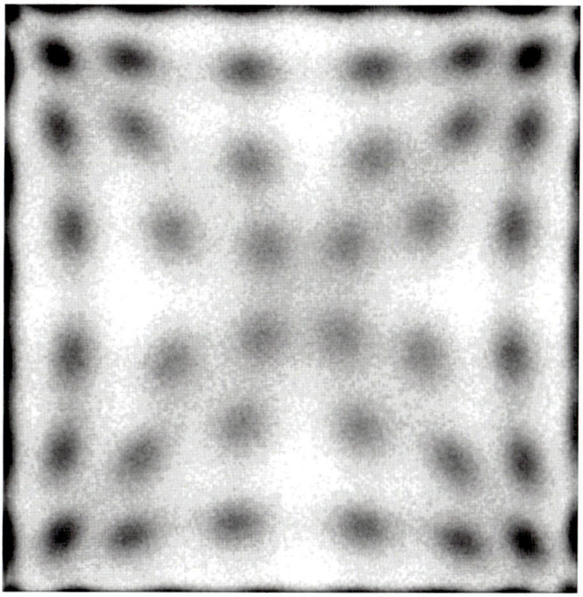

Fig. 13.1 Flood-field image obtained by uniformly irradiating a block detector with 511-keV annihilation photons. Individual block detector elements appear as distinct "blobs" in the image, allowing separation of events recorded within individual detector elements (Reproduced with permission from Physics in Nuclear Medicine; Fourth edition; Simon R. Cherry, James A Sorenson and Michael E. Phelps; Published 2012 by Elsevier Science)

position of an incident photon, a lookup table is used which translates the calculated positions into the actual positions. Again, in the past, this was often performed during a separate normalization procedure, whereas nowadays this is often part of the daily QC procedure.

Particularly during dynamic PET studies, high activity concentrations may occur. Even with the high count rate capability of current PET systems, detectors may still experience pulse pileup, i.e., the time between two pulses may be shorter than the duration of an individual pulse. Therefore specific data processing circuitry is used to minimize this effect. During normal operation of a PET/CT system, these techniques work reliably and will therefore not be discussed further.

PET/CT systems also experience dead time. Dead time is a consequence of the detection circuitry which can only process one event simultaneously. Thus, if a second event occurs during this time window, it will not be processed and the data is lost. Fortunately this dead time is very short. Also current PET/CT systems have a modular design which means that the detection circuitry only needs to handle the data of a few detectors. Nevertheless some dead time will always occur and may be considerable during the first minutes of a dynamic scan. Fortunately the relation between dead time and count rates is well known. Thus it can easily be corrected for. However, a potential source of error is that the correction is based on the total count rate of all detectors rather than on the count rate of each individual detector. This might be tested, for example, by performing a measurement with a small high activity source close to one of the detectors.

Apart from the energy and the line of coincidence, current PET/CT systems also record the time difference between the two detectors. The first purpose of this capability is to determine whether there is indeed a coincidence between the two detectors. However, in current PET/CT systems, this timing information is now so accurate that it can be used to estimate where on the line of response the annihilation occurred. This so-called time-of-flight information can be used during the reconstruction process and improves image quality considerably as will be discussed later. Obviously this requires that this time-of-flight information is correct and stable in time. Therefore this needs to be checked during the daily QC procedure.

Let us now assume for the moment that all detectors function properly and consider the different data corrections that are required in PET/CT systems.

13.3 Data Corrections Required in PET/CT

As mentioned above the sensitivity of the different detectors will be optimized during the daily QC procedure. However small differences will remain which must either be corrected before reconstruction or be taken into account during reconstruction. The same goes for differences in the time-of-flight information. Assuming that these problems are adequately handled, we must now consider the coincidences measured. Ideally, only true coincidences are measured. In reality, however, we will also measure scattered and random coincidences; see Fig. 13.2. The two annihilation photons created need to travel some distance through the tissue before reaching

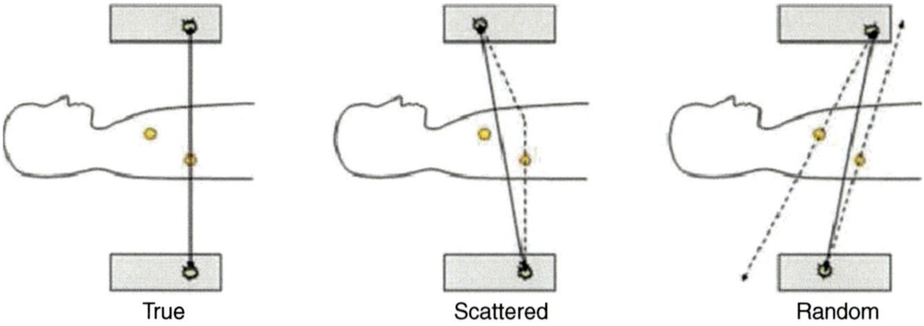

Fig. 13.2 True coincidence event (*left*), scatter coincidence event (*center*), and random or accidental coincidence (*right*) (Reproduced with permission of the IAEA from PET/CT Atlas on Quality Control and Image Artefacts; IAEA Human Health Series No. 27; ©IAEA; Published 2014)

the detectors. A photon can travel through the tissue without interaction, but it can also interact with the tissue.

If the interaction results in the absorption of the photon, a coincidence measurement is no longer possible. However, the interaction could also be in the form of a scattering event in which the photon loses some of its energy and changes direction. If the remaining energy of the photon is still within the energy window of the detector, it will be processed, but the resulting line of response does not longer coincide with the original positron decay. Therefore some form of scatter correction is required. In clinical applications, this is often performed using the so-called single scatter model. Given the radioactivity distribution and the electron density which follows from the CT scan, this model estimates the scatter based on the known probability of a photon to scatter with a specific angle. Since the scatter angle directly determines the energy of the scattered photon, this model can then predict which scattered photons will be within the energy window of the detector and thus be treated as an unscattered photon. As an example, the energy of a scattered photon is given by

$$E_{sc} = \frac{E_0}{1 + \frac{E_0}{0.511}\left(1 - \cos\theta\right)}$$

where E_0 = energy of the incident photon, E_{sc} = energy of the scattered photon, and theta = scatter angle.

For annihilation photons, $E_0 = 0.511$ MeV so the equation reduces to

$$E_{sc} = \frac{0.511}{1 + \left(1 - \cos\theta\right)} = \frac{0.511}{2 - \cos\theta}$$

So for an energy resolution of 20 %, it follows that θ is 41°. Even with an energy resolution of 10 %, θ is still 26°. Since scatter is mainly at small angles, this means that the majority of scattered photons will fall within the energy window and will be accepted.

The electron density is required since scattering is the result from an interaction of the annihilation photons with the electrons rather than the nuclei. Since the electron density also determines the absorption of photons through the photoelectric effect, it follows that the low-dose CT scan required for attenuation correction actually measures this electron density. The radioactivity distribution follows from the PET measurement. Since this will include scatter, the scatter correction will be slightly wrong (the amount of scatter will be slightly overestimated). However the scatter model does not include multiple scatter events, i.e., it slightly underestimates the amount of scatter. Since both errors are small and work in different directions, they will, in first-order approximation, compensate each other. For clinical practice, the current scatter correction is adequate. It remains to be seen whether more extended scatter models, up to Monte Carlo simulations, would have a significant influence on image quality. The ideal solution would be to prevent the detection of scatter events in the first place. Since all scattered photons have a lower energy than the incident photon, this would require a much higher energy resolution of the detectors as shown above. Unfortunately, there are currently no scintillation crystals available which offer the required energy resolution. It is well known that semiconductor devices have a much higher energy resolution. Particularly high-purity germanium detectors have a energy resolution well below 1 %. These detectors however require liquid nitrogen cooling and have a low sensitivity. Therefore, in practice, they are not alternative to current scintillation crystals.

Apart from true and scatter coincidences, we can also detect random coincidences. In this case, two unrelated photons are detected by two detectors within the coincidence time window. The amount of random coincidences is directly related to the singles count rate and for any detector pair given by

$$R_{\text{random}} = \Delta T * R_{\text{singles1}} * R_{\text{singles2}}$$

with ΔT being the coincidence time window and R_{singles1} and R_{singles2} being the singles count rate for detectors 1 and 2, respectively.

Fortunately, random coincidences can easily be corrected for using a delayed window technique. By their nature, on average the number of random coincidences is independent of the coincidence time window as long as the underlying activity distribution is constant. More specifically a typical coincidence time window may be in the order of 10 ns, and if we shift the coincidence time window to, e.g., 90–100 ns, the number of randoms should not change. Note that this is only true on average; therefore, the fluctuations will remain and slightly influence the signal-to-noise ratio of the final image.

After appropriate correction for scatter and randoms, the data can be reconstructed. However, part of the annihilation photons will be absorbed in the tissue. This attenuation effect depends on the specific shape and density of the patient and must be corrected for to ensure homogenous and quantitative valid images. Fortunately, in PET the attenuation for a single line of response does not depend on the exact position of the annihilation. Consider a subject with diameter D between the two detectors and the annihilation at some distance d from the center; cf. Fig. 13.3.

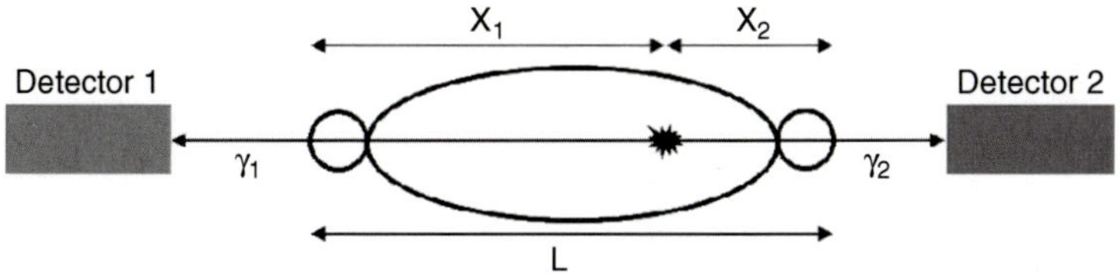

Fig. 13.3 Two photons (γ_1 and γ_2) are measured in coincidence between *detectors 1* and *2*. The "length" of the subject is *L*. The distance each photon has to travel to the tissue is x_1 and x_2, respectively

Assuming a constant attenuation coefficient, the transmission fraction to detector 1 is given by

$$T_1 = e^{-\mu x_1}$$

while the transmission to detector 2 is given by

$$T_2 = e^{-\mu x_2}$$

Since both photons need to be detected (coincidence detection), the total transmission is given by

$$T = T_1 * T_2 = e^{-\mu(x_1 + x_2)} = e^{-\mu L}$$

Thus, the transmission and consequently the attenuation are independent of the specific location on the line of response. Provided that the attenuation coefficients are available, the attenuation for each line of response can easily be calculated. As mentioned before, since CT is a transmission technique, the resulting Hounsfield units are directly related to these attenuation coefficients. A complicating factor is that the CT usually works in the 80–140 keV range, whereas PET needs the attenuation values for 511 keV. Therefore, the CT values must be translated which is usually done with a simple lookup table.

The use of the CT for attenuation correction has greatly improved PET scanning. First of all, it is very fast, and equally important, it has a high quality even though it is only a low-dose CT. However, care should be taken that there is no mismatch between the PET and CT data since this will introduce attenuation artifacts. Also, metal implants will strongly affect CT data and must be corrected before it is used for attenuation correction. Generally, it is a good clinical practice to also reconstruct the PET data without attenuation correction and inspect it in case of doubt.

13.4 Reconstruction Techniques

Although a description of different reconstruction techniques is beyond the aim of this manuscript, the specific reconstruction technique has a direct impact on image quality. Also some of the techniques which we'll discuss later are based on

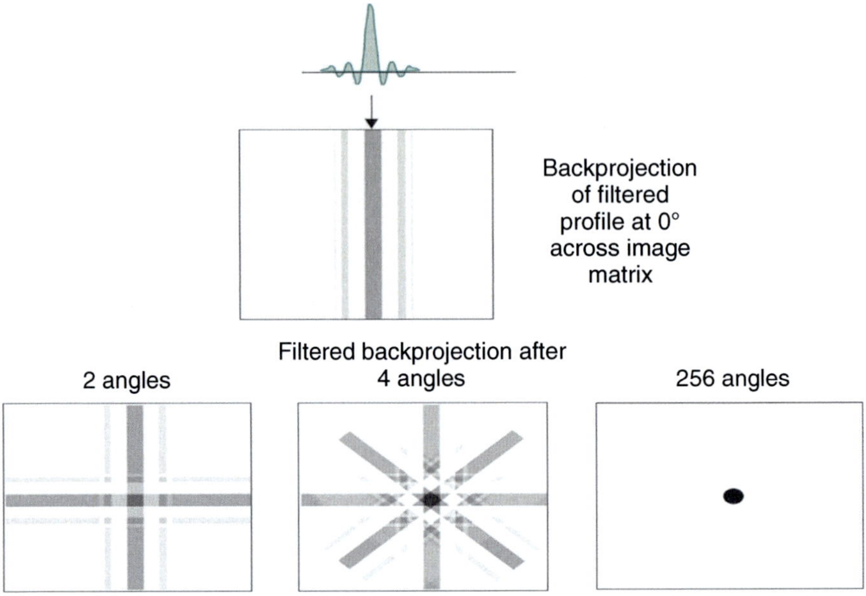

Fig. 13.4 Illustration of the steps in filtered back projection. The one-dimensional Fourier transforms of projection profiles recorded at different projection angles are multiplied by the ramp filter. After taking the inverse Fourier transform of the filtered transforms, the filtered profiles are back projected across the image, as in simple back projection (Reproduced with permission from Physics in Nuclear Medicine; Fourth edition; Simon R. Cherry, James A Sorenson and Michael E. Phelps; Published 2012 by Elsevier Science)

advanced reconstruction techniques. Therefore, we will very briefly describe the relevant reconstruction techniques with a focus on their potential impact on image quality.

The amount of activity between two detectors which is directly related to the count rate which will be measured by these detectors is given by the Radon transform. Based on the measurements between many groups of detectors, the original image can be reconstructed using the inverse Radon transform which is usually implemented as a filtered back projection. Importantly this technique starts by distributing the counts between two detectors over all image elements between those detectors. See Fig. 13.4. For high signal-to-noise ratio data such as CT, this technique works very well. However, for low signal-to-noise ratio data such as PET, the resulting image will also have a low signal-to-noise ratio. Another disadvantage of filtered back projection is that areas with high uptake, e.g., the bladder, are surrounded by strike artifacts. Consequently, this area cannot be interpreted. In the last decade, iterative reconstruction techniques have become the standard in PET. See Fig. 13.5.

In iterative reconstruction, an estimate of the image is forward projected, and the resulting projection is compared to the measured projection. From the differences,

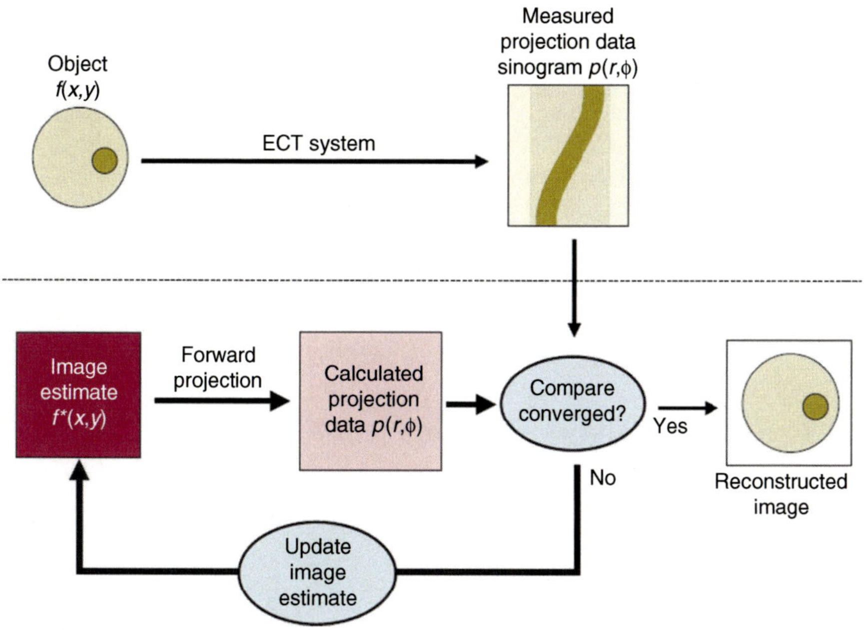

Fig. 13.5 Schematic illustration of the steps in iterative reconstruction. An initial image estimate is made, and projections that would have been recorded from the initial estimate then are calculated by forward projection. The calculated forward projection profiles for the estimated image are compared to the profiles actually recorded from the object, and the difference is used to modify the estimated image to provide a closer match. The process is repeated until the difference between the calculated profiles for successively estimated images and the actually observed profiles reaches some acceptably small level (Reproduced with permission from Physics in Nuclear Medicine; Fourth edition; Simon R. Cherry, James A Sorenson and Michael E. Phelps; Published 2012 by Elsevier Science)

an update is calculated, and a new estimate of the image is formed. With this technique, large low spatial frequency elements are generated first, and with each iteration, more high spatial frequency information is added. Since noise also has a high spatial frequency, a balance between accuracy and noise can be made by stopping the process after a fixed number of iterations. For clinical applications which only require visual analysis, this optimization can be performed visually. However more care is needed when some form of quantification is required since the apparent activity depends on the number of iterations. This is particularly the case for small lesions. To determine the number of iterations which are required to achieve convergence, a scan of a phantom with different-sized spheres can be performed and reconstructed with increasing number of iterations. By setting minimal levels for the convergence, say, 90–95 % of the final activity, the minimal number of iterations can be assessed. Notice that due to partial volume effect, to be discussed later, the activity in the smaller spheres will be lower than the actual activity. Convergence ensures that the measured activity no longer depends on the number of iterations, i.e., it sets a minimum value. When a dynamic PET scan is made for pharmacokinetic modeling, it also needs to be assured that the reconstruction is independent of the count rate. This is especially important since the count rate in the first few minutes of the scan can be much higher than those experienced during a standard whole-body scan. Note that if such a count rate dependency is found, it may also be caused by errors in the randoms, scatter, or dead-time corrections.

An additional advantage of iterative reconstruction is the possibility to "improve" the forward projector. The closer this projector models the actual system, the better the final reconstructed image will represent the real (unknown) image. Two improvements which have become available are time-of-flight and point spread function (PSF) modeling.

13.5 Time-of-Flight and PSF Compensation

As discussed above, the timing accuracy of current PET systems is so high that time-of-flight information is now available. This means that based on the time difference between two detectors, the position of the annihilation can be estimated. As an example, consider an event which occurred at a distance d from the center between the two detectors; cf. Fig. 13.6.

With D the distance between the detectors, the delay for detector one is given by

$$\Delta t_1 = (D/2 + d)/c$$

whereas the delay for detector two is given by

$$\Delta t_2 = (D/2 - d)/c$$

where c denotes the speed of light. Thus the difference between both detectors is given by

$$\Delta t = \Delta t_1 - \Delta t_2 = 2d/c$$

As an example when the accuracy in Δt equals 1 ns, the accuracy in the position d becomes

$$d = c * \Delta t / 2 = 3 * 10^8 \mathrm{m/s} * 10^{-9} s / 2 = 1.5\ 10^{-1} \mathrm{m} = 15 \mathrm{cm}$$

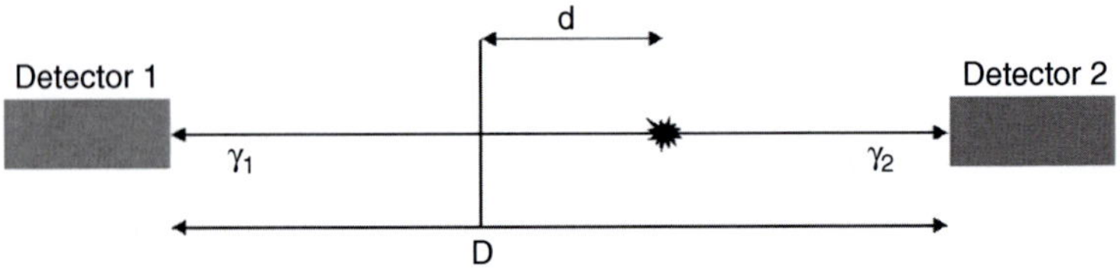

Fig. 13.6 Two photons (γ_1 and γ_2) are measured in coincidence between *detectors 1* and *2*. The distance between the detectors is D. The annihilation event takes place at distance d from the center

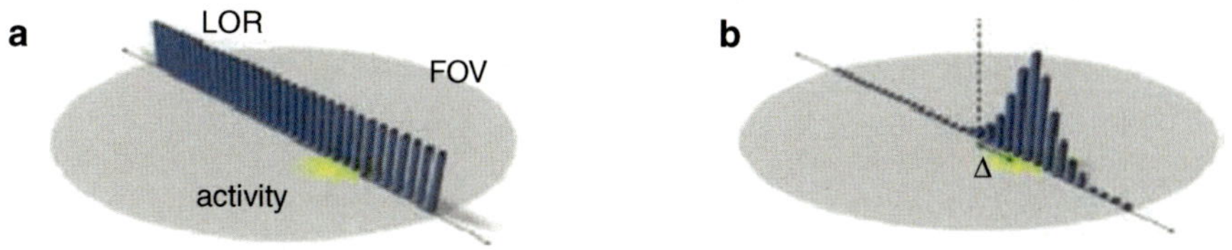

Fig. 13.7 (**a**) In ordinary PET, the counts in a line of response are assigned with equal probability to all of the pixels along the corresponding line in the image matrix. (**b**) In time-of-flight PET, the counts can be localized within a limited segment of the line of response. *FOV* field of view; *LOR* Line of response (Reproduced with permission of the IAEA from PET/CT Atlas on Quality Control and Image Artefacts; IAEA Human Health Series No. 27; ©IAEA; Published 2014)

Current PET/CT systems have an accuracy of about 500–800 ps. This means that the time-of-flight information is accurate within about 10 cm. Although this accuracy is much too low to allow a direct projection of the event, it can be used in the reconstruction process where it results in an improved signal-to-noise ratio. To understand this effect, consider a simple back projection strategy; cf. Fig. 13.7. Without time-of-flight information, the event would be distributed over the total line of response. With time-of-flight information, the distribution is over 10 cm only. This has the effect that the signal-to-noise ratio improves by the ratio of the diameter of the scanner to the accuracy of the time-of-flight information. In practice the improvements are related to the diameter of the patients and give a factor of about three to four. This is a major effect and is similar to an increase in either the dose given to a patient or the scan time of also a factor three or four. It is also clear that further improvements in the time-of-flight accuracy will have a direct and potentially substantial effect on the signal-to-noise ratio and thus the image quality.

Another innovation which has improved image quality considerably is the introduction of PSF information in the reconstruction process. The PSF describes the resolution of the PET/CT system. Previously the PSF was used in a deconvolution technique; however, with this approach, the noise is amplified. Consequently this technique is only suitable for high-quality phantom data and will not work for clinical data. By including this known response of the system in the forward projector of the iterative reconstruction process, the resolution of the resulting image can be improved without excessively increasing the noise. Originally, a fixed PSF was used. However since the resolution of the system is position dependent, the improvement is somewhat unpredictable. By measuring the actual resolution of the system in many positions, a position-dependent response correction was achieved. This has several effects. The first is a clear improvement in resolution of the system. Secondly, the resolution of the system becomes almost homogeneous over the total field of view. Finally the improved resolution results in a better recovery for small lesions and thus improves contrast with only a minor effect on the noise level. If this high resolution is not required, additional post-processing filtering may be applied to reduce noise as compared to a standard reconstruction without PSF information. In current clinical systems, this allows a resolution which is equal, or very close, to the theoretical optimum of half the dimension of the individual detector elements. Thus to improve the resolution of future systems, smaller detector elements need to be developed.

13.6 Partial Volume Effect and the Harmonization of Multicenter Trials

Even though the PSF reconstruction technique has improved the resolution of PET systems considerably, all structures smaller than, say, twice the resolution of the system will still be affected. Since PET measures activity concentrations, the limited resolution results in a reduction of the measured activity, the so-called partial volume effect. This partial volume effect also influences the visual interpretation since it directly reduces the image contrast. As an example, consider Fig. 13.8 which shows the effect in a simple 2-D simulation.

As can be seen, both the mean and maximum activity are affected particularly for small regions. The ratio between measured and actual activity is denoted as the recovery coefficient. Since the contrast is defined as the difference in tumor to

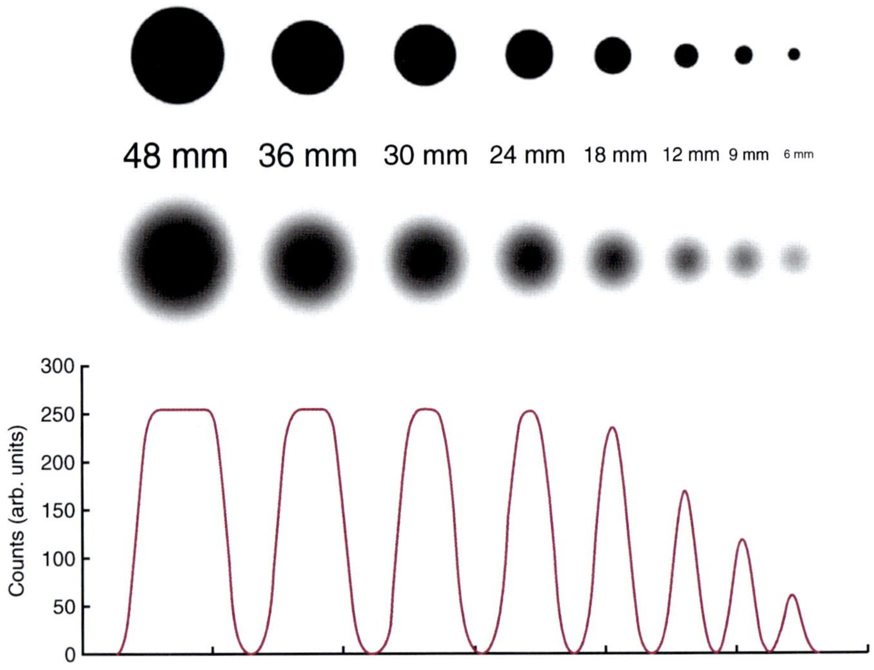

Fig. 13.8 Illustration of partial volume effect. The cylinders shown in the top row have diameters ranging from *48 mm* down to *6 mm*, and each contains the same concentration of radionuclide. The middle row shows a simulation of the images that would result from scanning these cylinders on a SPECT system with an in-plane spatial resolution of *12-mm* full width at half maximum. The cylinders are assumed to have a height much greater than the axial resolution. The bottom row shows count profiles through the center of the images. Although each cylinder contains the same concentration of radionuclide, the intensity, and therefore the apparent concentration, appears to decrease when the cylinder size approaches and then becomes smaller than the resolution of the SPECT system. The integrated area under the count profiles does, however, accurately reflect the total amount of activity in the cylinders (Reproduced with permission from Physics in Nuclear Medicine; Fourth edition; Simon R. Cherry, James A Sorenson and Michael E. Phelps; Published 2012 by Elsevier Science)

background activity divided by the background activity, the contrast is also reduced which is consistent with the visual impression. Thus, in clinical practice, both the detection of small lesions and their quantification are hampered by the partial volume effect. Provided that the reconstruction has reached convergence, the partial volume effect is a function of the effective resolution only. Note that the resolution is not only determined by the system's characteristics but also by the reconstruction filter and the matrix size. Especially the influence of the matrix size may easily be forgotten and may result in erroneous results when different matrix sizes are used.

Since the partial volume effect is an inherent characteristic of a PET system, the main aim should be to characterize it and to ensure that it is stable in time. For a given system and a particular reconstruction protocol, the recovery coefficient values can be determined using, for example, the NEMA image quality phantom. With regular quality control measurements, the stability of the system can be guaranteed. As an additional check, phantom scans can be repeated once or twice a year to ensure that the recovery coefficients remain the same. However, is this approach adequate if we want to use data from different machines or compare data between different machines? As an example, assume that literature indicates that the optimal therapy for patients depends on the SUV value with a cutoff value of, say, 3.3. To implement this knowledge in the own setting, one needs to ensure that the SUV value for a given lesion is independent of the site where it is measured or the specific type of PET/CT used. Vice versa to combine the data from different centers and/or different systems, some form of harmonization is paramount. Therefore, in Europe, for example, a guideline has been adopted by the european association of nuclear medicine (EANM) and is now implemented by the EANM research ltd. (EARL). Since this guideline is not only concerned with the reconstruction but also with the preparation of the patient, the acquisition protocol, and the analysis of the data, it greatly improves the consistency of patient data in multicenter trials.

13.7 Acceptance Testing

Now that we have a better understanding of some of the aspects which influenced the image quality of PET/CT systems, we should take one step back and consider the purchase and installation of a PET/CT system. The selection of a new PET/CT system is determined by many factors. The image quality is but one of them. Other factors are, for example, the price, the level of service available, and the ability to integrate the system in the local setting. Since these factors are unique in each case, the purchase, although extremely important for the image quality, will not be discussed further. So let us assume that a new system is installed and needs to be tested before patient scans can commence. To test the quality of the new system and to determine whether this quality is within the specifications of the manufacturer, acceptance tests need to be performed (International Atomic Energy Agency 2009). Most of the specifications are given according to the NEMA NU 2-2012 procedures. Since these tests often require specific phantoms and/or software to calculate the results, it is advisable to have the conduction of these measurements, either by the manufacturer or a third party, included in the contract. In most cases, the acceptance testing will only be performed once although sometimes it is recommended to also perform these tests after a major software or hardware update. In clinical practice, a simpler QC protocol is better suited. For example, a measurement of the NEMA image quality phantom could be performed to check the uniformity in the background and use the background also to check the calibration factor while the hot spheres can be used to calculate the stability of the recovery coefficients, the latter being an indirect measure of the system resolution. Generally it is not advisable to rely only on the daily QC procedure since these are generally very sensitive but not very specific.

13.8 Daily Quality Control

Once the system is accepted for clinical use, a quality control program is needed to ensure the day-to-day quality of the system. For PET a highly automated daily procedure is the norm. It generally consists of a scan of a homogeneous phantom which is sometimes combined with a number of line sources. The main advantage of a line source is that it has virtually no scatter and that it allows an easy check on the alignment of the PET and CT part of the system. The homogeneous phantom not only allows the quality control of the individual detectors but also enables the day-to-day calibration of the system. This is facilitated by the fact that the phantom is filled with a long-lived isotope, generally ^{68}Ge, and the actual activity at the moment of the QC can easily be calculated from some starting value and the decay. To calculate the relative uptake of a tracer, by the SUV, requires the system to be calibrated to the same dose calibrator which was used to determine the injected activity. Since the ^{68}Ge phantom is usually calibrated to the dose calibrator of its manufacturer, a cross calibration of a new source is required. Therefore, each PET system has its own protocol. Basically these protocols first calibrate the PET system with a known source, for example, a phantom filled with a known quantity of ^{18}FDG, and then determine the activity concentration in the new source and compare this value with the given activity concentration. From this a correction term can be calculated. The correction required is usually less than 5 %. Corrections of more than 10 % are suspicious and require a careful assessment of the procedure. The use of a ^{68}Ge phantom for daily QC and calibration has one potential drawback, i.e., it does not provide a daily control of the cross calibration factor between PET system and dose calibrator. If the sensitivity of the dose calibrator drifts in time, larger and larger errors will occur in the SUV values. To prevent this, the stability of the dose calibrator itself also needs to be checked with long-lived standard sources. In that case, the stability of the cross calibration between dose calibrator and PET only needs to be checked at few times a year. In our experience, current PET systems are very stable. For example, in Fig. 13.9, the calibration factor over a period of 12 months is given.

The daily QC procedure is very sensitive to errors in one of the detectors. Thus even minor problems will result in a failed QC rendering the system unsuited for clinical scans. It is difficult to predict the effect of, for example, a defect detector on image quality. Depending on the system, the specific problem, and the expertise of

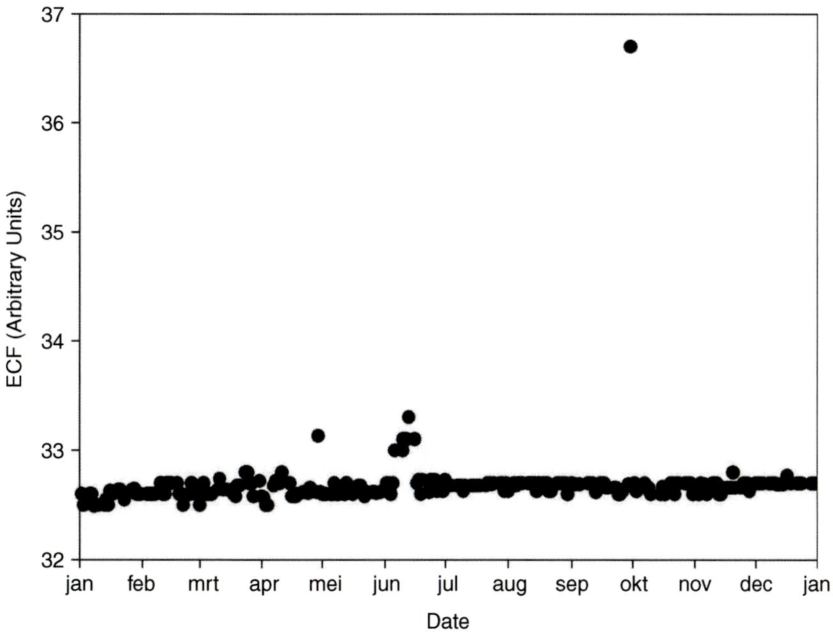

Fig. 13.9 The calibration factor (*ECF*) for a Siemens mCT PET/CT system over the period of 1 year. Generally, the calibration is very stable. Note that apart for the outlier in October, all values are within 2 % of the average value

its users, one may decide to continue scanning anyway. Obviously, in such a case, the responsibility is for the users and each scan must be carefully checked for potential artifacts.

13.9 End of Life

Although easily forgotten, the replacement of an old system with a new one requires special attention. An end of life should include a careful assessment of system QC data. Usually a backup of the daily QC results is a good start. Although generally not warranted, a number of acceptance tests may be repeated to document the quality of the system in more detail. Ideally, the quality of the system over its entirety is documented.

Since a new system will probably have improved specification, special care is needed with the transfer of (clinical) protocols from one system to another. As an example, an improved resolution will result in less partial volume effect which is not acceptable in longitudinal or multicenter studies. Consequently, for consistency, additional filtering may be required even if this means that the potential of the new system cannot be fully exploited. Of course, a better solution would be to create a cross calibration table which can translate the data in either direction. Generally, it is a good idea to carefully check all protocols to ensure consistency of data.

13.10 Future Perspectives

The image quality of PET/CT systems has improved considerably over the last 10 years. There is a reason to believe that these improvements will continue. However these improvements also required the system to be much more stable than previous ones. For example, the temperature dependency has increased considerably since the temperature not only influences the sensitivity of the detector but also its timing information. Since both are essential for the optimal performance of the system, cooling of the system is now much more critical. Thus the environment in which the system is used should also meet much stricter criteria.

Over the last years, the focus in PET development was on the construction of combined PET-MRI systems. The construction of these machines required the development of new PET detectors since the classical approach using photomultipliers could not be used due to the very high effect of magnetic fields on the photomultipliers. Therefore, the photomultiplier was replaced by a solid-state avalanche photdiode (APD) or Silicon photomultiplier (SiPM). It is envisioned that this technique will also be incorporated in a new generation of PET/CT systems. Now that this technique is available, one can speculate on its impact. For example, there are already SiPM-based detectors available which have an improved timing resolution. Further improvements in this aspect only would already improve image quality since the signal-to-noise ratio of ToF PET is directly related to the timing resolution as discussed before. Once mass production of these detectors is achieved, their price should drop and one can envision the construction of PET systems with a longer field of view. With an increased field of view, the number of positions required for a whole-body scan will drop which can either be translated into faster scanning and thus improved throughput or in an improved image quality due to a longer scan per bed position (Beyer et al. 2011). If all lines of responses are allowed, the increased field of view will also improve the sensitivity although at the costs of an even higher scatter fraction. With these improvements, the sensitivity to detect very small abnormalities will improve further. However, this also requires a more rigorous quality control.

References

Beyer T, Townsend DW, Czernin J, Freudenberg LS. The future of hybrid imaging-part 2: PET/CT. Insights Imaging. 2011;2(3):225–34.

Boellaard R, Delgado-Bolton R, Oyen WJ, Giammarile F, Tatsch K, Eschner W, Verzijlbergen FJ, Barrington SF, Pike LC, Weber WA, Stroobants S, Delbeke D, Donohoe KJ, Holbrook S, Graham MM, Testanera G, Hoekstra OS, Zijlstra J, Visser E, Hoekstra CJ, Pruim J, Willemsen A, Arends B, Kotzerke J, Bockisch A, Beyer T, Chiti A, Krause BJ. FDG PET/CT: EANM procedure guidelines for tumour imaging: version 2.0. Eur J Nucl Med Mol Imaging. 2015;42(2):328–54.

Cherry S, Sorenson J, Michael P. Physics in nuclear medicine. 4th ed. Philadelphia: Elsevier Health Sciences; 2012.

de Groot EH, Post N, Boellaard R, Wagenaar NR, Willemsen AT, van Dalen JA. Optimized dose regimen for whole-body FDG-PET imaging. EJNMMI Res. 2013;3(1):63.

International Atomic Energy Agency. Quality assurance for PET and PET/CT systems, IAEA human health series, vol. 1. Vienna: International Atomic Energy Agency; 2009. STI/PUB/1393. ISBN 978-92-0-103609-4.

International Atomic Energy Agency. PET/CT atlas on quality control and image artefacts, IAEA human health series, vol. 27. Vienna: IAEA; 2014. STI/PUB/1642. ISBN 978-92-0-101014-8.

Powsner RA, Powsner ER. Essential nuclear medicine physics. 2nd ed. Chichester: Wiley; 2006.

Patient Safety Considerations for Combined PET/MR Imaging

14

Michel Koole, Kristof Baete, Kwinten Porters, Ronald Peeters, and Koen Van Laere

14.1 Hybrid PET Imaging

Positron emission tomography (PET) is a valuable imaging tool for exploring a variety of cellular and molecular processes in vivo. A typical PET study involves the intravenous injection of a PET tracer (a compound labeled with a positron emitting isotope), which is delivered by arterial blood flow to the target tissue. While the PET tracer binds (ir)reversible to or is being trapped by its physiological target, the radioactive label will decay, emitting a positron which will annihilate with a nearby electron resulting in two simultaneous 511 keV photons in nearly opposite directions. These photon pairs are detected by the PET system as a pair of coincident annihilation photons within a predefined timing window (usually 6 ns – 10 ns) such that the line of response (LOR), along which the annihilation has occurred, can be determined. Therefore, PET is also being referred to as coincidence imaging. Over the total duration of the scan, data are acquired and corrected for physical effects such as attenuation, scatter, dead time, and detector response. These corrected data are binned into one or different time frames, and each time frame is reconstructed using an analytical or iterative reconstruction algorithm. This way a three-dimensional image of the radiotracer distribution is generated at one or various time points after tracer injection allowing an accurate quantification of the underlying physiological tissue characteristics such as blood flow, metabolism, cell proliferation, receptor density, or enzymatic activity. Because of its high sensitivity, only very low amounts of PET tracer activity need to be administered, and therefore pharmacological effects

M. Koole (✉) • K. Baete • K. Porters • K. Van Laere
Division of Nuclear Medicine, University Hospital Gasthuisberg/Catholic University Leuven, Leuven, Belgium
e-mail: michel.koole@uzleuven.be

R. Peeters
Division of Radiology, University Hospital Gasthuisberg/Catholic University Leuven, Leuven, Belgium

A.W.J.M. Glaudemans et al. (eds.), *Quality in Nuclear Medicine*,
DOI 10.1007/978-3-319-33531-5_14

and physiological changes are avoided. This way, PET can provide high-contrast and quantitative functional information about the disease state or therapy response, complementary to information provided by anatomical imaging modalities such as computed tomography (CT) or magnetic resonance imaging (MRI). On the other hand, PET suffers from the limited spatial resolution (typically 4–9 mm) and comparatively poor signal-to-noise ratio with regard to CT or MRI.

Over the past decade, stand-alone PET systems have ceased to be commercially available and have systematically been replaced by hybrid PET/CT systems. Combining functional PET information with the CT-guided localization of tumor lesions has made PET/CT the modality of choice for a vast majority of oncological indications. In addition, the CT data can be used to correct the PET data for attenuation effects.

New advances in PET detector hardware have led to integrated clinical PET/MRI systems allowing simultaneous acquisition of both PET and MR data. Hybrid PET/MRI systems are currently being introduced to the market with an install base that is constantly growing. While Philips currently offers a sequential in-room PET/MRI system combining standard PET and MRI technology, the detector technology of the Siemens and General Electric PET/MRI system allow for simultaneous PET and MR imaging. The Siemens mMR system uses avalanche photodiode (APD)-based PET detectors, and the GE Signa PET/MRI system uses silicon photon multipliers (SiPM)-based PET detectors. Both detector technologies are MR compatible and minimize the interference between the PET and MR components of these hybrid systems.

Improving the noise properties of PET imaging remains a permanent challenge and requires, in general, extended acquisition times or increased administered activity for sufficient statistics in the PET data. Longer acquisition times result in increased patient discomfort, while expanded dosing schemes yield an increased patient exposure, both of which are not acceptable in clinical PET imaging today. In terms of radiation exposure, hybrid PET/MRI substantially reduces the total radiation dose compared to PET/CT (Brix et al. 2005) since radiation exposure is limited to the PET component only. While this is desirable for all patients, this especially benefits pediatric patients and adult cancer patients with good prognosis but in need of frequent follow-up imaging. More personalized treatments could also result in multiple molecular imaging sessions with labeled antibodies. Since kinetics of antibodies are such that labeling with long-lived positron emitters such as zirconium-89 (^{89}Zr) and iodine-124 (^{124}I) is required for quantification, radiation exposure of the patient can become a critical aspect of the treatment.

In the next sections, patient safety considerations will be discussed for both PET and MR imaging. For PET imaging, patient safety issues are mainly related to the ionizing radiation of the administered PET isotopes, while for MR imaging, safety considerations are essentially related to nonionizing radiation.

14.2 Patient Safety Considerations for PET Imaging

As mentioned before for PET imaging, patient safety is generally related to the dosing of the radiopharmaceutical and the biological effects of the corresponding radiation exposure.

14.2.1 Biological Effects of Ionizing Radiation

Biological effects of radiation exposure can be subdivided into two categories. On the one hand, there are the deterministic effects where severity depends on the organ dose and where in general a characteristic threshold is applied to determine whether these effects will occur. On the other hand, radiation induces stochastic effects which present large uncertainties in terms of occurrence. For these effects, severity is independent of the organ dose and even a low radiation dose increases the probability of occurrence. According to the linear, non-threshold (LNT) hypothesis, one generally assumes that no threshold is applicable and that the probability of occurrence of these effects is proportional to the absorbed dose in the organ tissue (ICRP publication 103 2007). For PET imaging, the corresponding organ doses are well below the characteristic thresholds for deterministic effects, and therefore, only stochastic effects need to be taken into account. To put these stochastic effects into perspective, the term effective dose (ED) was introduced (SI unit: sievert or Sv). Stochastic effects have a probability of occurrence that is proportional to this ED, and as such, the ED can be used to assess the health risks related to stochastic effects of radiation exposure.

Several approaches exist to convert effective dose to absolute risk. One approach uses a risk coefficient for fatal cancer representing the sum of risk factors for all organs and tissue types. As such the average lifetime risk factor for cancer and leukemia caused by a low radiation dose is 0.05 Sv^{-1} (ICRP publication 60 1991). On the other hand, ICRP also proposed a concept for low doses and low dose tempos that is broader than fatal cancer and also includes nonfatal cancers and severe genetic effects. This resulted, for instance, in an average future lifetime probability of occurrence of 7.3 per 100,000 for the whole population, for an ED of 1 mSv and for all types of damage including fatal cancer, nonfatal cancer, and severe genetic effects. An alternative method to express absolute radiation risk is the loss of life expectancy (LLE) (Cohen 1991). This concept gives more contextual information rather than direct risk where risk earlier in life will have greater impact than risk during the last decades. An average population LLE for one radiation exposure is about 1year Sv^{-1} for high doses and high dose rate and smaller than 0.5 year Sv^{-1} for low diagnostic doses. To put effective dose into perspective, 1 mSv is actually the ICRP annual dose limit for public exposure. Compared with other "daily life" risks, 1 mSv corresponds to less than a year exposure to natural background at sea level, a few months exposure to natural background at high altitude, and a few hundreds of hours external exposure during transcontinental flights (Wilson et al. 1994).

14.2.2 Radiation Protection for Patients and Volunteers

In terms of patient care, medical imaging procedures involving ionizing radiation should be justified by adding valuable information for improved diagnosis and treatment while taking into account the individual health condition of the patient. On the other hand, even if imaging procedures involving ionizing radiation are fully justified in terms of patient care, the procedure needs to be optimized to such extent that

Table 14.1 Overview of the different WHO classes for healthy volunteers participating in clinical trials

Risk level	WHO class	ED (mSv)	Advantage required for approval
Trivial	I	<0.1	None
Small	IIa	0.1–1	Higher level of knowledge
Intermediate	IIb	1–10	Higher level of knowledge with the potential of providing better patient care and healthcare in the future
Moderate	III	>10	Substantial advantage for the volunteer him/herself

doses are "as low as reasonably achievable" (ALARA principle) for the patient, taking into consideration all costs and health factors.

In terms of clinical trials involving imaging procedures with ionizing radiation, ED is also used to create separate classes for the participation of healthy volunteers such that the risk and advantages can be evaluated by an independent board of experts (local ethics committees). Table 14.1 provides an overview of the different WHO classes. These WHO guidelines were also adopted by the ICRP guidelines (ICRP publication 62 1991) and by the EC (RP-99 1998). Approval will depend on the study design and protocol, the radiation burden, and informed consent. In general, WHO class IIb is applicable for healthy volunteers participating in clinical PET studies, allowing a maximum overall effective dose of 10 mSv (ICRP publication 62 1991). However, age is also taken into account when evaluating the radiation burden for patients and healthy volunteers. For volunteers aged 50 years or older, the detriment per unit dose is considered only one fifth to one tenth of that for younger adults, while for children the health detriment per unit dose is considered 2–3 times higher than for adults. In general, children and pregnant women are prohibited to participate in clinical trials involving ionizing radiation.

14.2.3 Fundaments of PET Tracer Dosimetry (Bolch et al. 2009; Zanotti-Fregonara and Innis 2012)

When a new PET tracer is considered for patient care or clinical trials, a dosimetry study needs to be performed to determine the effective dose. For this purpose, the Medical Internal Radiation Dose (MIRD) committee proposed a dosimetry scheme to model low dose and low dose rate radiation exposure specifically for diagnostic nuclear medicine, radionuclide therapy, and general internal contamination. It uses a source target model where on the one hand, the source organs with a significant uptake of radioactivity are identified and on the other hand, predefined target organs are receiving radiation from the source organs. The MIRD formalism can be described as

$$H_{\mathrm{T}} = \sum_{S} U_S \,\mathrm{SEE}\left(T \leftarrow S\right) \tag{14.1}$$

H_T represents the committed equivalent dose (SI unit: sievert or Sv) in target organ T, U_s denotes the time integral of the activity (SI unit: Bq-s) representing the total number of desintegrations in the source organ S, SEE is a characteristic function describing the energy deposition in organ T of the radiation originating from source organ S, and the index s represents a summation over all source organs.

The equivalent dose H_T actually represents a summation of all absorbed organ doses D_R in the target organ T for a specific type of radiation R multiplied by a radiation weighting factor w_R. The radiation weighting factor w_R was formerly known as a quality control factor Q (Valentin et al. 2003). As such the equivalent dose H_T can also be expressed as

$$H_T = \sum_R w_R D_R \tag{14.2}$$

For photons and electrons, the radiation weighting factor equals 1 for all energies, but this weighting factor can go up to 20 for alpha particles. Contrary to the absorbed dose, the equivalent dose H_T is a function of the incident radiation quality and dependent on the relative biological effectiveness (RBE) (Valentin et al. 2003). It allows comparison between different types of radiation but applies only to low dose and/or dose tempo for human organ absorbed doses.

In the context of dosimetry calculations, the term residence time τ_S, defined as the accumulated organ activity over the injected activity (SI unit: sec), is often used and can be considered as the virtual time during which the total injected activity resides in an organ to match the total accumulated activity in that organ. Using this concept, expression (14.2) for the equivalent organ dose H_T can be rewritten as:

$$H_T = A_0 \sum_S \tau_S \sum_R w_R S_R \left(T \leftarrow S\right) \tag{14.3}$$

In this expression, A_0 represents the total amount of injected activity and S_R the so-called S-factor representing the mean absorbed dose in the target organ T per unit activity from a uniform activity distribution in the source organ S.

Expression (14.1) and (14.3) are very similar, and both $\text{SEE}\left(T \leftarrow S\right)$ and $S_R\left(T \leftarrow S\right)$ depend on energy associated with the particular radiation type and the absorbed fractions (AF). The absorbed fraction represents the fraction of the total energy emitted by radiation of a particular type that is absorbed in the target organ. For beta and alpha particles, which have a short range in tissue, it can be assumed that all the energy will be deposited in the source organ, and other target organs will not be irradiated. For gamma-rays, however, specific absorbed fractions are generally derived using Monte Carlo simulations of radiation transport in mathematical models of the human body and its internal structures (organs, tumors, etc.) with average size and shape (Cristy and Eckerman phantom series: adult male and female; newborn; 1-, 5-, 10-, and 15-year-old child; pregnant woman).

Next to the absorbed fractions, the accumulated activity U_s or residence time τ_s of each source organ needs to be estimated accurately. Since the activity concentration in an organ is continuously changing over time due to various factors such as

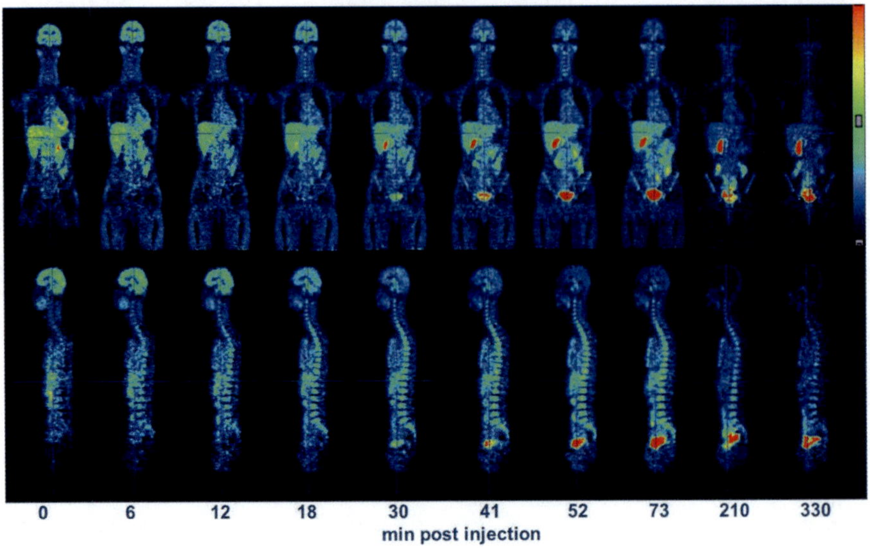

Fig. 14.1 Example series of ten whole-body scans acquired at different time point post injection for a ^{18}F-labeled radiopharmaceutical (physical half-life of 109.7 min) up to 330 min post injection. The *upper row* shows the coronal views while the *lower row* shows the sagittal views. First eight whole-body PET scans were acquired with the subject remaining positioned in the camera system, and while between the time point 8 and 9 and time point 9 and 10, the subject was allowed to get out of the camera system and empty the bladder

the uptake of the radiopharmaceutical, clearance from the organ, relevant excretion paths and physical decay, the cumulated activity U_s needs to be estimated as the area under curve (AUC) of a time activity curve (TAC). This TAC is generated by acquiring a series of whole-body PET scans at various time points after tracer injection (see Fig. 14.1). This way, the TAC represents the fraction of activity taken up by the source organs and the clearance due to the physical and biological properties of the PET tracer. The clearance rate is determined by the effective half-life which takes into account both the biological and physical half-life. For an accurate estimation of U_s for each source organ, one needs to catch the early uptake and washout phase while covering about three times the effective half-life of the radiopharmaceutical.

Once these series of whole-body PET scans are acquired, organs with significant uptake are identified and delineated using three-dimensional volume of interest (VOI) taking into account the corresponding CT-based structural organ definitions (see Fig. 14.2). This way the total organ activity can be estimated as function of time post injection (see Fig. 14.3). The AUC of the TAC of each source organ can be determined by the trapezoid rule where the integral is approximated by a series of trapezoids, and only physical decay is assumed after the last PET measurement point. On the other hand, the TAC can be modeled by a series of exponential terms,

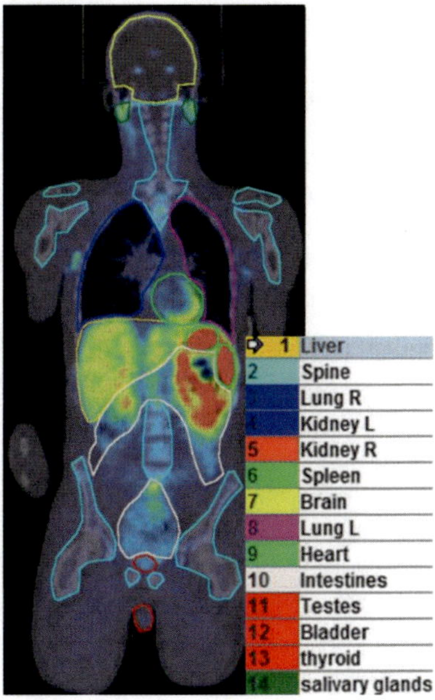

Fig. 14.2 Example of organ VOI delineations using both PET and CT information for organ definition

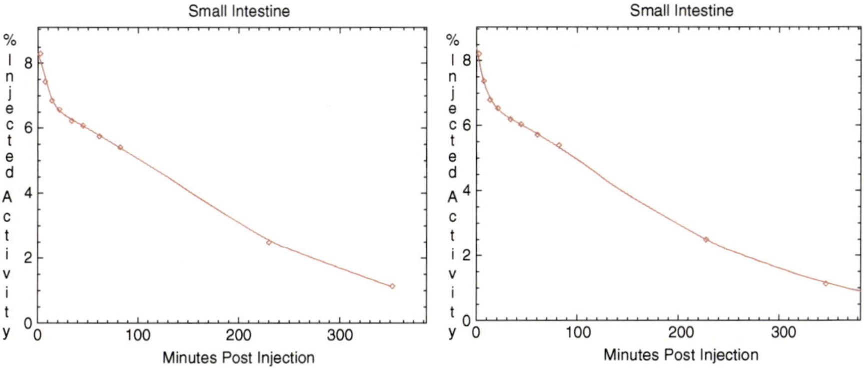

Fig. 14.3 Example time activity curve (*dots*) representing the percentage injected activity taken up by the small intestine at various time point posttracer injection. The solid line in the *left* figure represents a piece-wise linear interpolation while the solid line in the *right* figure represents a curve model fitted to the data points using a least squares approach

and this curve model can be fitted to the TAC data using a least squares approach. Once the curve model is fitted to the TAC data, the AUC can be estimated directly by integration of the mathematical expression describing the TAC. Only small differences were observed between a trapezoid approximation of the AUC and curve model fitting of the TAC data. For red marrow, the accumulated activity can be based either on the delineation of large bone structures or on time-dependent activity measures of blood samples assuming the red marrow to plasma activity ratio to be constant.

Once the organ equivalent doses are determined, the effective dose ED can be calculated as a weighted combination of the different organ equivalent doses:

$$\mathrm{ED} = \sum_{\mathrm{T}} w_{\mathrm{T}} H_{\mathrm{T}} \tag{14.4}$$

In this equation, w_{T} represents the tissue weighting factor which is higher for radiosensitive organs such as the lungs, reproductive system, red marrow, and gastrointestinal tract. These weighting factors are frequently being revised based on newly acquired knowledge about the radiosensitivity of different organ tissue types. The latest revised tissue weighting factors are available from the ICRP publication 103. As such the effective dose takes into account the radiosensitivity of different organs and expresses the dose estimates for several different organs as a single number related to overall radiation risk and the stochastic health detriment. This allows comparison of different procedures in nuclear medicine and of nuclear medicine procedures with other imaging modalities taking advantage of radiation such as diagnostic X-ray or computed tomography (CT).

This MIRD formalism, as described above, was implemented using MIRDOSE (Stabin 1996) which is software for calculating the absorbed organ doses and which was replaced by Organ Level Internal Dose Assessment (OLINDA) (Stabin et al. 2005). Based on the residence times for the different source organs, the isotope, and the mathematical model for the human body, equivalent organ doses are calculated for each radiation type, together with the fractional effective dose for each organ and total effective dose. Next to these calculations, two models are provided to account for relevant excretion paths. The gastrointestinal model allows estimation of the residence time for the stomach, small intestine, and upper and lower large intestine based on the fraction of injected activity entering the small intestine or entering and being absorbed by the stomach. This fraction of activity entering the small intestine can be estimated by delineating the abdominal area and quantifying the accumulated fraction in that volume of interest. On the other hand, the voiding bladder model allows to estimate the residence time for the urinary bladder based on the fraction of activity being cleared through the urinary tract together with biological half-life of this fraction and a bladder voiding interval. In general, a voiding interval of 2–4 h is used.

There are however several limitations inherent to the MIRD approach. First of all, it uses standard models instead of patient-specific models, and therefore it is not suited for risk evaluation for individual patients and should be considered as a population based risk assessment. It also assumes that the activity is distributed uniformly within each organ and that the energy is uniformly deposited throughout the organ. Finally, it is not really appropriate for situations involving radiation therapy as non-stochastic effects can be more important in this setting. For PET procedures however, the MIRD formalism presents a valid approach to estimate the effective dose.

14.2.4 Diagnostic Levels of Radiation Exposure for PET Procedures (ICRP 53 (Addendum 2 and 3) 2008; Bixler et al. 1999)

For ^{18}F-labelled radiopharmaceuticals (109.8 min half-life), the effective dose is generally in the range of 20–35 μSv/MBq, while for ^{11}C-labelled radiopharmaceuticals, the effective dose is generally lower than 9 μSv/MBq with an average 5.9 μSv/MBq (van der Aart et al. 2012; Gatley 1993). On the other hand, the effective doses for immuno-PET procedures are substantially higher. Immuno-PET aims at tracking monoclonal antibodies (mAbs) in vivo to improve diagnostic imaging and guide mAb-based therapies. Therefore, the half-life of the PET isotope needs to match the pharmacokinetics of mAbs (typically 2–4 d for intact mAbs) to achieve optimal tumor to non-tumor ratios. Suitable PET tracers for these PET procedures are ^{89}Zr with a half-life of 3.3 days, ^{124}I with a half-life of 4.2 days, and 64Cu with a half-life of 12.7 h. However, it has been shown that the total effective dose for immuno-PET with a ^{89}Zr-labeled monoclonal antibody can reach up to around 40 mSv for patients receiving an injected dose of 75 MBq (Börjesson et al. 2009). These high effective doses limit the repeated application of immuno-PET. Therefore, it remains one of the major challenges in the field of immuno-PET to further reduce the radiation dose of an immuno-PET procedure by improving the sensitivity of new PET scanners such that better-quality PET images with a lower dose of injected radioactivity can be acquired.

Next the fact that radiation exposure is inherent to PET imaging procedures, it is also mandatory to have the right dose for the right patient to reduce the radiation burden and patient risks. In this context, it is imperative that maintenance and quality control of dose monitors such as dose calibrators is assured and that patient weight is checked in case of weight-dependent dosing. In PET centers where imaging procedures with different PET tracers are performed, one needs to verify before injection that the appropriate tracer dose is prepared for each patient to avoid that the wrong PET tracer is administrated, the patient is exposed to radiation for no reason and the PET procedure needs to be rescheduled. Finally, special attention needs to be paid to the administration of the PET tracer in order to avoid paravenous tracer injection. Not only does the local deposit of high concentration of radioactivity induce patient discomfort (see Fig. 14.4), it also degrades the image quality of the PET scan since less tracer is available for specific uptake and hampers the quantification in terms of a biased standard uptake value (SUV).

14.3 Patient Safety Considerations for MR Imaging

MRI safety risks concern nonionizing radiation related to the main static magnetic field, the magnetic field gradients, radiofrequency pulses, and contrast media (Shellock and Crues 2004).

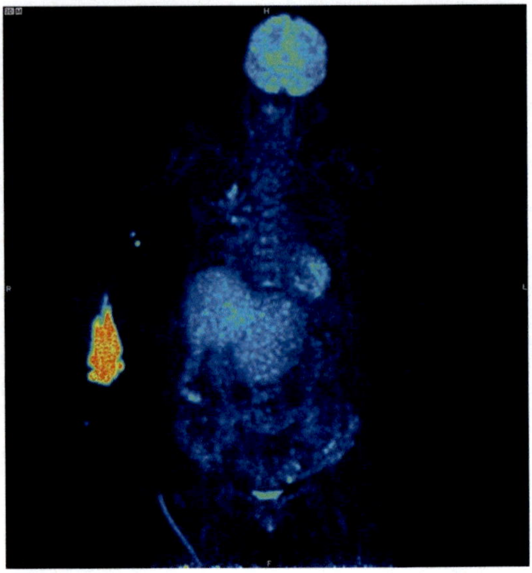

Fig. 14.4 Example of a paravenous injection of a PET tracer with the corresponding local deposit of high concentration of radioactivity in the right forearm

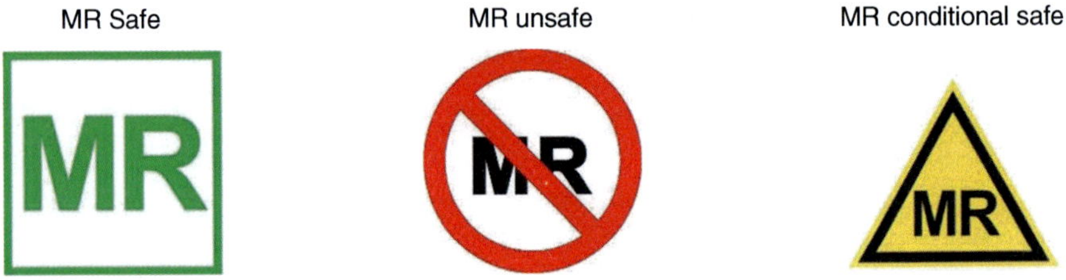

Fig. 14.5 Overview of the MR classification labels for devices

14.3.1 Static Magnetic Field

The field strength of a static magnetic field ranges from 1 to 11.7 Tesla, with typically field strengths for clinical systems 1.5 or 3 Tesla. Although there is no proof for short- and long-term biological health risks, the main magnetic field attracts ferromagnetic material (clips, keys, coins, phones, tools, gas cylinders, wheel chairs, beds, etc.), can also interfere with electronic devices (pacemakers, neurostimulators, etc.) and magnetic media (bank cards, badges, etc.) (Kanal et al. 2015; Shellock 2002a, b). For this purpose, objects can be classified as MR safe, MR unsafe, and MR conditional (safe under strict conditions, for instance, the distance to the magnet should be sufficient that the static field experienced by the equipment is lower than 200 mT) (Shellock et al. 2009) (see Fig. 14.5). MR safe means that normal use should not cause any problems in a static magnetic field, which is different from MR compatible which means that the equipment is not only MR safe but that it also causes minimal artifacts in the MR images. On the other hand, MR unsafe means that the object should not be introduced in a static magnetic field at all; it should be kept outside of the 0.5 mTesla line. Clinical MRI scanners make use of superconducting coils to generate the static magnetic field which is always present. In case of an emergency, this can be removed by pressing an emergency stop button which basically means the superconductive system is stopped by local heating and quenching the MRI magnet, inducing a rapid boil off of the liquid helium. While this is not toxic, it can present a risk since it is very cold and can displace the oxygen in the room when the quench tube is not functioning correctly.

14.3.2 Magnetic Field Gradients

While the main static magnetic field is continuously present, the magnetic field gradients are only used during the actual image acquisition. They generate strong and fast fluctuating changes of the magnetic field in all 3 directions at frequencies up to 5 kHz. These gradients produce considerable acoustic noise levels and can induce electrical currents in closed conducting circuits (Vogt et al. 2004). The maximum noise level from switching magnetic field gradients can go up to around 115 db(A), which can induce temporary hearing loss. In general, hearing protection is recommended for noise levels over 80 db(A), while hearing protection is mandatory for noise levels over 85 db(A). Therefore, hearing protection is obligatory for all people present in the MRI room during image acquisition. In terms of noise attenuation, ear plugs reduce the noise by 10–15 db(A) and head phones by 15–30 db(A), while ear plastics damp the noise level with 15–25 db(A). As such personnel and patients are advised to use MR compatible headphones and/or ear plugs while for pediatric patients earplugs and MiniMuffs® are recommended.

In terms of the electrical currents induced by the magnetic field gradients, the risk for patients include peripheral nerve stimulation (Zhang et al. 2003) and electrical currents in closed wired circuits such as pacemakers or neurostimulators. Therefore correct patient positioning or patient posture is critical to avoid closed body circuits with the extremities (feet, hands, or knees touching each other or the torso) (see Fig. 14.6).

14.3.3 RF Pulsing

The radiofrequency pulses are also used only during scanning; these radiofrequency pulses at the precession frequency of the water protons change the energy state of these protons, which relax back to their steady state after the RF pulse at different speed for different tissue types to generate the endogenous contrast in the MR images. The energy deposition of these RF-pulses in the body is quantified as specific absorption rate (SAR) and can cause local heating of body parts. SAR limits are applicable such as a maximum of 4 W/kg as average for 15 min whole-body acquisition, a maximum of 3 W/kg as average for 10 min head acquisition, and a maximum of 10 W/kg as average for 5 min acquisition of the extremities.

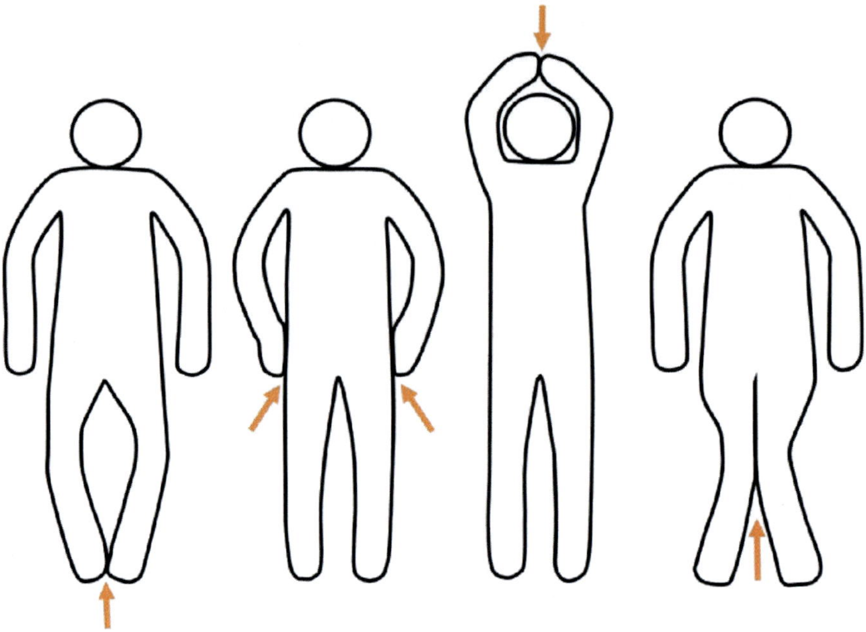

Fig. 14.6 Overview of patient postures which can be critical for inducing closed body circuits

SAR limits are imposed by the acquisition of soft- and hardware but also rely on the patient's weight which needs to be entered accurately. Persons inside the room (e.g., anesthesiologists during the scans of pediatric patients next to the MRI system are at a much larger distance from the RF antenna than patients, and therefore the RF pulse have minimal effects while outside of the MRI room). RF radiation is fully shielded off by the cage of faraday in which the MR machine is positioned. The RF fields can also cause heating in conducting wires like, e.g., pacemaker leads or the receive antenna cables which can cause local burns if not isolated from the patient.

14.3.4 Contrast Media

When contrast media are administered (mostly gadolinium-based chelates) to generate exogenous contrast, patients risks are mostly limited with small side effects such as redness and itching in less than 5 % of the patients and very rare serious side effects (shock reaction) in 1 out of 150,000 cases. Patients with kidney insufficiency on the other hand have a risk for nephrogenic systemic fibrosis (NSF) when exposed to gadolinium-based contrast agents causing disturbed organ function, swollen extremities, and possible death (Shellock and Spinazzi 2008a). To assess kidney function, estimated glomerular filtration rate (eGFR) or creatine can be measured. If eGFR values are below 60 or creatine is higher than 120 μmol/l, the use of gadolinium-based contrast agents need to be considered carefully, and the amount used should be as little as possible.

14.3.5 Contraindications

Finally, patients themselves can present risks in terms of claustrophobia or implanted devices which are not MR safe. Some devices are an absolute contraindication for MR such as most ICD's (intracardiac defibrillator), while other devices are conditional MR safe such as several types of pacemakers and some neurostimulators. Conditional MR safe means that patients with these devices can be safely scanned in an MRI machine when certain device-specific conditions are met like MR conditional pacemakers and also lead certain maximum static field strengths, specific maximum gradient strength, and certain maximum SAR levels. Also small metal parts in, e.g., tattoos (Tope and Shellock 2002), surgical clips, or medicinal patches can induce small currents and cause local heating and burns. If possible, these should be removed and if necessary cooling with a wet towel needs to be applied. In this context, screening of patients by experienced staff members before entering the MRI suite is mandatory to reduce patient risks (Shellock and Spinazzi 2008b; Boutin et al. 1994; Murano et al. 2011).

14.4 Patient Safety Considerations for Combined PET/MR Imaging

Until now, little is known about possible synergistic effects of combined PET/MR imaging (Brix et al. 2009). Since PET imaging is a fairly standard imaging procedure using the exogenous contrast, PET tracer characteristics, injection, and handling are critical. On the other hand, MRI generally relies on the endogenous contrast that is generated during the imaging procedure with limited use of standard contrast agents. As such, operation of the MR imaging system is the crucial part of the imaging procedure (Calamante et al. 2015). Therefore, both imaging procedure pose different patient safety risks in term of imaging, even when both imaging procedures are combined. On the other hand, mild hyperthermia, caused by the RF pulses, can change tissue and tumor physiology, increasing local oxygenation and having a radio sensitizing effect (Song et al. 2001; Horsman and Overgaard 2007). Meanwhile the static and low-frequency magnetic fields might cause oxidative stress and genetic mutations (Ghodbane et al. 2013), while other data suggest that magnetic field exposure enhances DNA repair (Chow and Tung 2000). Therefore, further studies are mandatory to assess the biological effects of simultaneous exposure to both ionizing radiation and electromagnetic fields taking into account realistic exposure levels and scanning procedures. This way, health risks can be determined for combined and simultaneous PET/MR imaging and imaging procedures can be optimized to reduce health damaging synergistic effects.

References

Bixler A, Springer G, Lovas R. Practical aspects of radiation safety for using fluorine-18. J Nucl Med Technol. 1999;27(1):14–6; quiz 18–9.

Bolch WE, Eckerman KF, Sgouros G, Thomas SR. MIRD pamphlet No. 21: a generalized schema for radiopharmaceutical dosimetry--standardization of nomenclature. J Nucl Med. 2009;50(3):477–84.

Börjesson PKE, Jauw YWS, de Bree R, Roos JC, Castelijns JA, Leemans CR, van Dongen GAMS, Boellaard R. Radiation dosimetry of 89Zr-labeled chimeric monoclonal antibody U36 as used for immuno-PET in head and neck cancer patients. J Nucl Med. 2009;50(11):1828–36.

Boutin RD, Briggs JE, Williamson MR. Injuries associated with MR imaging: survey of safety records and methods used to screen patients for metallic foreign bodies before imaging. Am J Roentgenol. 1994;162(1):189–94.

Brix G, Lechel U, Glatting G, Ziegler SI, Münzing W, Müller SP, Beyer T. Radiation exposure of patients undergoing whole-body dual-modality 18F-FDG PET/CT examinations. J Nucl Med. 2005;46(4):608–13.

Brix G, Nekolla EA, Nosske D, Griebel J. Risks and safety aspects related to PET/MR examinations. Eur J Nucl Med Mol Imaging. 2009;36 Suppl 1:S131–8.

Calamante F, Faulkner WH, Ittermann B, Kanal E, Kimbrell V, Owman T, Reeder SB, Sawyer AM, Shellock FG, van den Brink JS. MR system operator: recommended minimum requirements for performing MRI in human subjects in a research setting. J Magn Reson Imaging. 2015;41(4):899–902.

Chow KC, Tung WL. Magnetic field exposure enhances DNA repair through the induction of DnaK/J synthesis. FEBS Lett. 2000;478(1–2):133–6.

Cohen BL. Catalog of risks extended and updated. Health Phys. 1991;61(3):317–35.

RP-99: Guidance on medical exposures in medical and biomedical research. European Commission. Luxembourg; 1998.

Gatley SJ. Estimation of upper limits on human radiation absorbed doses from carbon-11-labeled compounds. J Nucl Med. 1993;34(12):2208–15.

Ghodbane S, Lahbib A, Sakly M, Abdelmelek H. Bioeffects of static magnetic fields: oxidative stress, genotoxic effects, and cancer studies. BioMed Res Int. 2013;2013.

Horsman MR, Overgaard J. Hyperthermia: a potent enhancer of radiotherapy. Clin Oncol. 2007;19(6):418–26.

Kanal E, Froelich J, Barkovich AJ, Borgstede J, Bradley W, Gimbel JR, Gosbee J, Greenberg T, Jackson E, Larson P, Lester J, Sebek E, Shellock FG, Weinreb J, Wilkoff BL, Hernandez D. Standardized MR terminology and reporting of implants and devices as recommended by the american college of radiology subcommittee on MR safety. Radiology. 2015;274(3):866–70.

Murano T, Minamimoto R, Senda M, Uno K, Jinnouchi S, Fukuda H, Iinuma T, Tsukamoto E, Terauchi T, Yoshida T, Oku S, Nishizawa S, Ito K, Oguchi K, Kawamoto M, Nakashima R, Iwata H, Inoue T. Radiation exposure and risk-benefit analysis in cancer screening using FDG-PET: results of a Japanese nationwide survey. Ann Nucl Med. 2011;25(9):657–66.

ICRP publication 53 (Addendum 2) Radiation dose to patients from radiopharmaceuticals. Ann ICRP. 1998;28(3):1–126.

ICRP Publication 53 (Addendum 3). Radiation dose to patients from radiopharmaceuticals. ICRP Publication 106. Approved by the Commission in October 2007. Ann ICRP. 2008;38(1-2):1–197.

ICRP publication 62. Radiological protection in biomedical research. A report of committee 3 adopted by the International Commission on Radiological Protection. Ann ICRP. 1991;22(3):1–28; v–xxiv.

ICRP publication 60. Recommendations of the international commission on radiological protection. Ann ICRP. 1991;21(1–3):1–201.

Shellock FG. Magnetic resonance safety update 2002: implants and devices. J Magn Reson Imaging. 2002a;16(5):485–96.
Shellock FG. Biomedical implants and devices: assessment of magnetic field interactions with a 3.0-tesla MR system. J Magn Reson Imaging. 2002b;16(6):721–32.
Shellock FG, Crues JV. MR procedures: biologic effects, safety, and patient care. Radiology. 2004;232(3):635–52.
Shellock FG, Spinazzi A. MRI safety update 2008: Part 1, MRI contrast agents and nephrogenic systemic fibrosis. Am J Roentgenol. 2008a;191(4):1129–39.
Shellock FG, Spinazzi A. MRI safety update 2008: part 2, screening patients for MRI. Am J Roentgenol. 2008b;191(4):1140–9.
Shellock FG, Woods TO, Crues JV. MR labeling information for implants and devices: explanation of terminology. Radiology. 2009;253(1):26–30.
Song CW, Park H, Griffin RJ. Improvement of tumor oxygenation by mild hyperthermia. Radiat Res. 2001;155(4):515–28.
Stabin MG. MIRDOSE: personal computer software for internal dose assessment in nuclear medicine. J Nucl Med. 1996;37(3):538–46.
Stabin MG, Sparks RB, Crowe E. OLINDA/EXM: the second-generation personal computer software for internal dose assessment in nuclear medicine. J Nucl Med. 2005;46(6):1023–7.
ICRP publication 103. The recommendations of the international commission on radiological protection. Ann ICRP. 2007;37(2–4):1–332.
Tope WD, Shellock FG. Magnetic resonance imaging and permanent cosmetics (tattoos): survey of complications and adverse events. J Magn Reson Imaging. 2002;15(2):180–4.
Valentin J, Cox R, Kellerer AM. Relative biological effectiveness (RBE), quality factor (Q), and radiation weighting factor (wR). Ann ICRP. 2003;33(4):1–117.
van der Aart J, Hallett WA, Rabiner EA, Passchier J, Comley RA. Radiation dose estimates for carbon-11-labelled PET tracers. Nucl Med Biol. 2012;39(2):305–14.
Vogt FM, Ladd ME, Hunold P, Mateiescu S, Hebrank FX, Zhang A, Debatin JF, Göhde SC. Increased time rate of change of gradient fields: effect on peripheral nerve stimulation at clinical MR imaging. Radiology. 2004;233(2):548–54.
Wilson OJ, Young BF, Richardson CK. Cosmic radiation doses received by Australian commercial flight crews and the implications of ICRP 60. Health Phys. 1994;66(5):493–502.
Zanotti-Fregonara P, Innis RB. Suggested pathway to assess radiation safety of 11C-labeled PET tracers for first-in-human studies. Eur J Nucl Med Mol Imaging. 2012;39(3):544–7.
Zhang B, Yen YF, Chronik BA, McKinnon GC, Schaefer DJ, Rutt BK. Peripheral nerve stimulation properties of head and body gradient coils of various sizes. Magn Reson Med. 2003;50(1):50–8.

Standardization of Imaging Biomarkers: The FDG PET/CT Example

15

Ronald Boellaard

Abstract

In this book chapter, requirements and solutions for using fluorodeoxyglucose positron emission tomography/computed tomography (FDG PET/CT) as a quantitative imaging biomarker are explained. Requirements for the use of (any) medical imaging modality as imaging biomarker are being discussed and, in particular, the implications for use of quantitative FDG PET/CT studies in a multicenter setting are summarized. Moreover, future developments, new quantitative metrics, and international efforts to implement medical imaging as validated imaging biomarkers are highlighted.

15.1 Introduction

Positron emission tomography/computed tomography (PET/CT) using [^{18}F]-fluorodeoxyglucose (FDG) has become one of the most important imaging modalities for diagnosis and staging in oncology (Brady et al. 2008). Moreover, FDG PET/CT can be used as prognostic factor and to predict treatment response (Geus-Oei et al. 2007; Czernin and Schelbert 2007; Kobe et al. 2012; Zhang et al. 2012; Scheffler et al. 2013). In particular, metabolic changes may occur earlier during treatment than anatomical (tumor size) changes (Weber 2005a, b). With new emerging targeted (cytostatic) drugs, such as thymidine kinase inhibitors, tumor size reduction may not be observed at all or only very late during the course of

R. Boellaard, PhD
Department of Radiology and Nuclear Medicine, VU University Medical Center, Amsterdam, The Netherlands

Department of Nuclear Medicine and Molecular Imaging, University Medical Center Groningen/University of Groningen, Groningen, The Netherlands
e-mail: r.boellaard@umcg.nl

A.W.J.M. Glaudemans et al. (eds.), *Quality in Nuclear Medicine*,
DOI 10.1007/978-3-319-33531-5_15

treatment, and FDG PET/CT may play an important role for assessing the efficacy of these drugs early during treatment (Zander et al. 2011). Quantitative reads of FDG PET/CT examinations could further facilitate its use as imaging biomarker thereby providing an observer-independent measurement of tracer uptake (Hoekstra et al. 2000; Itti et al. 2013).

The potential use of FDG PET as a quantitative biomarker was already recognized in 1999 when Young et al. (1999) published the European Organization for Research and Treatment of Cancer (EORTC) guideline for treatment response assessment. More recently, Wahl et al. (2009) recommended PET response criteria, called positron emission tomography response criteria in solid tumors (PERCIST), and indicated specific acquisition and analysis procedures to quantitatively determine and classify treatment response. Despite the clear potentials of FDG PET/CT as a quantitative imaging biomarker tool, its widespread introduction and acceptance is still hampered by the lack of standardized imaging and data analysis procedures.

In the majority of published studies, quantification of FDG PET/CT is based on the so-called standardized uptake value (SUV) as a quantitative index of tracer uptake. However, SUV-based quantification is not trivial and influenced by many factors. In various publications, these factors have been described extensively and their impact on SUV has been identified. Yet, a large variability in applied imaging procedures still exists. Graham et al. (2011) performed a survey among academic sites in the United States and observed large variations in imaging procedures. Similar observations were made by Beyer et al. (2011) among imaging sites across the world. Both authors indicate a large variability in, e.g., used FDG activities, image reconstruction parameters, data analysis procedures, and uptake times.

In order to enhance the use of FDG PET/CT as imaging biomarkers, several guidelines have been published. Already in 1998 Schelbert et al. (1998) published procedure guidelines for FDG PET imaging. Since then several updates and new guidelines have been published, which were reviewed by Boellaard (2009). Most recently, it has become clear that minimal performance standards alone are not sufficient, and that rigorous harmonization of imaging procedures is essential for accurate and reproducible quantification of FDG PET/CT studies. The latter is of utmost importance in multicenter studies and, therefore, to qualify FDG PET/CT as imaging biomarker.

In this chapter a review will be provided explaining the requirements for using FDG PET/CT as imaging biomarker and the performance standards that need to be met in order to obtain reproducible quantitative reads from FDG PET examinations.

15.2 Requirements for a Quantitative Imaging Biomarker

A definition for a biomarker was presented by the "Biomarkers definition working group" in 2001 as "a characteristic that is objectively measured and evaluated as an indicator of normal biologic processes, pathogenic processes, or pharmacologic responses to a therapeutic intervention" (Biomarkers Definitions Working Group 2001). Biomarkers should have a high feasibility, precision, and accuracy. A biomarker is thus a parameter representing (patho-)physiological processes and should be suitable as indicator to diagnose and treat patients. A biomarker should be objective and quantitative.

From these definitions it is clear that first of all (quantitative) reads from any imaging biomarker should have diagnostic, prognostic, and/or predictive value, i.e., its clinical use and impact on patient management for both patient care and in trials should have been established. As indicated before, the clinical use of FDG PET/CT has been established and is described in many publications and summarized by Fletcher et al. (2008), and its cost-effectiveness for staging of lung cancer has been shown by, e.g., Van Tinteren et al. (2002). The SUV, as a quantitative measure for FDG uptake, may be used at various stages of patient care, may facilitate further the concept of personalized medicine, and can be used in trials. Both for personalized medicine and in trials, there are similarities in using FDG PET/CT. Some examples of potential applications of SUV or its relative change for patient care or in clinical studies are illustrated in Fig. 15.1.

Secondly, an imaging biomarker should have sufficient accuracy, repeatability, and reproducibility. A high accuracy means that the imaging biomarker provides an index that correlates and/or corresponds with (the severity or magnitude of) the (patho-)physiological process. Repeatability indicates the ability of an imaging biomarker to provide the same (quantitative) read when examining the same patient under identical conditions. Usually for FDG PET/CT, this is evaluated using the so-called test-retest (TRT) studies where the patient is scanned using the same PET/

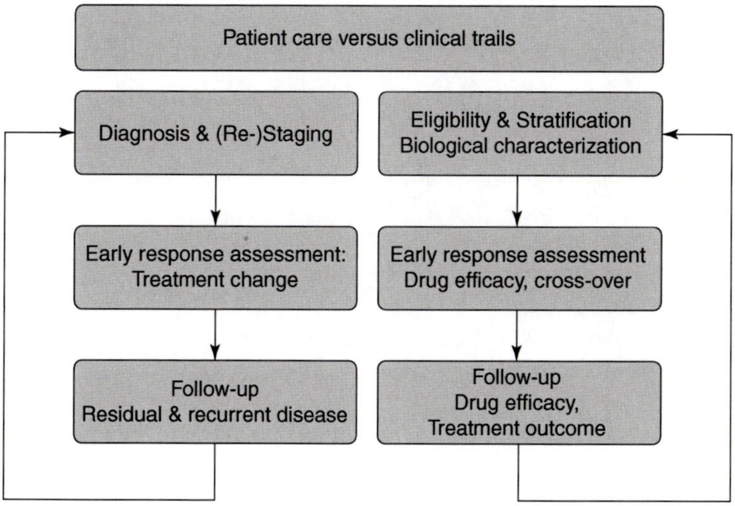

Fig. 15.1 Schematic overview of some applications of quantitative FDG PET/CT for both patient care and in clinical trials. The figure does not provide a complete overview but attempts to illustrate similarities in these applications between patient care and trials

CT system and imaging procedures within a short time interval (e.g., within 1 week) such that no changes in tracer uptake and distribution can be expected. The test-retest (TRT) performance has been studied extensively, and a recent meta-analysis showed that TRT performance equals 10–15 % (1 SD). This high repeatability was also seen in a multicenter TRT study published by Velasquez et al. but the authors also indicated that in about 25 % of the studies, quality of the PET data was not sufficient for quantitative analysis. Besides repeatability, reproducibility is an essential requirement. Reproducibility is the ability to provide the same result when scanning the same patient on different PET/CT systems and at different imaging sites. The latter implies that not only the same imaging procedure is used but, in fact, also that the same scanner performance or quantitative image characteristics, data analysis, and interpretations are applied across all imaging sites. Harmonization of these aspects, rather than defining minimal standards alone, is thus required to guarantee sufficient reproducibility. The European guideline for quantitative FDG PET/CT oncology imaging in multicenter studies, published in the European Journal of Nuclear Medicine and Molecular Imaging in 2010 (Boellaard et al. 2010), is particularly providing recommendations and performance standards aiming at harmonization of quantitative FDG PET/CT measurements.

15.3 Harmonization of FDG PET/CT Studies

The various factors affecting SUV and giving rise to SUV uncertainties have been well identified and are frequently classified as technical, physical, and biological factors. A detailed overview of these factors and their impact on SUV uncertainty are given in (Boellaard 2009) and will not be extensively replicated here. Below a short overview of some of the activities and precautions needed to arrive at reproducible quantitative FDG PET/CT reads will be given. This overview aims at describing these steps or actions in a chronological order. In general the following phases or steps may be defined:

1. The phase prior to performing quantitative FDG PET/CT examinations ("start-up phase")
2. Patient preparation phase
3. Actual image acquisition and reconstruction
4. Image analysis
5. Interpretation and longitudinal analysis – assessment of treatment response or follow-up/recurrent disease

During the start-up phase (phase 1), actions required prior to scanning patients to set up for quantitative examinations can be taken care of. During this phase sites should take care of mitigating the negative effects of technical factors, such as ensuring proper PET/CT system calibration and verification of clock synchronization. Moreover, quantification is determined by applied region of interest methodology in combination with image characteristics, such as image noise and contrast recovery. The interplay between contrast recovery, noise, and data analysis method is illustrated in Fig. 17.2, and an example of the effects of changing acquisition and reconstruction parameters in combination with data analysis approaches is illustrated in Fig. 17.3. Contrast or SUV recovery is a function of (iterative) reconstruction settings, such as applied number of iterations and subsets, matrix size, and image filters. Contrast recovery can be varied by changing these parameters. Therefore, it is of utmost importance to first harmonize scanner performance with respect to applied SUV method, i.e., max or mean SUV, and contrast recovery coefficients. To this end, the combination of reconstruction parameters, which result in SUV recoveries within a specified bandwidth, should be first determined. This can be done by studying SUV recovery coefficients in, e.g., the NEMA NU2 2007 Image Quality phantom by varying reconstruction settings. By changing these settings, it is possible to derive an acquisition and reconstruction protocol that results in harmonized SUV recoveries across different imaging sites and systems. To ensure sufficient image quality, PET/CT system accreditation programs have been set up by several organizations (Makris et al. 2013). One of these accreditation programs is offered by the European Association of Nuclear Medicine (EANM) Research Limited, EARL, aiming at achieving harmonized quantitative PET/CT system performance by performing several quality control experiments. Over the last 2 years, EARL has shown that this accreditation program substantially reduces PET/CT system performance within the specified performance criteria and that it is feasible across more than 75 sites having PET/CT systems of all three major vendors.

When a patient is planned for an FDG PET/CT examination (phase 2), it is essential that patients have fasted properly. Current guidelines recommend a fasting period of 4–6 h prior to administration of FDG. With exceptions for diabetic patients, fasting ensures low and reproducible plasma glucose levels (4–7 mmol/l), thereby ensuring reproducible and sufficient uptake of FDG. Moreover, strenuous exercise should be avoided about 24 h prior to the PET study. More precautions and patient preparations can be found in Boellaard et al. 2010. Patient weight should be measured at the department using a calibrated scale at each time a patient will undergo a PET/CT examination. The FDG activity should be adjusted based on patient weight to ensure a minimal PET image quality over a wide range of patient weights. A recent study has shown that adjusting the FDG activity based on the square of the patient weight rather than the weight itself may further harmonize image quality, specifically for heavy weight (>100 kg) patients (de Groot et al. 2013). However, rather than increasing FDG activities to extreme levels, scan duration should be prolonged instead, and FDG activities should generally remain below 500 MBq. The correct net injected activity and measured patient weight should be entered into the PET/CT system so that subsequent SUV calculation uses the right information.

After administration of FDG and an uptake period of 60 min, a patient undergoes the actual FDG PET/CT examination (phase 3). The minimal scan duration should be chosen in combination with the administered activity and body weight. Upon or already during acquisition, the projection data is reconstructed providing images representing the tracer distribution in vivo. For quantitative evaluations in a multicenter study, the harmonized reconstruction method and settings should be chosen, as determined before or during an accreditation procedure. For visual interpretation different local reconstruction preferences may be chosen. At present the only option to combine these two sets of (different) reconstruction settings is to perform a second reconstruction although this may not be convenient. Another option would be to use a higher spatial resolution dataset and perform an offline image filter to arrive at the required harmonized image characteristics (Lasnon et al. 2013). This functionality is, however, not yet routinely provided with the PET/CT systems, but efforts are now being undertaken by the vendors to support harmonized FDG uptake quantification.

Once reconstructed images have become available, the FDG uptake is usually assessed visually. Specific criteria for visual assessment of tracer uptake in, e.g., lymphoma have been provided by the Deauville criteria, where tracer uptake is rated using a 5-point scale using liver and mediastinal blood pool uptake as reference. The validity of this approach has been shown by an international validation study by Biggi et al. (2013). Although the use of the Deauville criteria resulted in more consistent reads across imaging sites and readers, limitations of visual reads have been discussed as well. One of the limitations arises from the human visual system where estimation of intensity is affected by local background, as illustrated in Fig. 17.4. Quantitative assessment of tracer uptake could result in a more objective read (Itti et al. 2013) and may outperform visual read, as shown by Itti et al. Moreover, SUVs are provided on a continuous scale allowing for a more differentiated categorization. Consequently, the use of SUV for evaluation of uptake (at interim PET) or response (relative to baseline) has gained interest, not only in lymphoma studies. Recently, Zander et al. (2011) showed that changes in tracer uptake based on SUV can be used as early prediction of Erlotinib treatment response.

The first step in deriving SUV is the definition of a region (2D) or volume (3D) of interest (phase 4). Next, the maximum or average uptake, SUVmax or SUVmean, respectively, in this region of volume of interest is determined. Another alternative is the so-called SUVpeak, which is based on the average uptake in a 1 ml spherical volume of interest. The volume of interest is positioned such that SUVpeak represents the highest value across all possible positions within the tumor. The various volumes of interest have their particular advantages and limitations. For now, one should consider that SUV data change when changing the volume of interest method used to analyze tracer uptake. It is therefore important to realize that reproducible quantification requires the use of a specific combination of image characteristics and data analysis methods. Changing any of these factors will cause a systematic change in SUV, as illustrated in Figs. 15.2, 15.3, and 15.4.

SUV provides an objective quantitative index of FDG uptake. Yet, these data still need to be correctly interpreted (phase 5). Confounding factors are, e.g., increased uptake due to inflammation or reduced uptake due to increased blood glucose levels. Also other clinical symptoms, tumor location, and patient history need to be considered. During interpretation a quality control of the PET data should be considered. Studying liver uptake may help in the identification of (large) errors in, e.g., injected activity or other error sources. In unaffected livers, SUV usually equals around 1.5–2.0, slightly depending on, e.g., PET/CT system. Liver SUV outside the range of about

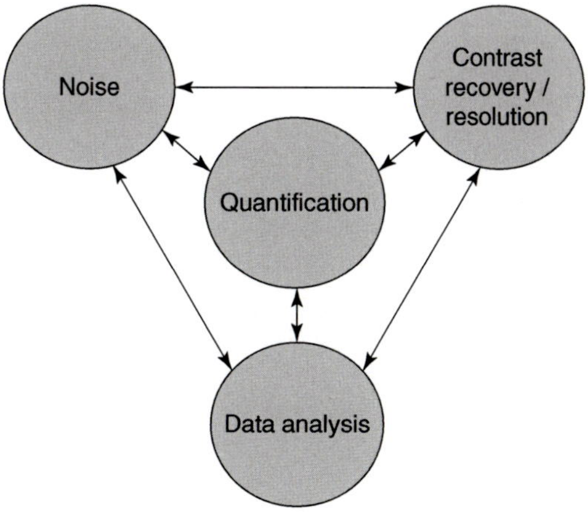

Fig. 15.2 Interplay between noise, data analysis method, and contrast recovery and their effect on quantification. Changing any of these factors independently will change the quantitative results of an FDG PET/CT study

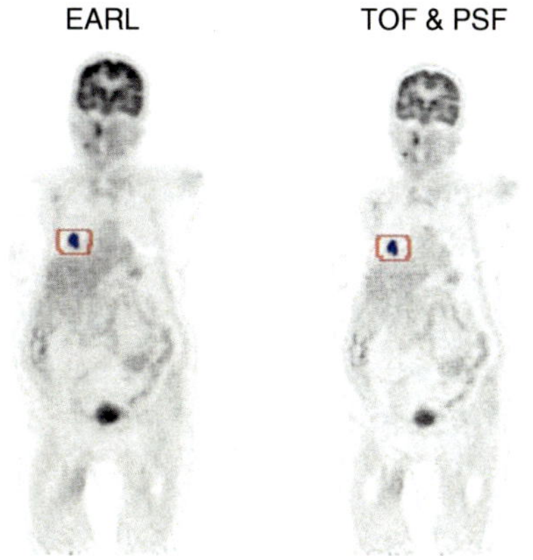

Parameter				Difference (%)
SUV_{max}	=	9.9	13.8	+39
SUV_{peak}	=	7.9	10.2	+29
SUV_{mean}^{liver}	=	2.8	2.5	−11
SUV_{max}^{liver}	=	4.1	4.0	−2.5
MATV (A50%)	=	4.7	4.1 ml	−13

Fig. 15.3 Example on change in quantitative results when changing image characteristics and data analysis method. Picture on the left was obtained by using EARL compliant reconstruction settings, and the picture on the right was generated using the vendor provided point spread function (*PSF*) reconstruction method. Below the impact on SUV_{max} and SUV_{peak} for the lesion (*blue* area within the *red* contour) and liver are shown. By simply changing reconstruction settings, a large change in SUV and a moderate change in metabolically active tumor volume (*MATV*), in particular for the lesion, can be observed (Data was provided by S. Stroobants, UZA, Antwerp, Belgium)

1.2–2.3 may indicate poor quantitative accuracy. Yet, one should be aware that factors, such as granulopoiesis-stimulating factors (GSFs) or disease, could affect liver uptake, and in these cases deviating liver uptake should not be interpreted as poor PET image quality. The magnitude of SUV itself or its relative change contains

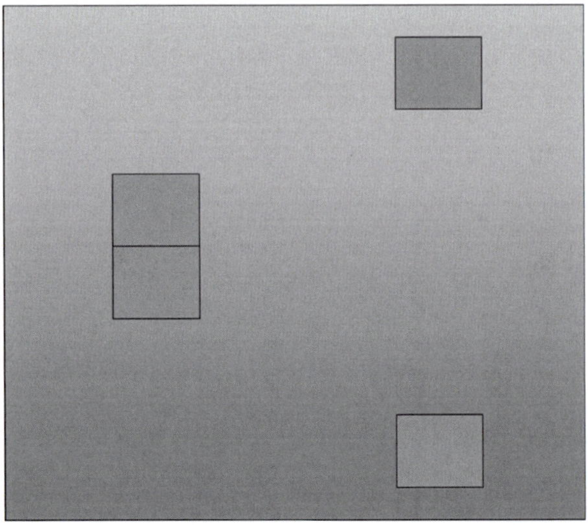

Fig. 15.4 Misleading intensity observation caused by the human visual system. All small squares within the large background area have *exactly* the same gray level. By changing the background gray level surrounding the small square, the visually apparent gray level of that smaller square seems to change. The figure demonstrates that visual assessment of tracer uptake intensity may be misled by the human visual system and may emphasize the need for more quantitative (objective) reads

prognostic or predictive information. The challenge for using FDG PET/CT as a quantitative imaging biomarker first relies on performing the studies in a standardized manner and, subsequently, deriving quantitative cutoffs for diagnosis and/or response assessment. Response criteria have been proposed by the EORTC (Young et al. 1999) and, more recently, Wahl et al. (2009) proposed the PERCIST criteria. In both cases the suggested change in SUV to reflect a true metabolic response was about 30%. For both criteria, this value seems to be based on observed test-retest repeatabilities (de Langen et al. 2012), suggesting that SUV changes beyond 30% are likely to reflect true changes in tumor metabolic activity. Yet, larger SUV changes may be required in specific cases for a clinically meaningful change. For example, Lin et al. (2007) suggest that an SUV decrease of ~65% can be used to differentiate between good and poor responders for lymphoma patients. Yet, Zander et al. (2011) showed that PERCIST criteria may be a good system for solid cancers. Now that the basic components, guidelines, and an accreditation program have been realized, these criteria can and should be further validated and developed.

15.4 Other Quantitative Metrics Than SUV

Apart from quantifying tracer uptake by means of SUV measured at a certain uptake period, full quantitative analysis can be performed based on dynamic imaging, collection of (arterial) input function, and compartment analysis. The full quantitative approach has certain advantages over simple uptake measures, although large-scale clinical applicability is limited due to limited axial coverage, overall scanner occupation, and data analysis complexity. On the other hand, SUVs do not take tracer uptake kinetic behavior into account (Vriens et al. 2010). One of the first papers describing the change of SUV over time, published by Lowe et al. (1995), showed that some lesions may have a higher uptake than other lesions at early time points (<60 min) but can have lower uptake at later time points. Clearly, evaluation of tracer uptake at a fixed uptake time will not be able to take differences in kinetics into account. Moreover, input functions, describing the availability of the radiotracer in plasma over time, may be different between subjects and/or can change during therapy. This has been observed by Freedman et al. (2003), Doot et al. (2007) and Cheebsumon et al. (2011a) where changes in SUV were smaller than changes in quantitative measures of glucose consumption. These papers demonstrate that full quantitative analysis may play a role in the (early) validation of simplified quantitative measures, such as SUV, for response assessment, as was also discussed by Lammertsma et al. (2006) For other tracers, full quantitative analysis may be required to determine which simplified analysis approach, such as SUVs with different normalizations or tumor to background ratios, can be used best as surrogate for full quantitative analysis.

As suggested above various other quantitative metrics may be derived from an FDG PET/CT study. A very good correlation between SUV and glucose consumption is usually observed, but in some specific situations, other parameters, such as tumor to blood ratios, may be more suitable as surrogate for full quantitative analysis, as was also shown by van den Hoff et al. (2013). Moreover, recently it has been demonstrated that metabolically active tumor volumes have prognostic and/or predictive value (Zhang et al. 2012) and research is dedicated to derive more accurate and precise PET-based tumor delineation methods (Cheebsumon et al. 2011b). Tumors may also show specific intratumoral tracer uptake distributions, and methods are being developed to characterize tracer uptake texture and heterogeneity (Cook et al. 2013; Lambin et al. 2012; van Velden et al. 2011). It is not fully clear yet what the clinical value of tracer uptake heterogeneity measures are, although there are some initial reports suggesting potential added value as prognostic value.

PET/CT offers opportunities to derive various quantitative data, which may be helpful in the clinic and for trials. In all cases robust quantitative measures can be derived only when the PET/CT are collected in a standardized manner. When these quantitative measures meet the basic requirements for a biomarker, being accurate, repeatable, and reproducible, their clinical value can be assessed and subsequently use for patient care.

15.5 Application for Other Tracers and Future Developments

The principles for PET/CT harmonization are the same for most radiotracers and radioisotopes. Likely future guidelines will be developed, and accreditation programs will be expanded to include long-lived isotopes, such as ^{89}Zr. However, different radiotracers measure different biological characteristics, and consequently, issues related to biological factors are different. Patient study preparation and optimal uptake time are radiotracer specific and should be adjusted. Moreover, some of the technical factors, such as calibration of the systems, require additional verification. Dose calibrators may have different sensitivities for measuring different radioisotope than ^{18}F, and PET/CT system should correctly compensate for differences in positron abundance, etc. It is therefore mandatory to verify correct cross-calibration between dose calibrators and PET/CT systems for each positron-emitting isotope being used. For some radioisotopes, such as ^{89}Zr, this is relatively straightforward, as was recently shown by Makris et al. (2014). However, for radioisotopes that emit prompt gammas, such as ^{124}I, ensuring accurate quantification and calibration of systems is more challenging. Also differences in positron range may affect SUV recovery coefficients. Yet, calibration and image quality harmonization procedures similar to those applied for FDG by EARL can be applied to optimize harmonized quantification in multicenter studies. In other words, the basic principles are independent on the radioisotope being used, but specific adaptations in image processing and data analysis procedures may be required.

The publication of guidelines also triggered research on further improving quantitative accuracy and image quality. For example, the European guideline suggest to adjust the amount of FDG activity linearly with patient weight, although it has been recognized that other relationships may be needed to obtain more uniform image quality across patients with different weights. Recently, Groot et al. (2013) showed that a quadratic relationship between activity and weight may further improve harmonization of image quality and this relationship could be considered in future guidelines. Further refinements in accreditation programs may also be the inclusion of (minimal) performance criteria for image noise levels. Specific quality control procedures and measurements may be designed to determine the minimal amount of activity in combination with scan duration and patient weight for each system, such that optimization of minimal activity is based on the actual system performance. In this way new developments that improve image quality can be translated into adjustment of overall scan duration and/or lowering activity to reduce radiation dose.

Quantitative image analysis is still mostly based on SUVmax measurements. SUVmax may suffer from upward bias due to image noise and other volume of interest approaches may be considered. SUVpeak, defined as the average SUV in a 1 ml spherical volume of interest located such that it represents the highest value across the tumor, could be an attractive alternative. SUVpeak is not only less sensitive to image noise, but it is also able to mitigate the effects of (small residual) differences in image characteristics on quantification (Makris et al. 2013). However, it may also suffer more from partial volume effects in case of small lesions (<1 cm diameter) than SUVmax. Moreover, to date SUVpeak is still not widely available, as was observed in a recent survey among EARL-accredited sites where less than 50% of the imaging sites are able to provide SUVpeak results (data not shown). SUVmean is based on the average SUV in an irregularly drawn volume of interest. At present, there are many different 3D volume of interest methods implemented and developed, and there is not yet a consensus which of these methods could be used as standards. Therefore, further exploring use of SUVpeak may be a good first extension of current guidelines and accreditation programs.

New applications beyond oncology are foreseen to become more and more incorporated within multicenter studies and/or as part of routine clinical workup. FDG and/or amyloid brain imaging may be one of these candidates. The Alzheimer's Disease Neuroimaging Initiative, ADNI, has collected numerous PET neuroimaging data across many sites in order to further introduce and validate, e.g., FDG PET as imaging biomarker in diagnosis and for treatment response evaluation in Alzheimer's disease (AD) (Cummings 2010). Several collaborative groups and scientific organizations are now developing PET system validation/accreditation programs specifically to support multicenter FDG brain imaging.

15.6 International Efforts for Harmonizing Imaging Biomarkers

The need for standardization and harmonization has been recognized by several organizations and collaborative groups. Scientific societies and organizations, such as the Society of Nuclear Medicine and Molecular Imaging (SNMMI), European Organization for Research and Treatment of Cancer (EORTC), American College of Radiology (ACR), European Association of Nuclear Medicine (EANM), European Society of Radiology (ESR), and various collaborative groups and national societies have developed guidelines and/or are running accreditation programs. Several years ago the Radiological Society of Northern America (RSNA) took the initiative to organize round table discussion of the various stakeholder involved or interested in quantitative biomarker imaging. The RSNA started the Quantitative Imaging Biomarkers Alliance (QIBA), led by Daniel Sullivan, with the aim of validating and qualifying several imaging biomarkers (Buckler et al. 2011). QIBA initially focused on 3 imaging biomarkers, namely, volumetric computed tomography (CT), dynamic contrast-enhanced magnetic resonance imaging (DCE-MRI), and FDG PET/CT. For each of these imaging biomarkers, committees were formed with representatives from the various scientific societies, experts or opinion leaders, and display software and imaging equipment manufacturers. The main goal of these committees was to generate a so-called QIBA profile, a document that in detail recommends actions, requirements, and specifications where users and equipment should comply with in order to achieve the defined required imaging biomarker performance. The profile for FDG PET/CT can be found at the QIBA/RSNA web page. Together with drafting the profile, which mainly addresses performance of equipment, an international consensus imaging procedure guideline was drafted as well. This effort is referred to uniformity of protocol in clinical trials (UPICT). The FDG PET/CT UPICT document can be found at the abovementioned website as well. The UPICT protocol is derived from various published guidelines or scientific paper and tries to develop an internationally supported consensus imaging guideline. Both documents, the QIBA profile and UPICT protocol, have been reviewed ("public comment") and have been published. It is anticipated that by this international effort, users, scientific organization, and vendors collectively support and realize FDG PET/CT imaging as a validated and qualified imaging biomarker.

References

Beyer T, Czernin J, Freudenberg LS. Variations in clinical PET/CT operations: results of an international survey of active PET/CT users. J Nucl Med. 2011;52(2):303–10.

Biggi A, Gallamini A, Chauvie S, et al. International validation study for interim PET in ABVD-treated, advanced stage hodgkin lymphoma: interpretation criteria and concordance rate among reviewers. J Nucl Med. 2013;54:683–90.

Biomarkers Definitions Working Group. Biomarkers and surrogate endpoints: preferred definitions and conceptual framework. Clin Pharmacol Ther. 2001;69:89–95.

Boellaard R. Standards for PET image acquisition and quantitative data analysis. J Nucl Med. 2009;50 Suppl 1:11S–20.

Boellaard R, O'Doherty MJ, Weber WA, et al. FDG PET and PET/CT: EANM procedure guidelines for tumour PET imaging: version 1.0. Eur. J Nucl Med Mol Imaging. 2010; 37:181–200.

Brady Z, Taylor ML, Haynes M, et al. The clinical application of PET/CT: a contemporary review. Australas Phys Eng Sci Med. 2008;31:90–109.

Buckler AJ, Bresolin L, Dunnick NR, Sullivan DC. A collaborative enterprise for multi-stakeholder participation in the advancement of quantitative imaging. Radiology. 2011;258:906–14.

Cheebsumon P, Velasquez LM, Hoekstra CJ, et al. Measuring response to therapy using FDG PET: semi-quantitative and full kinetic analysis. Eur J Nucl Med Mol Imaging. 2011a;38:832–42.

Cheebsumon P, Yaqub M, van Velden FH, Hoekstra OS, Lammertsma AA, Boellaard R. Impact of [(1)(8)F]FDG PET imaging parameters on automatic tumour delineation: need for improved tumour delineation methodology. Eur J Nucl Med Mol Imaging. 2011b;38:2136–44.

Cook GJ, Yip C, Siddique M, et al. Are pretreatment 18F-FDG PET tumor textural features in non-small cell lung cancer associated with response and survival after chemoradiotherapy? J Nucl Med. 2013;54:19–26.

Cummings JL. Integrating ADNI results into Alzheimer's disease drug development programs. Neurobiol Aging. 2010;31:1481–92.

Czernin J, Schelbert HR. PET/CT in cancer patient management – introduction. J Nucl Med. 2007;48:2S–3.

de Groot EH, Post N, Boellaard R, Wagenaar NR, Willemsen AT, van Dalen JA. Optimized dose regimen for whole-body FDG-PET imaging. EJNMMI Res. 2013;3:63.

de Langen AJ, Vincent A, Velasquez LM, et al. Repeatability of 18F-FDG uptake measurements in tumors: a metaanalysis. J Nucl Med. 2012;53:701–8.

den HJ V, Oehme L, Schramm G, et al. The PET-derived tumor-to-blood standard uptake ratio (SUR) is superior to tumor SUV as a surrogate parameter of the metabolic rate of FDG. EJNMMI Res. 2013;3:77.

Doot RK, Dunnwald LK, Schubert EK, et al. Dynamic and static approaches to quantifying 18F-FDG uptake for measuring cancer response to therapy, including the effect of granulocyte CSF. J Nucl Med. 2007;48:920–5.

Fletcher JW, Djulbegovic B, Soares HP, et al. Recommendations on the use of F-18-FDG PET in oncology. J Nucl Med. 2008;49:480–508.

Freedman NM, Sundaram SK, Kurdziel K, et al. Comparison of SUV and Patlak slope for monitoring of cancer therapy using serial PET scans. Eur J Nucl Med Mol Imaging. 2003;30:46–53.

Geus-Oei LF, van der Heijden HF, Corstens FH, Oyen WJ. Predictive and prognostic value of FDG-PET in nonsmall-cell lung cancer: a systematic review. Cancer. 2007;110:1654–64.

Graham MM, Badawi RD, Wahl RL. Variations in PET/CT methodology for oncologic imaging at U.S. academic medical centers: an imaging response assessment team survey. J Nucl Med. 2011;52:311–7.

Hoekstra CJ, Paglianiti I, Hoekstra OS, et al. Monitoring response to therapy in cancer using [18F]-2-fluoro-2-deoxy-D-glucose and positron emission tomography: an overview of different analytical methods. Eur J Nucl Med. 2000;27:731–43.

Itti E, Meignan M, Berriolo-Riedinger A, et al. An international confirmatory study of the prognostic value of early PET/CT in diffuse large B-cell lymphoma: comparison between Deauville criteria and DeltaSUVmax. Eur J Nucl Med Mol Imaging. 2013;40:1312–20.

Kobe C, Scheffler M, Holstein A, et al. Predictive value of early and late residual 18F-fluorodeoxyglucose and 18F-fluorothymidine uptake using different SUV measurements in patients with non-small-cell lung cancer treated with erlotinib. Eur J Nucl Med Mol Imaging. 2012;39:1117–27.

Lambin P, Rios-Velazquez E, Leijenaar R, et al. Radiomics: extracting more information from medical images using advanced feature analysis. Eur J Cancer. 2012;48:441–6.

Lammertsma AA, Hoekstra CJ, Giaccone G, Hoekstra OS. How should we analyse FDG PET studies for monitoring tumour response? Eur J Nucl Med Mol Imaging. 2006;33 Suppl 1:16–21.

Lasnon C, Desmonts C, Quak E, et al. Harmonizing SUVs in multicentre trials when using different generation PET systems: prospective validation in non-small cell lung cancer patients. Eur J Nucl Med Mol Imaging. 2013;40(7):985–96.

Lin C, Itti E, Haioun C, et al. Early 18F-FDG PET for prediction of prognosis in patients with diffuse large B-cell lymphoma: SUV-based assessment versus visual analysis. J Nucl Med. 2007;48:1626–32.

Lowe VJ, DeLong DM, Hoffman JM, Coleman RE. Optimum scanning protocol for FDG-PET evaluation of pulmonary malignancy. J Nucl Med. 1995;36:883–7.

Makris NE, Huisman MC, Kinahan PE, Lammertsma AA, Boellaard R. Evaluation of strategies towards harmonization of FDG PET/CT studies in multicentre trials: comparison of scanner validation phantoms and data analysis procedures. Eur J Nucl Med Mol Imaging. 2013;40:1507–15.

Makris NE, Boellaard R, Visser EP, et al. Multicenter Harmonization of 89Zr PET/CT Performance. J Nucl Med. 2014;55:264–7.

Scheffler M, Zander T, Nogova L, et al. Prognostic impact of [18F]fluorothymidine and [18F] fluoro-D-glucose baseline uptakes in patients with lung cancer treated first-line with erlotinib. PLoS One. 2013;8:e53081.

Schelbert HR, Hoh CK, Royal HD, et al. Procedure guideline for tumor imaging using fluorine-18-FDG. Society of nuclear medicine. J Nucl Med. 1998;39:1302–5.

van Tinteren H, Hoekstra OS, Smit EF, et al. Effectiveness of positron emission tomography in the preoperative assessment of patients with suspected non-small-cell lung cancer: the PLUS multicentre randomised trial. Lancet. 2002;359:1388–92.

van Velden FH, Cheebsumon P, Yaqub M, et al. Evaluation of a cumulative SUV-volume histogram method for parameterizing heterogeneous intratumoural FDG uptake in non-small cell lung cancer PET studies. Eur J Nucl Med Mol Imaging. 2011;38:1636–47.

Vriens D, Visser EP, de Geus-Oei LF, Oyen WJ. Methodological considerations in quantification of oncological FDG PET studies. Eur J Nucl Med Mol Imaging. 2010;37:1408–25.

Wahl RL, Jacene H, Kasamon Y, Lodge MA. From RECIST to PERCIST: evolving considerations for PET response criteria in solid tumors. J Nucl Med. 2009;50 Suppl 1:122S–50.

Weber WA. Use of PET for monitoring cancer therapy and for predicting outcome. J Nucl Med. 2005a;46:983–95.

Weber WA. PET for response assessment in oncology: radiotherapy and chemotherapy. Br J Radiol. 2005b;78:42–9.

Young H, Baum R, Cremerius U, et al. Measurement of clinical and subclinical tumour response using [18F]-fluorodeoxyglucose and positron emission tomography: review and 1999 EORTC

recommendations. European organization for research and treatment of cancer (EORTC) PET study group. Eur J Cancer. 1999;35:1773–82.
Zander T, Scheffler M, Nogova L, et al. Early prediction of nonprogression in advanced non-small-cell lung cancer treated with erlotinib by using [18F]fluorodeoxyglucose and [18F]fluorothymidine positron emission tomography. J Clin Oncol. 2011;29:1701–8.
Zhang H, Wroblewski K, Liao S, et al. Prognostic value of metabolic tumor burden from [18F]-FDG PET in surgical patients with non-small-cell lung cancer. Acad Radiol. 2012;39:27–38.

Medical Imaging Informatics in Nuclear Medicine

16

Peter M.A. van Ooijen and Wiard Jorritsma

Abstract

Medical imaging informatics is gaining importance in medicine both in clinical practice and in scientific research. Besides radiology, nuclear medicine is also a major stakeholder in medical imaging informatics because of the variety of available imaging modalities and the imaging-oriented operation of this specialization. The amount of data produced by imaging modalities and other diagnostic devices per exam is growing steadily together with the number of exams performed, resulting in a data explosion that provides major opportunities for data analytics and data mining in big data projects. However, it can also fuse problems in storage, distribution, review, and interpretation of the enormous amounts of clinical (image) data while maintaining high-quality patient care. To tackle these problems, standardization, structuring, and automation are crucial. As one of the major producers of medical imaging data, nuclear medicine should stay at the forefront of these developments.

P.M.A. van Ooijen, MSc, PhD (✉)
Department of Radiology, University Medical Center Groningen,
University of Groningen, Groningen, The Netherlands

Center for Medical Imaging North East Netherlands,
University Medical Center Groningen, University of Groningen,
Groningen, The Netherlands
e-mail: p.m.a.van.ooijen@umcg.nl

W. Jorritsma, MSc
Department of Radiology, University Medical Center Groningen,
University of Groningen, Groningen, The Netherlands

A.W.J.M. Glaudemans et al. (eds.), *Quality in Nuclear Medicine*,
DOI 10.1007/978-3-319-33531-5_16

16.1 Data Management and the Nuclear PACS

Because of the data explosion of the past decades in the area of medical imaging in general, data management in healthcare is of growing concern and interest. This involves many different topics such as archiving, workstation review, reporting, telemedicine, and clinical workflow. Each of these topics has their own challenges and heavily depends on the advances in Medical Imaging Informatics research.

In the early years of Picture Archiving and Communication Systems (PACS) in the 1980s, nuclear medicine was one of the pioneering fields together with radiology in which these new systems were first developed and deployed (Lemke 2011). Because of this an extensive library of publications can be found regarding the digitalization of the nuclear department and the Nuclear PACS (Parker et al. 1983; Bian et al. 2009; Lemke 2011). Parker et al. already mentioned fully digital nuclear medicine department achieved as early as 1983, over 10 years before the first fully digital radiology departments were reported (Parker et al. 1983). However, with respect to becoming integrated with the rest of the hospital including workflow optimization and proper support of image display and analysis, nuclear medicine started legging behind. This trend was broken when PET-CT became more mainstream requiring a better integration with radiology and the rest of the healthcare enterprise (Zemariame et al. 2011).

When archiving data, several issues are of major importance, such as the adequate storage, the lifetime guarantee of the archive, and the safety of the archive. However, in medical imaging, an image archive is not "dead" data, and therefore image search and retrieval also have to be guaranteed over the years including the readability of old media within the archive. This is already made clear in the generally used name for these image archives, Picture Archiving and Communication System (PACS), which clearly shows that in medical imaging, it is not only about the archiving of (image) data but also about the communication of that data. To achieve this communication, standards have been developed including the Digital Imaging and Communication in Medicine (DICOM) standard to ensure the storage of data in a standardized image format and the proper communication with and operation of the digital image archive. The main focus in these developments has been on radiology and not nuclear medicine. However, nuclear medicine is forced to achieve integration and seamless connectivity with the more general archiving systems generally developed for radiology which gives rise to a number of challenges and problems (Wallis 2004).

16.2 The PACS Core

The Picture Archiving and Communication System (PACS) is a complex system of different tools and services that together take care of the storage, distribution, and display of medical imaging data. To achieve this, the PACS core generally consists of a number of basic components.

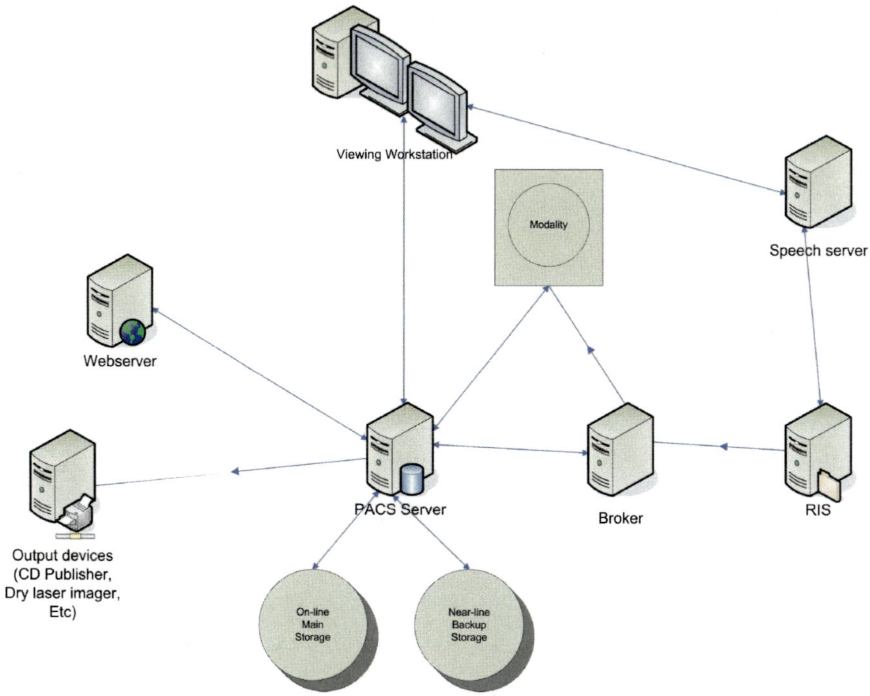

Fig. 16.1 General components of a Picture Archiving and Communications System

The different basic components of a PACS are shown in Fig. 16.1. The communication between the different components is possible through a network. In most current implementations, this network is set up in a star configured switched network, typically with network speeds of 1 Gbit/s or higher.

The main PACS consists of one or more servers that take care of the distribution of image-related data and the database service of the PACS. The PACS stores the images it receives from imaging modalities or other sources (e.g., secondary captures from postprocessing workstations) and distributes them towards the online main storage and the near-line backup storage. Upon request of a viewing workstation, the image data is transmitted to the viewing workstation. In some cases, the data will also be transmitted to a separate web server providing images to departments outside the imaging department.

Different output devices are still available to distribute the image data to other entities such as patients or other health institutions, for example, by publishing CDs or by printing films on a dry laser imager.

The core of the PACS consists of a system that receives incoming DICOM images, distributes DICOM images to different locations, and sends DICOM images to different systems upon request. In most cases this PACS core consists of multiple servers covering the different tasks. Some of the tasks can be performed on multiple servers to ensure availability by having redundancy. Furthermore, the use of multiple servers for the same task can also increase the capacity of the system by having them all fully operational and balancing the load between them. The PACS core also contains the database that holds all the information on what is stored in the entire PACS. This database is a crucial part of the system because the inability to access the database will completely block the access to the image data.

16.3 DICOM

In 1983 the ACR (American College of Radiology) and the NEMA (National Electrical Manufacturers Association) defined a standard for the interconnection of medical imaging devices, known as ACR-NEMA Version 1.0. The standard included a list of required data elements and a specification of the physical hardware for connecting the devices. This first version was released at the RSNA in 1985, followed by Version 2.0 at the RSNA in 1988. Up until then only point-to-point networking was specified. However, in 1990 work was started to add a network standard. This resulted in a combination of these network standards and the ACR-NEMA Version 2.0 to lay the foundation of the current Digital Image Communication in Medicine (DICOM) standard (version 3.0) [Hindel 1994].

The three main goals of the DICOM standard are defined as (Pelanek 1997):

1. Establish a standard for communication in a networked environment.
2. Set minimum requirements for claiming performance to the standard.
3. Allow interoperability, not just interconnection, between multiple vendors' equipment.

To meet these main goals, DICOM is defined to conform with layer 7 (application level) of the OSI (Open System Interconnect) reference model.

So in summary, DICOM is a standard for handling, storing, printing, and transmitting information in medical imaging. It includes a file format definition and a network communication protocol. The communication protocol is an application protocol that uses TCP/IP to communicate between systems. DICOM files can be exchanged between two entities that are capable of receiving image and patient data in DICOM format following a fixed set of communication rules.

A DICOM data object (or file) consists of a number of attributes, including items such as name, patient ID, etc., and also one special attribute containing the image pixel data. A single DICOM file can only contain one data instance (e.g., an image). An image instance may have multiple frames, allowing the storage of cine loops or other multiframe data into one single DICOM file (e.g., used for conventional coronary angiography cine loops). The image data can either be uncompressed or compressed. Compression can be done both lossless and lossy using a variety of compression standards including JPEG, JPEG lossless, JPEG 2000, and run-length encoding (RLE). Although in most cases the DICOM file body consists of a medical image, it can also contain other information objects such as medical reports or even audio recordings. The header of a DICOM file consists of patient information (name, ID, birthdate, sex, etc.), study information (referring physician, accession number, study instance UID (=Unique Identifier), etc.), series information (series description, series instance UID, etc.), and the instance (image) information (row/column size, photometric interpretation, etc.).

In DICOM, dedicated file structure is defined for each Acquisition Modality including those involved in nuclear medicine such as NM and PET.

Since nuclear medicine modalities were originally digital imaging modalities, the field developed its own alternatives to standards such as DICOM at an early phase and thus was reluctant to adopt to these standards dictated from other imaging specialties such as radiology where images were mainly two-dimensional, static and monochrome (Somer 2006).

A topic not directly playing a role in nuclear medicine is relating to the acquisition of nuclear medicine data that is the requirement to define the Gross Tumor Volume for Radiotherapy (Sattler et al. 2010). This requires dedicated support and standardization to allow proper formatting and storage of this data. To support this a dedicated addition was developed to the DICOM standard resulting in the DICOM RT information object definitions (IOD) regulating the proper storage and processing of radiation therapy planning. The RT structure set consists of several DICOM RT object such as RT-Plan, RT-Struct, RT-Dose, and RT-Image. If measurements are made on workstations outside the radiotherapy domain, the DICOM RT IODs should be properly supported by the workstation and the PACS in order to ensure that the RT object can be imported into the systems at radiotherapy. If measurements are made at dedicated image-processing workstations at the radiotherapy department, CT, MR, and PET data can be transferred to those workstations using standard IODs. However, to store and retrieve the RT IODs, they should be supported by the general PACS.

16.4 DICOM Conformance Statement

A DICOM Conformance Statement has to be made available by the vendor for each imaging modality, workstation, or other DICOM node that is claimed to support DICOM. The conformance statement describes the DICOM capabilities and features of the product in a standardized, defined, manner. These documents are the most commonly used specifications relating to the DICOM standard and provide key information to determine interconnectivity and interoperability between two DICOM nodes. The DICOM Conformance Statement is a public document, which means that all vendors have their DICOM Conformance Statements publicly available, in most cases directly accessible on their respective websites.

When purchasing new equipment, the DICOM Conformance Statements can be used to assess whether the required functionality for interoperability with existing, already running, DICOM compatible equipment is supported adequately. In case of nuclear medicine devices, for example, the PET and NM Information Object Definitions (IODs) should be present and Service Class User/Provider pairs should be available for storage and query/retrieval.

16.5 Integration Problems in Nuclear Medicine and PACS

In the first few decades of PACS, the systems were dedicated to a single department or group of modalities, and subsystems were installed throughout the hospitals in order to satisfy the unit or department storage needs. This led to a diversity of systems that were pretty much stand alone and unable to communicate with each other (the so-called mini-PACS). However, the back end of these systems was very similar, and when conforming to standards such as DICOM and IHE, they were in principle universally applicable in all imaging departments and to all DICOM-enabled modalities. This eventually led to a more centralized storage into a radiology or ICT PACS of the data originating from different departments resulting in enterprise wide systems. All these developments were originating from the radiology departments that aimed at a centralized, multimodality, departmental PACS which would be the platform for all imaging modalities. However, because of this focus on radiology, specific issues concerning nuclear medicine modalities were not tackled. These issues would arise because of proprietary information stored in private fields by the manufacturer of NM acquisition devices and poor support of NM modalities in the DICOM standard (Somer 2006). One of the reasons for this poor support of NM modalities in the DICOM standard was the fact that nuclear medicine had already developed its own file format standard with the INTERFILE format developed by the Working Group 1 of the European project COST-B2 on quality assurance of nuclear medicine software (Todd-Pokropek et al. 1992). This project aimed to develop an appropriate mechanism to allow nuclear medicine data interchange between systems of different vendors and achieved this by defining an intermediate file format (INTERFILE). This format was widely adopted and specifically designed for use in nuclear medicine. It provided all required properties and possibilities, which was not the case with DICOM which was a broad multimodality standard encompassing the file format and communication standards.

Possible challenges one could run into when connecting nuclear medicine modalities to a DICOM-based PACS are (Wallis 2004):

- NM images can be stored into the PACS, but the data cannot be used to its full possibilities when retrieving the images back to a nuclear medicine system.
- Quantitative measurements are not possible anymore after retrieving PET images from the PACS.
- Data presentation of nuclear medicine images on the PACS workstation is incomplete.
- Data presentation of nuclear medicine images on the PACS workstation is not usable for nuclear medicine viewing and interpretation.

Common causes for the challenges presented are the aforementioned inclusion of proprietary, vendor-specific, information into private fields of the DICOM header. Most PACSs conserve these proprietary fields and thus also include them when images are retrieved. However, some PACS vendors are internally not keeping the

DICOM files but copy them into a proprietary format reassembling the DICOM files upon export. In this case, if the PACS is not configured to properly handle the proprietary information, it will get lost and not be present in the reassembled DICOM files. A similar loss of information can be caused by the modality archiving the data because of the use of incorrect DICOM header elements when storing data to a PACS (e.g., using the NM Information Object Definition for PET images). These issues have a great impact on the quality of patient care and thus are the subject of debate. This leads to the intention to better develop the implementation of the DICOM standard into nuclear medicine.

Therefore, to tackle these issues and to move into the era of DICOM, the Society of Nuclear Medicine (SNM) created a taskforce in 2000 that had to evaluate digital communication issues in nuclear medicine. This leads to the founding of the SNM DICOM Working Group whose goal was to improve the DICOM connectivity and interoperability for nuclear medicine (Wallis 2004). However, to fully allow the interoperability and connectivity to flourish in nuclear medicine, the mere implementation of standards like DICOM is not sufficient. This also requires to achieve consensus on how to utilize the defined standards for the integration between information systems conforming to these standards. Therefore, the SNM turned to the Integrating the Healthcare Enterprise (IHE) organization to start the design and implementation of workflow profiles for nuclear medicine that aim to achieve this consensus and allow proper interoperability.

A further boost to improve interconnection with other systems and departments within the hospital started when PET-CT became more mainstream requiring a better integration with radiology and the rest of the healthcare enterprise (Zemariame et al. 2011). The multimodality imaging approach required the implementation of DICOM Modality Worklist features, the ability to compare studies (recent and old), the support of PET and CT on a single workstation, and the ability to access the electronic medical record (EMR). This had a high impact on the clinical workflow of nuclear medicine and the way the nuclear medicine workstations were designed and implemented.

16.6 Clinical Workflow: IHE in Nuclear Medicine

In 1999 the Radiological Society of North America (RSNA) and the Healthcare Information and Management Systems Society started a collaborative project called Integrating the Healthcare Enterprise (IHE). The aim of this IHE initiative was to create profiles that specify in detail how standards, such as DICOM and HL-7, could and should be used to exchange information between different systems (actors) in a variety of scenarios (Zemariame et al. 2011) to improve interoperability among healthcare systems. The IHE profiles are not regarded as standards and thus are not obligatory to be used by vendors; the compliance to IHE profiles must be requested by the user on voluntary basis. This implied that IHE profiles should be requested by the users though inclusion into purchase RFPs (request for proposals) and contracts when buying new or upgrading equipment.

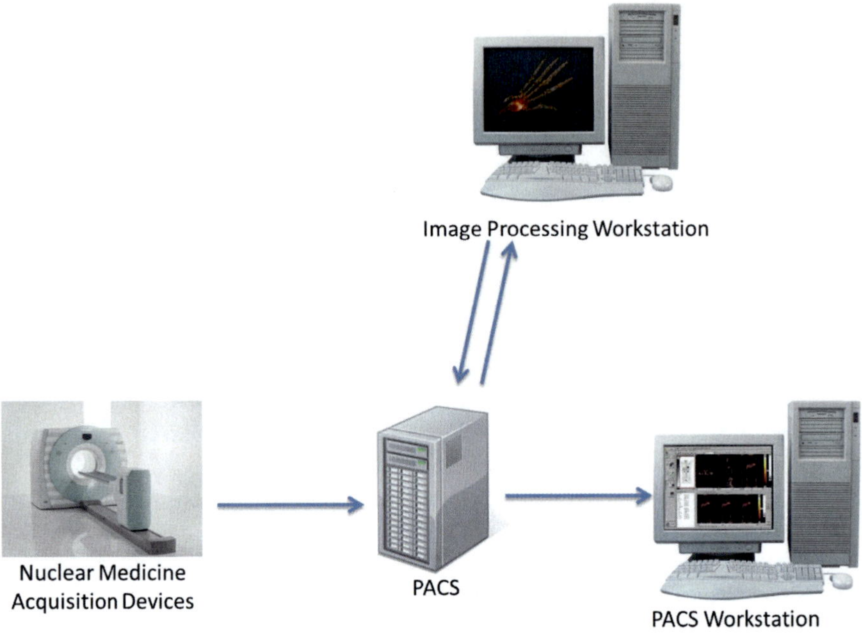

Fig. 16.2 The actors involved in the NM profile. The acquisition devices (Acquisition Modality actor), the PACS (Image Archive/Manager actor), the Image Processing Workstation (Evidence Creator actor), and the PACS Workstation (Image Display actor)

The IHE integration profiles for nuclear medicine were originally based on the, already mentioned, work of the SNM procedure guideline and include dedicated nuclear medicine profiles such as the NM Image Profile. The actors involved are the Acquisition Modality as creator of the original data, the Image Archive/Manager (PACS), the Evidence Creator (e.g., a postprocessing workstation) as creator of result images after postprocessing, and the Image Display (e.g., a general PACS workstation) (Fig. 16.2). In this setup, the Evidence Creator could also be partly integrated into the acquisition device. The main goals of the nuclear medicine profile are first to highlight the unusual characteristics of nuclear medicine images and second to define a set of requirements for dealing with nuclear medicine images and to increase interoperability with respect to nuclear medicine data (Wallis 2004). By doing this, the NM profile provides a set of specifications that define how NM systems and other systems such as PACS should interact when dealing with nuclear medicine data. Figure 16.3 shows how this is presented in the IHE profile documentation. This schematic introduces the actor modalities, PACS systems, display systems, and workstation each with their own set of possible transactions (such as for example Create, Query, Retrieve, Store). A modality may create, store, and transmit NM images. A PACS system (Image Archive/Manager actor) may store, manage, and/or display NM images. The display systems used by physicians such as radiologists and cardiologists may query, retrieve, and display NM images. The

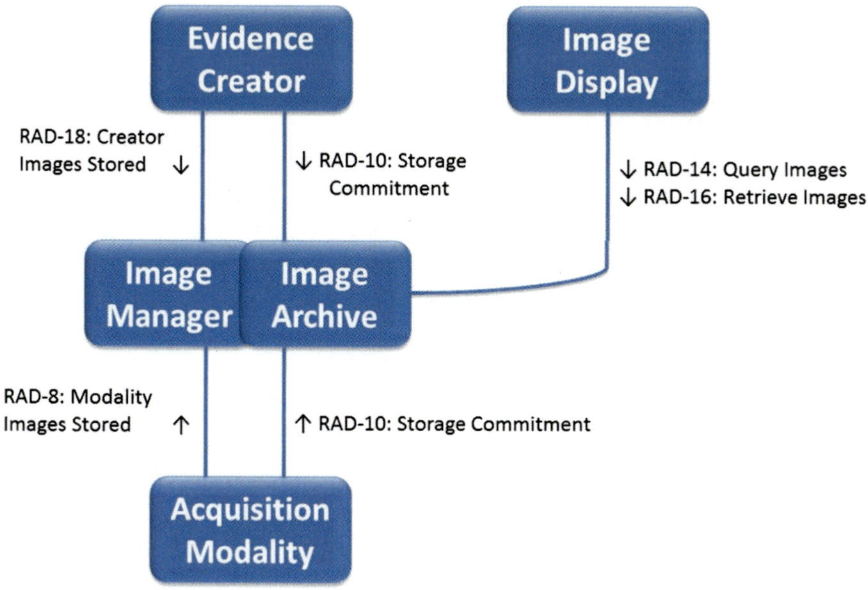

Fig. 16.3 Actors and transactions of the IHE Nuclear Medicine Image Profile (IHE Wiki 2013)

workstations (or Evidence Creators), typically used by nuclear medicine physicians, may retrieve, process, and display NM image and are able to create evidence documents (images). This process is summarized in Fig. 16.3.

To improve the image display, requirements were also defined to create dedicated display profiles for practical display of nuclear medicine images. An example of the dedicated specification for nuclear medicine is the implementation of independent control of upper and lower levels instead of the, in radiology used, window and level setting. The image display includes General NM Image Option, a Cardiac NM Option, a Result Screen Export Option, and an MPR (Multiplanar Reformation) Option. After the adoption of the initial IHE nuclear medicine profile, a profile for image fusion of PET/CT data was soon added.

The major benefits in complying to the IHE profiles specified for nuclear medicine are for the nuclear medicine physician who will be able to distribute images with the confidence that quality will be maintained by ensuring the storage of image data in a manner that will allow fully functional retrieval and also ensuring the quality of display of those images. The profiles will also provide aid in displaying nuclear medicine images in a proper way at the general workstation and are thus also beneficial to other physicians such as the radiologists and cardiologist.

Some of the profiles available in IHE are general profiles that can be applied to all image data-producing departments including radiology and nuclear medicine. An example of such a profile closely related to quality management in both radiology and nuclear medicine is the IHE REM (Radiation Exposure Monitoring) profile (see Fig. 16.4) that was introduced at the connectathon in 2009. Several commercial

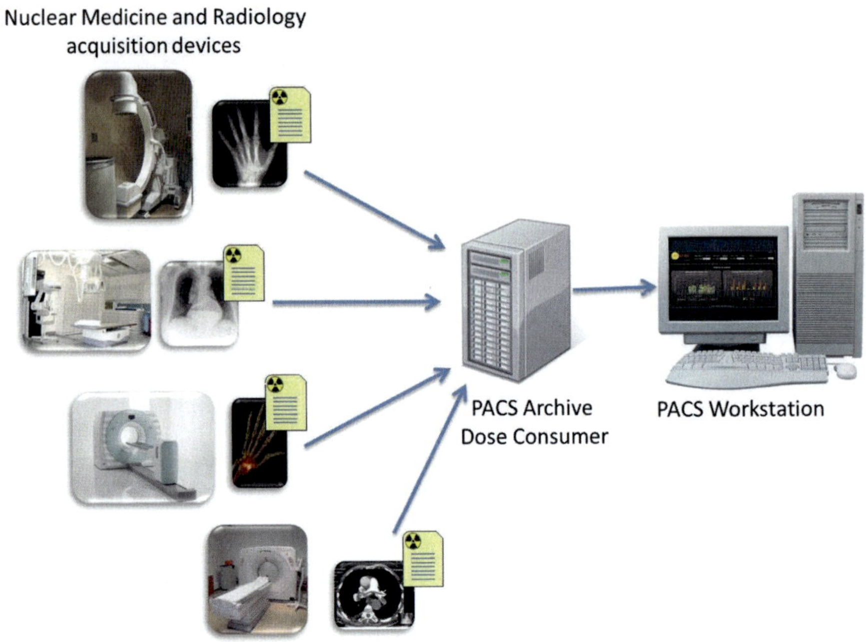

Fig. 16.4 Schematic of the IHE workflow profile for Radiation Exposure Monitoring (REM)

and open-source software tools are currently available for dose reporting that support the REM profile. A major problem still current in dose reporting is the fact that all modalities have their own method for export of dose information including MPPS (Modality Performed Procedure Step), images, secondary captures of screen information, and RDSR (Radiation Dose Structured Report). Data collection is hampered by this variety of data structures and also by the fact that to get information out of images or secondary captures, character recognition and interpretation are required which are prone to failure and thus could introduce inconsistency in the data. Furthermore, to obtain valid dose information from a DICOM header requires correct interpretation and completion of all required header items by the acquisition devices as well as by the dose consumer.

Another profile developed for general radiology use, but expected to be most used in nuclear medicine, is the Image Fusion Profile (Wallis 2006). To comply to the Image Fusion Profile, systems have to support DICOM objects especially created for image fusion. These DICOM objects are the registration object, defining how to images are aligned, and the blending presentation state, defining how the fused image data should be presented on screen including all image settings and the registration object. The same actors as defined in Figs. 16.2 and 16.3 are involved, with the addition of the dedicated DICOM objects.

The IHE profiles are tested in a so-called connectathon that allows cross-testing with other vendors during live networking sessions. At such a connectathon, companies that have implemented IHE profiles come together and test their compliance to the IHE profiles by connecting to a central test infrastructure and with each other's implementation. When the tests are successful, this is listed as such on the IHE connectathon website, and the respective companies can claim that they are IHE compliant for the specific IHE profiles they successfully tested. These connectathons are organized and refereed by the IHE in several places around the world.

Of the 37 companies that evaluated the NM Image Profile at the connectathons of the IHE (Connectathon 2013), the majority focused on support of the Image Manager actor (32/37 = 86.5 %); the other three actors are less supported. Acquisition Modality was only supported by 3 (8.1 %), Evidence Creator by 5 (13.5 %), and Image Display by 14 (37.8 %). Most vendors only supported one of the actors (28/37 = 75.7 %), four supported two actors (10.8 %), two supported three actors (5.4 %), and three supported all four actors defined (8.1 %). The limited support of the Acquisition Modality actor can be explained by the fact that there are not that many modality companies involved in NM. However, the limited support of the Evidence Creator and especially the Image Display actors shows that implementation of IHE profiles in nuclear medicine is still very limited. When querying the IHE connectathon result database for the Image Fusion Profile, the result of this query shows that only one vendor has tested and is indicated to support this profile for the Acquisition Modality. No other vendors have demonstrated this profile at a connectathon yet.

16.7 The Nuclear Medicine Workstation

The unique part of each imaging department is not in the PACS core, but in the viewing application since every medical specialty has its own specific demands with respect to image display, visualization, and processing. Therefore, a current trend is visible towards large, institution wide, PACS systems with dedicated viewing applications or workstations for the different specialties as was also shown earlier in the section on IHE.

Nuclear medicine cannot use standard workstations provided by a (radiology) PACS vendor because of the specific requirements for the evaluation of NM exams. Most of these radiology workstations are optimized for viewing and handling CT and MR images which might be awkward or even impossible to use for nuclear medicine examinations. Therefore, the full PACS workstations are mostly limited to the radiology department and some kind of Webclient is made available for the rest of the hospital. However, these Webclients are mainly provided for integration in electronic patient records (EPR) to allow different physicians a quick and easy access to the imaging data and are in most cases also too basic for the specific needs of NM. Therefore, the workstations in NM should receive extra attention and should be made dedicated for the tasks at hand. Besides the ability to merely display and evaluate nuclear medicine imaging data, the advent of multimodality examinations that really took flight with the introduction of the integrated PET-CT modalities that allow simultaneous acquisition of both PET and CT introduces additional requirements for image interpretation, navigation, and communication software. As mentioned before, the profiles as specified by IHE aim to achieve a more dedicated nuclear medicine workstation with improved quality of patient care.

Within the field of nuclear medicine, many of the studies will be multimodality combining the acquired data of different imaging modalities to obtain adequate information on the condition of the patient and to allow diagnosis. A typical requirement in a viewer suitable for nuclear medicine work up is the ability to support both CT and NM images (Im et al. 2010). This involves both the support of basic functionality such as window/level, zoom, pan, scroll, maximum intensity projection (MIP), etc. and the support of more dedicated capabilities such as pseudo-coloring, region of interest (ROI) identification with the ability to display standardized uptake values (SUV). However, software developed as general PACS workstation viewer will not provide adequate support of multimodality display and evaluation of imaging data. Therefore, in many cases, multimodality data such as PET-CT results are stored as secondary captures or snapshots of already fused images generated by the nuclear medicine physician. This limits the use of these results since the secondary captures are fixed, and manipulations such as independent interaction with the different datasets, realignment of the two datasets, and adjustment of the amount of blending are impossible.

Another main issue is the registration and simultaneous, fused, display of CT and PET or CT and SPECT imaging. A partial solution for the problem is the display ready production of secondary captures of pre-fused data from the modality itself. However, in this case the adjustment of image properties such as the thresholding and fusion opacity is not possible anymore resulting in nonoptimal display (Somer 2006). One possible solution proposed to obtain a more convenient visualization of image fusion on a PACS workstation that does not support "real" image fusion is called SADS (Sliced alternating DICOM series) (Vogel et al. 2005). With this solution the images from – for example – CT, PET, and already fused images are combined into a single series with alternating presentation. When scrolling through a series in a standard PACS viewer, the user will be presented with the CT, PET, and fused image of the same location in sequence (Fig. 16.5). When the PACS viewer is capable of standard display of three images of one series simultaneously side by side, the CT, PET, and fused images can be viewed per location at the same time. Although the limitation of reduced interaction possibilities still

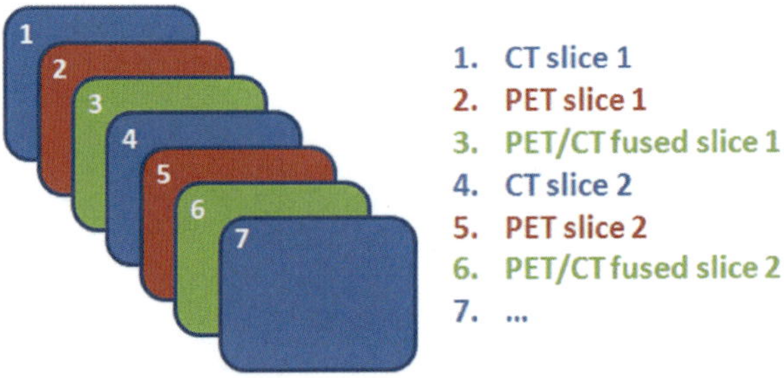

Fig. 16.5 SADS principle

exists, this method could provide a proper display with easy anatomical correlation of multimodality data.

However, when preregistered data is not available, the problem with fused multimodality imaging is the difference in data properties with respect of voxel size, slice thickness, field of view, and matrix size of the two modalities that need to be fused. With separate acquisition of CT and PET/SPECT, this requires a first step of image registration and a second step of fusion. With newer PET-CT modalities, the registration is no longer required, but proper fusion is still a must.

An issue that could occur in general PACS workstations is the inability to deal properly with the powerful image format of the Nuclear Medicine Information Object Definition of the DICOM standard (Wallis 2004). A variety of different information object such as different views, phases, and multienergy can be encapsulated into a single DICOM image. The implementation of general PACS workstations is frequently not properly executed to handle such complex instances and thus fails in the correct interpretation and display of these images.

The issues described clearly demonstrate that dedicated viewing software is required for display of nuclear medicine acquisitions. This is also illustrated by the fact that both the Society of Nuclear Medicine (SNM) and the American Heart Association (AHA) have included reference standards for minimum display functionality into their guidelines. The SNM has defined the minimum display functionality for remote nuclear medicine viewing systems (Parker et al. 2002); the AHA has provided a reference standard for the display of myocardial perfusion imaging (Cerqueira et al. 2002).

Based on published literature, the following are the basic capabilities required by a nuclear medicine workstation in order to obtain high-quality data assessment and diagnosis (Barbaras et al. 2007; Im et al. 2010; Haraguchi et al. 2011):

- *Must have*:
  - Navigation capabilities for paging through image sequences
  - Simultaneous display of native and fused image sequences
  - Multiplanar Reformation (MPR) capabilities for native and fused data
  - Adjustable color and transparency
  - Ability to link sequences for simultaneous scrolling or cine-mode viewing
  - Cursor linking in all displays
  - Manual drawing and/or outline tools to define regions of interest (ROIs)
  - Semiquantitative analysis of activity by calculating the maximum and mean standardized uptake value (SUV_{max}, SUV_{mean}) for an ROI
  - Ability to compare PET, CT, and fused series from different dates simultaneously
- *Nice to have*:
  - Maximum intensity projection (MIP)
  - Ability to copy images from one study to another
  - Ability to rotate and mirror images
  - Export of cine loops to avi-file format
  - Adding pointers and text annotations

Because of the requirement for dedicated tools for evaluation of nuclear medicine data, a multitude of commercial and noncommercial solutions are available for image review.

16.8 Usability

Besides the technical specifications of a nuclear medicine workstation, the usability of the workstation is also very important. Usability refers to the effectiveness, efficiency, and satisfaction with which users can interact with the workstation (Cockton et al. 2003; ISO 1998). Because computer software plays a vital role in the workflow of many healthcare professionals, including those in nuclear medicine, usability studies are becoming increasingly common in the medical domain (Jaspers 2009). Most of these studies (e.g., Bakhshi-Raiez et al. 2012; Menon et al. 2012; Chan et al. 2011) evaluate a single system and aim to improve its usability. These types of studies are very important, because they lead to software that is more consistent with the physical and cognitive capabilities of its end users and thereby allows them to interact with the software more effectively, efficiently, and enjoyably.

There are also studies (e.g., Bazak et al. 2000; Boehm et al. 2004; Jorritsma et al. 2014) that compare the usability of multiple systems. This approach is useful in a software selection process, where the hospital has to choose between software packages of different vendors. Including a usability evaluation in this process ensures that the hospital buys a system that not only meets its functional requirements but also allows end users to work with it in an effective and efficient manner.

16.9 Structured Reporting

Reporting is traditionally based on the dictation of an unstructured report by a physician. This allows the physician to express freely and precise but on the other hand results in, possibly ambiguous, reports that cannot be processed easily by a computer. In his overview Reiner (2009) states that a report of sufficient quality should comply to the eight Cs, namely Clarity, Correctness, Confidence, Concision, Completeness, Consistency, Communication, and Consultation. With the conventional method for reporting in free text, it is difficult to adhere to and implement proper validation of these required properties. In addition to the eight Cs, Reiner defines two additional requirements, timeliness and standardization. Of these two the standardization could help comply to the eight Cs mentioned before. Therefore, in recent years, the call for increased structure and standardization has become louder. Structured reports improve the information transmission between the interpreting and the referring physician (Reiner 2009; Barbosa et al. 2010; Schwartz et al. 2011) and allow for easier and more elaborate data mining of the report database (Zimmerman et al. 2011), which can be used as input for decision and workflow support systems and to obtain business information. However, structured reporting is also believed to restrict the expression of the reporting physician and thus possibly lead to incomplete reports.

In an extensive study with the purpose to determine the differences in opinion and expectations of radiologists and referring clinicians with respect to the radiology reports, Bosmans et al. showed that preferences of the provider and consumer of radiology reports diverge fundamentally from the way radiology is practiced and taught today (Bosmans et al. 2011). In their paper they clearly showed the importance of the report as an indispensable tool requiring the specific expertise of the imaging specialist. They also showed that itemized reporting is preferred by clinicians (84.5 %) and radiologists (65.7 %). These findings would indicate that structured reporting is the definite solution for all problems achieving high level of structure, accuracy, and readability. However, structured reporting can be implemented in different ways ranging from itemized reports with free text entry to fully guided digital forms.

In general, the trends that are visible in radiology and nuclear medicine are an increase in structure of reporting, coding of examinations, findings and conclusions, and automation.

16.10 Structure

Structured reporting can be achieved in two ways: by having physicians report according to some form of a standardized structured format or by using natural language processing (NLP) techniques to convert free text into a structured format.

A variety of implementations exist to provide a standardized, structured, format. The one extreme is providing a set template for dictation, just providing the headings that need to be addressed in the report allowing entry or dictation of free text for each heading. The other extreme is a fully guided report based on drop boxes, checklists, and guided entry of measurements. Multiple studies have been performed by different groups with conclusions ranging from the meaning that structured reports have significantly better content and greater clarity than free text reports (Schwartz et al. 2011) to the statement that although structured reporting has potential benefits, it cannot be assumed to improve report accuracy or completeness (Johnson et al. 2009). This diversity in findings indicates that the success of structured reporting relies heavily on the method and tools used and maybe also on the local situation.

The approach of converting free text into a structured format could be beneficial since it does not require extra effort from the physician, but current NLP systems are not capable yet of accurately and reliably converting free text to structured reports. However, there have been very promising results with NLP in radiology (e.g., Do et al. 2013; Esuli et al. 2013), and a hybrid approach to report structuration, in which the physician and an NLP system work together to create the structured report, seems realistic in the near future in both radiology and nuclear medicine.

16.11 Coding

To utilize medical information contained in health information systems for multiple purposes, it is essential that this medical information is stored in an understandable and structured manner. To achieve this, the use of coding, classification, and medical terminology is advised since by the introduction of coding and classification, the possibility arises to uniformly index and retrieve information from information sources. This includes reports as provided by nuclear medicine. Proper coding could reduce miscommunication, allow data mining of reports, and facilitate scientific research.

Using a coding system, codes are connected to procedures, findings, conclusions, and anatomical descriptions. These codes can be used for a wide variety of applications in the entire imaging workflow (Fig. 16.6).

16.11.1 Imaging Examination Request

The coding of examination and patient-related information could be employed to facilitate the implementation of decision support in the imaging examination request. The names of the examinations will be consistent throughout the hospital, and patient information can be structured facilitating the application of clinical guidelines and workflows to guide the examination request.

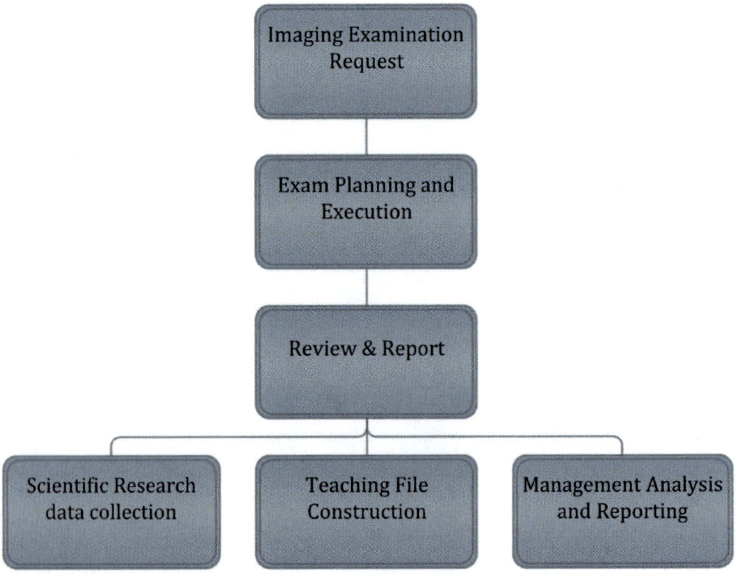

Fig. 16.6 Imaging workflow of a typical radiology or nuclear medicine department. Coding could be employed at all different steps of this typical workflow

16.11.2 Exam Planning and Execution

Examinations are fitted with descriptions for the studies and series included in the examination. These descriptions are often provided by the vendor of the acquisition device by their default protocols or entered manually by the operator of the specific device. In exam planning, coding of examinations allows for the implementation of vendor-independent protocols for complex examinations. This is achieved by consistent use of codes for examinations and procedure steps, thus ensuring the same coding for the same examination across all modalities and allowing for easy determination of relationships between different examinations.

16.11.3 Review and Report

To obtain an optimal workspace for review of nuclear medicine examinations, the presentation of the image data on the computer screen is of utmost importance. This presentation is usually based on a display protocol that describes which series from which study should be shown at what position on the computer screen. However, the implementation of such display protocols is often hampered by the different use of examination (study and series) description by different modalities or even within one modality. The use of proper coding for each examination as mentioned in the previous section would therefore greatly increase the successful implementation of display protocols.

This standardization of the examination descriptions also allows automated inclusion of information about imaging techniques and sequences used into the report, thus avoiding repetitive dictation or writing of large blocks of text. Dictation can be further improved using the information about the examination (anatomic region, modality, etc.) as input parameters to improve speech recognition.

The application of coding and thus standardized terms during the reporting process also introduces the ability to provide context guided decision support. Using the standard terms, relevant information such as checklists, differential diagnosis, relevant PubMed publications, or internet pages can be automatically provided, if needed, during the dictation process. An example is provided in figures 7 and 8. During the dictation the term lymphoma would be linked to a RadLex code of RID3840 providing the ability to automatically link to the information on the web as shown in Fig. 16.7. From this information, further information can be obtained by, for example, clicking on a reference image and automatically gaining access to the publication from which this reference image originates (Fig. 16.8).

16.11.4 Scientific Research Data Collection

The collection of data for retrospective scientific research is often cumbersome because of the inability to properly search the IT systems for the required subset. Standardization and coding facilitate collection of data based on specific

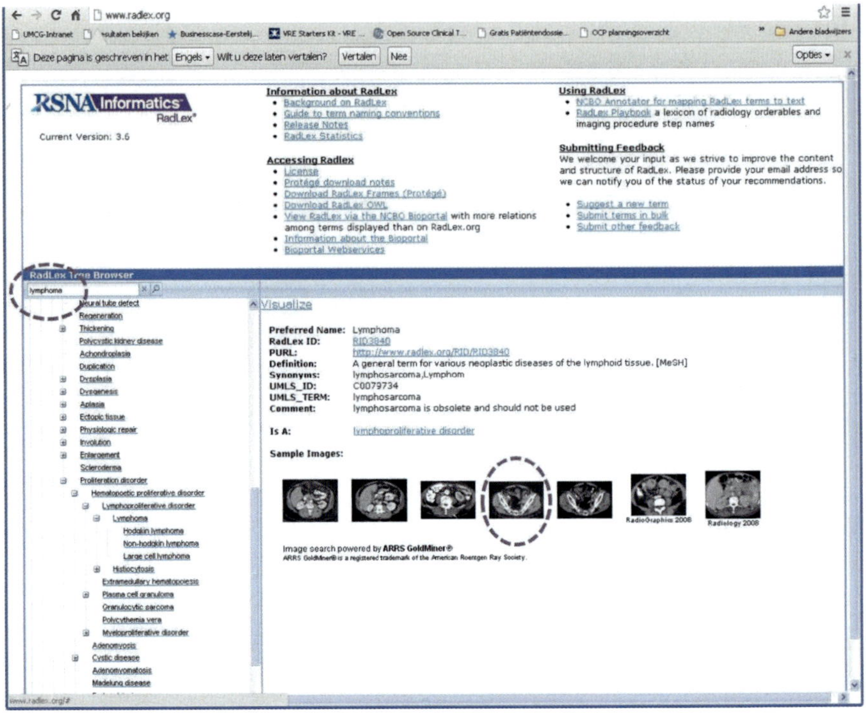

Fig. 16.7 Screenshot of the RadLex webpage showing the RadLex information on lymphoma

(examination) techniques, clinical question, disease, or any single-coded parameter or a combination of coded parameters from the report.

16.11.5 Teaching File Construction

The use of standardized terminology in radiology reports and examination descriptions facilitates the easy selection of teaching file cases from the entire database of clinical cases contained in the Electronic Health Record. Furthermore, structuring and indexing of the teaching file become an easy task when all cases included are coded in a standardized manner.

16.11.6 Management Analysis and Reporting

Measurement of production numbers with adequate subdivision to specific types of examination or other parameters is difficult when dealing with unstructured data. When coding and standardization are properly integrated into the whole imaging workflow, standardized terms can be connected to any report. Based on these standardized terms, databases can be queried easily and management information about the department can be obtained.

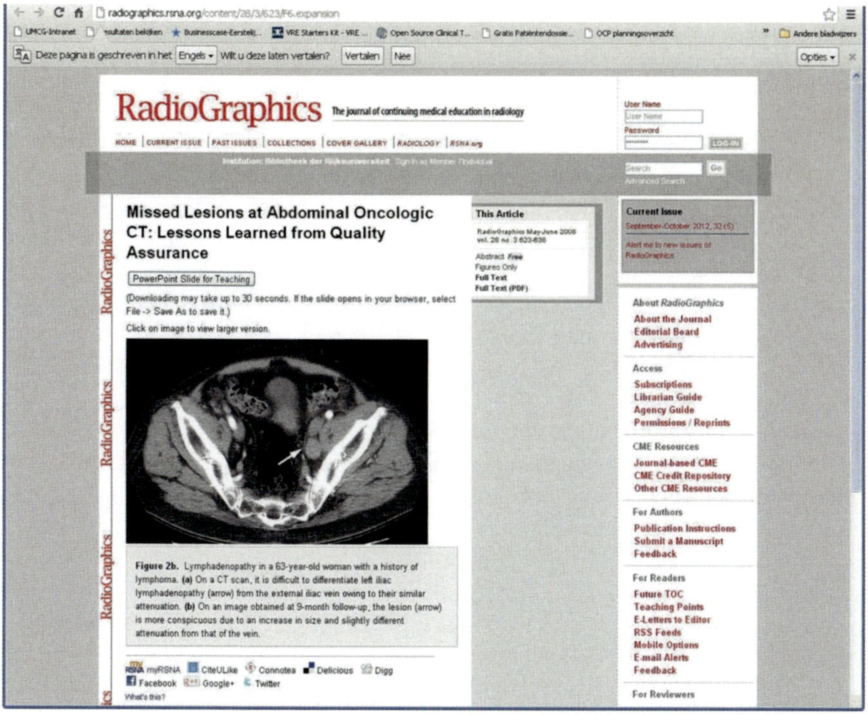

Fig. 16.8 Screenshot of the radiographic journal reference of the image circled in Fig. 16.7 demonstrating the easy integration of teaching using the coding system

16.12 Automation

As mentioned previously, the introduction of standardization and coding will also provide the ability to automate processes. As shown, the possibilities for workflow support are especially interesting from the interpreting physician's perspective, because it would allow all kinds of relevant information to be added to the report automatically. For example, when the physician measures a nodule, the system could retrieve the size of this nodule from previous reports, calculate the change in size, and automatically integrate this information into the report without intervention of the user.

16.13 Tele-Nuclear Medicine

The technological developments on computing and networking in the past decade facilitated the advent of telemedicine. Telemedicine involves a wide spectrum of applications where the healthcare provider and healthcare customer are at a geographically different location and use modern devices and communication networks to exchange health-related information. In case of medical imaging, this relationship shifts in tele-radiology and tele-nuclear medicine since in this case the healthcare consumer is not only the patient but can also be a colleague requesting review and reporting of imaging data from an expert located somewhere around the globe.

Tele-radiology was defined in 2006 by the European Society of Radiology as a telemedicine service which involves the electronic transmission of radiographic images from one geographical location to another for the purpose of interpretation and consultation. It has developed alongside the gradual shift in medical imaging from film-based to digital imaging-based technologies. Well-structured professional organizations and early establishment of standards have supported this development. Tele-radiology can help healthcare facilities to cope with peak workloads, ensure round-the-clock services, reduce waiting lists for specific examinations, and, above all, cut costs.

A similar definition holds for tele-nuclear medicine for which a procedure guideline for tele-nuclear medicine version 1.0 was already published by Parker et al. in 2002. The purpose of this guideline was "to assist nuclear medicine practitioners in using tele-nuclear medicine for interpretation and consultation of nuclear medicine studies" (Parker et al. 2002). In this publication, tele-nuclear medicine is defined as *Tele-nuclear medicine refers to nuclear medicine interpretation or consultation at a location distant from that at which the data are acquired. There is a continuum of separation between the physical location of the acquisition and interpretation, but tele-nuclear medicine is meant to imply that the interpretation is relatively remote as compared with the typical interpretation* (Parker et al. 2002).

Common indications for tele-nuclear medicine are the desire to provide timely interpretation of routine studies at a remote location or emergency studies in an on-call setting or to provide the ability of remote consultation.

The main technical challenges of telemedicine are presented by the confirmation of patient data security and safety, quality control of remote displays used by the expert, and sufficient network speed to allow a fast and adequate response by the expert.

For the quality of the tele-nuclear interpretation, the availability of the information about the patient and the examination at the site of interpretation is crucial. This information includes background and historical information on the patient, details about the current examination, and relevant prior examinations including their related information and details. Furthermore, with remote access to imaging data, the quality of the displays used and their responding quality insurance protocols including frequent calibration and testing are of concern as well as the environmental conditions (e.g., lighting) in which those displays are used.

An important challenge for tele-nuclear medicine is to ensure that it develops in a manner that benefits patient care and ensures overall patient safety and does not in any way reduce the quality of nuclear medicine services provided to the citizen. Therefore, urgent action needs to be taken to obtain legal clarity including assurance of high quality in patient care. Although technically tele-nuclear medicine can be employed, the physical distance between expert and patient can be a significant problem (Als and Bischof 2007). Therefore, one of the clinical challenges of tele-nuclear medicine is to provide sufficient insight in the clinical condition of the patient to the expert to allow proper evaluation and diagnosis.

16.14 Artificial Intelligence Applications

Artificial intelligence is becoming more ubiquitous in the medical domain. It is most often applied in the shape of support systems, which assist clinicians in some aspect of their work. This support can range from a suggestion of the most effective scanning protocol based on the patient's clinical information to the detection and diagnosis of lesions in a patient's images. Artificial intelligence techniques are also essential for the interpretation of the large and ever-increasing amounts of data generated in the modern hospital. The following sections will discuss some applications of artificial intelligence that are relevant for nuclear medicine.

16.15 Diagnostic Support

Intelligent systems that assist physicians during medical image diagnosis are often referred to as computer-aided diagnosis (CAD) systems. A distinction can be made between computer-aided detection (CADe), which focuses on the *detection* of abnormalities, and computer-aided diagnosis (CADx), which focuses on the *diagnosis* of abnormalities. Note that this distinction is not always clear, because CADe systems sometimes provide an evaluation of the detected abnormalities, and CADx systems often detect abnormalities first and subsequently use them as the basis for their diagnosis.

CADe systems use sophisticated image-processing and artificial intelligence techniques to detect abnormal regions in a medical image. These regions are marked on the image and the marked image is presented to physicians after they have reviewed the image on their own (Fig. 16.9). In this way, CADe aims to reduce perceptual oversight by drawing physicians' attention to abnormalities they might have missed.

CADe is a hot research topic in radiology, and it has been applied in a wide variety of domains, including mass and microcalcification detection in mammography, nodule detection in chest CT, and polyp detection in colonography. CADe has already found its way into clinical practice and its usage is increasing rapidly. In 2004, CADe was used in 39% of screening mammography studies in the United States, which increased to 74% in 2008 (Rao et al. 2010).

CADe has not received as much attention in nuclear medicine, but promising CADe systems in this discipline do exist, for example, for the detection of abnormalities in bone scintigraphy (Huang et al. 2007) (Fig. 16.9), the detection of interval changes on successive bone scintigrams (Shiraishi et al. 2007), and tumor detection in PET (Li et al. 2009). The high stand-alone performance of these systems indicates that they can be useful to nuclear medicine physicians and have the

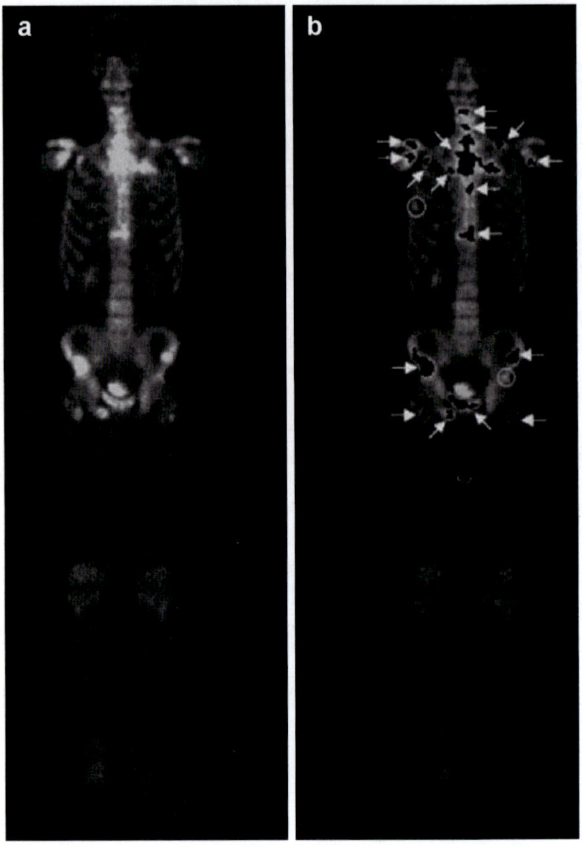

Fig. 16.9 Original whole-body bone scan (*left*, (**a**)) and the marks made by the CADe system developed by (Huang et al. 2007) (*right*, (**b**)). The arrows indicate true positive marks and the circles indicate false positive marks (Reprinted from Huang et al. (2007). Copyright 2007 by IEEE. Reprinted permission must be acquired)

potential to increase their detection performance. However, to the best of our knowledge, no observer studies with physicians using CADe have currently been conducted in nuclear medicine.

In contrast with CADe, CADx focuses on the diagnosis of abnormalities, rather than on their detection. CADx systems extract information from an image and use this information to reach a diagnosis, which can be used by physicians as a second opinion. Various forms of CADx exist. For example, there are systems that classify images as being normal or abnormal, systems that calculate a degree of malignity for abnormalities, and systems that provide a pathological classification of abnormalities.

In nuclear medicine, CADx has been used for a variety of diagnostic tasks, including the diagnosis of coronary artery disease, ischemia, and infarction in myocardial perfusion SPECT (Ezquerra et al. 1993; Tägil et al. 2008) and the differentiation of benign from malignant pulmonary nodules in PET/CT (Nie et al. 2006). Observer studies in nuclear medicine have shown that CADx improves physician's diagnostic performance and decreases interobserver variability (Sadik et al. 2009; Tägil et al. 2008).

16.16 Clinical Support

We define clinical decision support systems (CDSSs) as intelligent systems that assist clinicians in any clinical task that is not directly related to diagnosis. There are many kinds of tasks for which CDSSs can be useful. For example, they can be used for patient monitoring to warn when changes in the patient's condition occur, to check for dosage errors and drug-drug interactions, and to suggest the most optimal imaging procedure for a specific patient.

A typical CDSS consists of a medical knowledge base, a mechanism that extracts patient information, a rule-based inference mechanism that draws patient-specific conclusions based on these two sources of information, and a user interface that presents the conclusions to the clinician in a meaningful way (Fig. 16.10). There are also machine learning approaches to CDSS, which means that the system is trained on an extensive amount of clinical examples and learns to draw valid conclusions on its own. This results in a much more flexible system and eliminates the need to explicitly define all relevant medical knowledge and inference rules (which is a very time-consuming and sometimes virtually impossible task). A downside of using machine learning techniques is that it is more difficult to present the rationale behind the system's conclusions in a way that is meaningful to the clinician.

In order for any CDSS to provide accurate and useful support, it needs to have access to high-quality information. Ideally, all information should be available in a structured and standardized format, such that it can be easily interpreted by a computer. The advent of the Electronic Health Record and structured reporting and the increasing usage of image quantification provide rich sources of information that can be used to increase the quality of CDSSs.

Much research has been done to evaluate the effectiveness of CDSSs in clinical practice, but the results are still inconclusive. A recent review showed that 57 % of CDSS studies found a significant improvement in practitioner performance, and only 30 % found a positive effect on patient outcomes (Jaspers et al. 2011).

Kawamoto et al. (2005) identified four features that are strongly associated with the effectiveness of a CDSS in clinical practice: (1) decision support provided automatically as part of clinician workflow, (2) decision support delivered at the time and location of decision-making, (3) actionable recommendations provided, and (4)

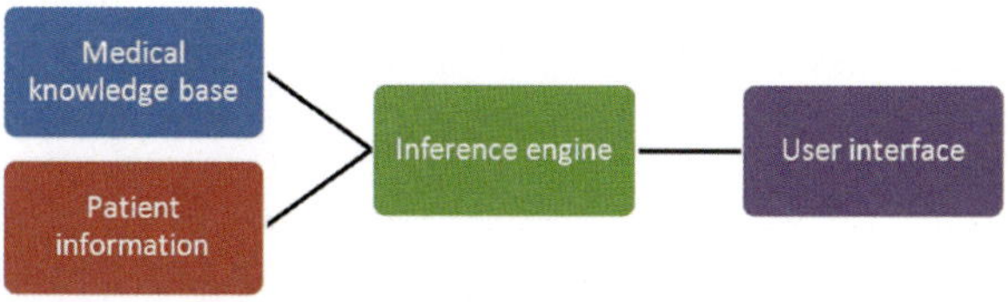

Fig. 16.10 General framework of a typical CDSS. The system consists of a medical knowledge base, a mechanism that extracts patient information, a rule-based inference mechanism that draws patient-specific conclusions based on these two sources of information, and a user interface that presents the conclusions to the clinician in a meaningful way

computer-based generation of support. These factors are all related to usability, indicating that a primary goal in the development of a CDSS should be to optimize the interaction between clinicians and the CDSS.

16.17 Quality Control

One of the main issues in quality control that gained a lot of public interest is radiation protection. The public and political debate on this issue led to the trend, and sometimes legislative requirement, of minimizing the radiation dose administered to a patient by looking at meaningful use of imaging: avoiding unnecessary examinations on the one hand and minimizing the amount of radiation administered when imaging is performed on the other (ALARA principle – As Low As Reasonably Achievable). Furthermore, the requirement of generating a full report of the incremental radiation administered to a patient over his or her lifetime is currently being advocated, implemented, and – in some cases – legislated.

Generating a patient-specific radiation report requires the extraction of radiation dose information from different databases and information systems. This can be difficult within a healthcare institution, but when a patient has been imaged at different locations or even countries, this task becomes increasingly challenging. Another problem is that the DICOM tag values relevant for radiation dose can be missing, inconsistent, or inappropriate. There can also be important information in the secondary screen captures stored by the acquisition device (e.g., the exam protocol screenshot usually generated by computed tomography includes information such as the CT dose index (CTDI) and dose-length product (DLP) for individual series and total examinations).

Intelligent systems, such as the one described in (Wang et al. 2011), can be very useful in this area. They can automatically extract radiation information from different sources, normalize information from different vendors and modalities, compensate for missing or inappropriate information, perform dose calculations, and integrate the results in a patient-specific dose report. These systems can also provide alerts, for example, when a CT perfusion scan exceeds predetermined values of mA, seconds, or kVp.

As shown earlier IHE tries to tackle the problem of data gathering for dose computation by the IHE REM (Radiation Exposure Monitoring) profile introduced at the connectathon in 2009.

16.18 Summary and Conclusion

It is essential that nuclear medicine is fully integrated into the mainstream (imaging) workflow of the healthcare enterprise. To achieve this, nuclear medicine imaging equipment and workstations should be compatible with the DICOM standard and more specifically with the DICOM nuclear medicine IOD. Furthermore, to ensure and facilitate integration, the IHE nuclear medicine profiles should also be adopted throughout the nuclear medicine department. A key focus in medical imaging for the coming years will be interoperability including the exchange of imaging data using a standardized methodology.

Further developments and trends show a growing interest in nuclear medicine in medical imaging informatics topics such as usability, structured reporting, and artificial intelligence methods such as computer-aided diagnosis. Promising results and useful applications have already emerged from these areas, and the near future will show even more scientific and technological developments and a wider acceptance and implementation of advanced medical imaging informatics systems in the nuclear medicine work environment.

References

Als C, Bischof Delaloye A. Clinical quality management in telenuclear medicine. Eur J Nucl Med Mol Imaging. 2007;34:1727–8.

Bakhshi-Raiez F, de Keizer NF, Cornet R, Dorrepaal M, Dongelmans D, Jaspers MWM. A usability evaluation of a SNOMED CT based compositional interface terminology for intensive care. Int J Med Inform. 2012;81:351–62.

Barbaras L, Tal I, Palmer MR, Parker JA, Kolodny GM. Shareware program for nuclear medicine and PET/CT PACS display and processing. AJR. 2007;188:W565–8.

Barbosa F, Maciel LMZ, Vieira EM, De Azevedo Marques PM, Elias J, Muglia VF. Radiological reports: a comparison between the transmission efficiency of information in free text and in structured reports. Clinics. 2010;65(1):15–21.

Bazak N, Stamm G, Caldarone F, Lotz J, Leppert A, Galanski M. PACS workstations 2000: evaluation, usability and performance. 18th international EuroPACS conference. Graz; 2000. p. 133–42.

Bian J, Topaloglu U, Lane C. EIR: enterprise imaging repository, an alternative imaging archiving and communication system. Conf Proc IEEE Eng Med Biol Soc. 2009;2009:2168–71.

Boehm T, Handgraetinger O, Link J, Ploner R, Voellmy DR, Marincek B, et al. Evaluation of radiological workstations and web-browser-based image distribution clients for a PACS project in hands-on workshops. Eur Radiol. 2004;14:908–14.

Bosmans JML, Weyler JJ, De Schepper AM, Parizal PM. The radiology report as seen by radiologists and referring clinicians: results of the COVER and ROVER surveys. Radiology. 2011;259(1):184–95.

Cerqueira MD, Weissman NJ, Dilsizian V, Jacobs AK, Kail S, Laskey WK, Pennell DJ, Rumberger JA, Ryan T, Verani MS. Standardized myocardial segmentation and nomenclature for tomographic imaging of the heart: a statement for healthcare professionals from the Cardiac Imaging Committee of the Council on Clinical Cardiology of the American Heart Association. Circulation. 2002;105:539–42.

Chan J, Shojania KG, Easty AC, Etchells EE. Usability evaluation of order sets in a computerised provider order entry system. BMJ Qual Saf. 2011;20:932–40.

Cockton G, Lavery D, Woolrych A. Inspection-based evaluations. In: Jacko JA, Sears A, editors. The human-computer interaction handbook. Mahwah: Lawrence Erlbaum; 2003. p. 1119–38.

Connectathon Results Browser. http://connectathon-results.ihe.net. Accessed 19 Nov 2013.

Do BH, Wu AS, Maley J, Biswal S. Automatic retrieval of bone fracture knowledge using natural language processing. J Digit Imaging. 2013;26(4):709–13.

Esuli A, Marcheggiani D, Sebastiani F. An enhanced CRFs-based system for information extraction from radiology reports. J Biomed Inform. 2013;46(3):425–35.

Ezquerra N, Mullick R, David Cooke C, Krawczynska EG, Garcia EV. PERFEX: an expert system for interpreting 3D myocardial perfusion. Expert Syst Appl. 1993;6(4):459–68.

Haraguchi D, Kim J, Kumar A, Constantinescu L, Wen L, Fang DD. A web-based image viewer for multiple PET-CT follow-up studies. 2011. 22nd annual international conference of the IEEE EMBS. Boston. August 30–September 3, 2011:5279–82.

Hindel R. Implementation of the DICOM 3.0 standard – a pragmatic handbook. 1994. Radiological Society of North America, Oak Brook.

Huang J-Y, Kao P-F, Chen Y-S. A set of image processing algorithms for computer-aided diagnosis in nuclear medicine whole body bone scan images. IEEE Trans Nucl Sci. 2007;54(3):514–22.

IHE Wiki – Nuclear Medicine Image. 2013. http://wiki.ihe.net/index.php?title=Nuclear_Medicine_Image. Accessed 22 August 2013, Page last modified at August 31, 2011.

Im KC, Choi IS, Ryu J-S, Eo GS, Kim JS, Moon DH. PET/CT fusion viewing software for use with picture archiving and communication systems. J Digit Imaging. 2010;23(6):732–43.

ISO 9241-11. Ergonomic requirements for office work with visual display terminals (VDTs) -- Part 11: Guidance on usability. 1998. Geneva: International Organization for Standardization.

Jaspers MWM. A comparison of usability methods for testing interactive health technologies: methodological aspects and empirical evidence. Int J Med Inform. 2009;78:340–53.

Jaspers MWM, Smeulers M, Vermeulen H, Peute LW. Effects of clinical decision-support systems on practitioner performance and patient outcomes: a synthesis of high-quality systematic review findings. JAMIA. 2011;18(3):327–34.

Johnson AJ, Chen MYM, Swan JS, Applegate KE, Littenberg B. Cohort study of structured reporting compared with conventional dictation. Radiology. 2009;253(1):74–80.

Jorritsma W, Cnossen F, van Ooijen PM. Merits of usability testing for PACS selection. Int J Med Inform. 2014;83:27–36.

Kawamoto K, Houlihan CA, Balas EA, Lobach DF. Improving clinical practice using clinical decision support systems: a systematic review of trials to identify features critical to success. BMJ. 2005;330:765.

Lemke HU. Short history of PACS (part II: Europe). Eur J Radiol. 2011;78:177–83.

Li Z, Li Q, Yu X, Conti PS, Leahy RM. Lesion detection in dynamic FDG-PET using matched subspace detection. IEEE Trans Med Imaging. 2009;28(2):230–40.

Menon A, Korner-Bitensky N, Chignell M, Straus S. Usability testing of two e-learning resources: Methods to maximize potential for clinician use. J Rehab Med. 2012;44:338–45.

Nie Y, Li Q, Li F, Pu Y, Appelbaum D, Doi K. Integrating PET and CT information to improve diagnostic accuracy for lung nodules: a semiautomatic computer-aided method. J Nucl Med. 2006;47(7):1075–80.

Parker JA, Royal HD, Uren RF, et al. An all-digital nuclear medicine department. J Digital Imaging. 1983;16(1):5–10.

Parker JA, Wallis JW, Jadvar H, Christian P, Todd-Pokropek A. Procedure guideline for telenuclear medicine 1.0. J Nucl Med. 2002;43(10):1410–3.

Pelanek GA. A DICOM cardiology exchange. In: Kennedy TE, Nissen SE, Simon R, Thomas JD, Tilkemeier PL, editors. Digital cardiac imaging in the 21st century: a primer. Bethesda: Cardiac and Vascular Information Working Group; 1997.

Rao VM, Levin DC, Parker L, Cavanaugh B, Frangos AJ, Sunshine JH. How widely is computer-aided detection used in screening and diagnostic mammography? J Am Coll Radiol. 2010;7(10):802–5.

Reiner BI. The challenges, opportunities, and imperative of structured reporting in medical imaging. J Digit Imaging. 2009;22(6):562–8.

Sadik M, Suurkula M, Höglund P, Järund A, Edenbrandt L. Improved classifications of planar whole-body bone scans using a computer-assisted diagnosis system: a multicenter, multiple-reader, multiple-case study. J Nucl Med. 2009;50(3):368–75.

Sattler B, Lee JA, Lonsdale M, Coche E. PET/CT (and CT) instrumentation, image reconstruction and data transfer for radiotherapy planning. Radiother Oncol. 2010;96:288–97.

Schwartz L, Panicek D, Berk A, Li Y, Hricak H. Improving communication of diagnostic radiology findings through structured reporting. Radiology. 2011;260(1):174–81.

Shiraishi J, Li Q, Appelbaum D, Pu Y, Doi K. Development of a computer-aided diagnostic scheme for detection of interval changes in successive whole-body bone scans. Med Phys. 2007;34(1):25.

Somer EJ. PACS man: questioning nuclear medicine and PET integration. Nucl Med Commun. 2006;27:601–2.

Tägil K, Bondouy M, Chaborel JP, et al. A decision support system improves the interpretation of myocardial perfusion imaging. Eur J Nucl Med Mol Imaging. 2008;35(9):1602–7.

Todd-Pokropek A, Cradduck TD, Deconinck F. A file format for the exchange of nuclear medicine image data: a specification of Interfile version 3.3. Nucl Med Comm. 1992;13(9):673–99.

Vogel WV, Oyen WJG, van Dalen JA, Huisman H, Karssemeijer N. Sliced alternating DICOM series: convenient visualization of image fusion on PACS. Eur J Nucl Med Mol Imaging. 2005;32(2):247–8.

Wallis JW. Nuclear PACS: problems, solutions. Decis Imaging Econ. 2004;6:21–5.

Wallis JW. PET/CT image fusion headed for PACS. Decisions in imaging economics. Allied Media LLC: Kansas, USA; 2006.

Wang S, Pavlicek W, Roberts CC, Langer SG, Zhang M, Hu M, Morin RL, Schueler BA, Wellnitz CV, Wu T. An automated DICOM database capable of arbitrary data mining (including radiation dose indicators) for quality monitoring. J Digit Imaging. 2011;24(2):223–33.

Zemariame N, Knight N, Siegel EL. Redesigning the nuclear medicine reading room. Semin Nucl Med. 2011;41:463–71.

Zimmerman SL, Kim W, William W. Automated structured reporting of imaging findings using the AIM standard and XML. RadioGraphics. 2011;31:881–7.

Part IV

Preclinical Quality Issues

Preclinical Testing of Novel Radiotracers for Positron Emission Tomography (PET)

17

Aren van Waarde, Jürgen W.A. Sijbesma, Janine Doorduin, Philip H. Elsinga, and Erik F.J. de Vries

Abstract

Preclinical tests of novel radiotracers in experimental animals are required to move tracer candidates from the stage of in vitro testing to the stage of toxicity testing and finally studies in human volunteers. Such preclinical tests are aimed at demonstrating: (1) specific in vivo interaction of the tracer with its target, (2) adequate kinetics and metabolic stability of the tracer after it has been injected into living mammals, and (3) sensitivity of tracer uptake to changes of target expression. Possible strategies to reach these aims are discussed, including specific animal models which are used in our institution. These include pharmacological treatment of healthy animals, target gene knockout, tumor growth, brain lesions resulting in loss of myelin, viral infection, sterile inflammation, and xenografting of inflammatory cells.

17.1 Introduction

Changes in receptor availability, enzyme activity, or transporter function can be early biomarkers of human disease or indicators of the therapeutic success (Aronson 2005; Biomarker Definitions Working Group 2001; Duffy and Treasure 2011; Puntmann 2009; Strimbu and Tavel 2010). A major, worldwide research effort of imaging centers is therefore focused on the development of novel radiotracers that can visualize and quantify such changes in living subjects (Backer and Backer 2012; Brooks and Pavese 2011; Eckelman et al. 2008; Nordberg 2011; Palumbo et al. 2014; Richter 2006; Wu et al. 2013). Before a novel tracer can be applied in humans,

A. van Waarde (✉) • J.W.A. Sijbesma • J. Doorduin • P.H. Elsinga • E.F.J. de Vries
Department of Nuclear Medicine and Molecular Imaging, University of Groningen, University Medical Center Groningen, Hanzeplein 1, Groningen 9713 GZ, The Netherlands
e-mail: a.van.waarde@umcg.nl

A.W.J.M. Glaudemans et al. (eds.), *Quality in Nuclear Medicine*,
DOI 10.1007/978-3-319-33531-5_17

it should be thoroughly tested (Honer et al. 2014; Ingvar et al. 1991). The testing of a radiotracer for positron emission tomography (PET) imaging proceeds in three distinct phases:

1. It should be demonstrated that the probe binds preferentially to the chosen target, not only in cells in vitro but also in intact animals in vivo. The target may be a receptor, a protein aggregate, an ion channel, an enzyme, or a transporter protein. The tracer should have adequate plasma and tissue kinetics, resulting in high-contrast images within the time frame dictated by the short-lived isotope. Radioactive metabolites of the injected tracer should not enter the tissue of interest to a significant extent. Only the unchanged probe should get there. Because a PET camera cannot distinguish between radioactivity originating from the parent tracer and its metabolites, the presence of radiometabolites in the region of interest should be avoided (Pike 2009).
2. It should be demonstrated that the binding of the probe is sensitive to changes in target expression. Such changes may, e.g., be caused by disease or by an applied therapy. Changes of the binding of a sensitive probe will be an accurate reflection of changes of target concentration in the tissue of interest. Before a PET probe is tested in a disease or an intervention model, it may be necessary to assess reproducibility of the target measurements by performing a "test-retest study" in healthy animals (Alexoff et al. 2003; Dandekar et al. 2007; Kroll et al. 2014; Lamoureux et al. 2012; Thackeray et al. 2013; Tseng et al. 2005). Subtle changes of target expression associated with a disease or a therapeutic intervention will only be detectable when the test-retest reproducibility of the PET measurements is good.
3. It should be demonstrated that the radiation dose of the tracer (both to the whole body and to vital organs) is acceptable. Finally, it should be demonstrated that the probe is not toxic, teratogenic, or mutagenic (even at high doses) so that it can be safely applied for scanning purposes in humans (Aboagye et al. 2002; Doze et al. 2000a; Marzin 1998; Silberstein 2000). For obvious reasons (Nuremberg Code and Declaration of Helsinki), animal studies and toxicity tests are always required before novel imaging probes can be applied in humans. Guidelines for toxicity testing of novel PET tracers that will be applied in microdose concentrations in humans have been issued by the European Medicines Agency.

17.2 Why PET Probes Should Be Tested in Experimental Animals

The radiotracers which are developed in our institution are aimed at targets (receptors, transporters, enzymes, ion channels, protein aggregates) which play an important role in the pathophysiology of neurodegenerative diseases (Alzheimer disease, Parkinson's disease, multiple sclerosis), psychiatric disorders, cardiovascular disease (atherosclerosis, heart failure), infections (or inflammation), and cancer.

Suitable PET tracers for these targets will result in greater understanding of the physiology and biochemistry of the human body in health and disease and will provide important diagnostic information. They may also allow evaluation of the impact of novel treatment strategies and their use can result in the development of patient-tailored therapy (or "personalized medicine"). Moreover, such PET probes may be used in drug development (e.g., early clinical studies of novel therapeutic drugs), and they can be applied for longitudinal studies in experimental animals, resulting in a reduction of animal use (Fischman et al. 2002; Jacobson and Chen 2013; Kramer-Marek and Capala 2012; Lancelot and Zimmer 2010; Pomper and Lee 2005; Vanderheyden 2009). Preclinical tests of novel radiotracers are required in radiotracer development to move tracer candidates from the stage of in vitro testing to the stage where they can be tested in humans (patients and healthy control subjects).

Candidate PET tracers are selected based on the results from in vitro tests. In studies using membrane fragments or cells grown in culture, they should bind with high affinity and high selectivity to their intended target (Ametamey et al. 2008; Eckelman 1994; Eckelman 1998; Eckelman and Mathis 2006; Laruelle et al. 2003; van Waarde et al. 2004c), and during incubation with blood plasma, liver microsomes, or hepatocytes, they should show a reasonable metabolic stability (Ametamey et al. 2008; Giron et al. 2008; Laven et al. 2004; Ma et al. 2001, 2002a, b, 2003; Moerlein et al. 1993). They should also have appropriate physicochemical characteristics, e.g., proper lipophilicity for passage through the blood-brain barrier and low hydrogen bonding in the case of tracers for targets in the central nervous system (Dishino et al. 1983; Laruelle et al. 2003; Levin 1980; McCarthy et al. 2009; Moerlein et al. 1985; Waterhouse 2003).

Although potential imaging probes are subjected to extensive in vitro screening before they are tested in experimental animals (Patel and Gibson 2008; Wong and Pomper 2003), in vivo testing remains necessary because of the complexity of the mammalian body. The probe may bind not only to its intended target but also to plasma proteins and to tissue components (protein, phospholipids) which are structurally different from the target. The probe may accumulate in tissue because of a specific target interaction but also because of its general physical properties (e.g., trapping of a protonated form of the tracer molecule in lysosomes). Labeled metabolites may be formed in the liver and in other tissues (lungs, blood cells); these radioactive compounds will be released into the blood and they can be taken up by the tissue of interest. Many of such processes are combined in the living organism, resulting in an unpredictable amount of non-displaceable tracer binding. If the non-displaceable binding is strong, it may totally obscure the binding of the probe to its target (Honer et al. 2014). Probe kinetics should be evaluated as well. The rates of tracer clearance from the circulation and tracer accumulation in target tissue should match. The clearance of non-bound tracer from target and nontarget tissues should be sufficiently rapid and occur within the time span of the PET measurement. Diffusion barriers – such as the blood-brain barrier and the blood-testis barrier – may hamper the transport of the probe to the tissue of interest (Doze et al. 2000b; Ishiwata et al. 2007; Passchier et al. 2000). An imaging probe for a target in the brain may fail because it does not pass the blood-brain barrier in the living organism, and a probe for a target in tumors may fail because its entry into tumor tissue is too slow.

A candidate PET tracer which has passed in vitro screening procedures is thus subsequently subjected to a number of preclinical tests in experimental animals. In each step of preclinical evaluation, the tracer may fail to pass a test. If the tracer candidate passes the preclinical tests, it will undergo toxicological screening, and in the case of proven absence of toxicity, it will proceed to "first-in-man" studies in human volunteers. The three steps of preclinical testing are aimed at: (1) demonstrating specific in vivo interaction of the tracer with its target, (2) demonstrating adequate kinetics and metabolic stability of the tracer after it has been injected into a living mammal, and (3) demonstrating sensitivity of tracer uptake to changes of target expression. Such changes can be related to disease or to a specific intervention.

17.3 Proving Specificity of Probe Binding

Some generally accepted criteria are used to identify specific target binding. Association of the probe should occur with: (1) high affinity, (2) high specificity (including stereoselectivity), (3) saturability, (4) appropriate kinetics (Eckelman et al. 2009; Giron 2009), and (5) a regional tissue distribution that is related to target expression and/or the physiological target response (Eckelman 1991; Gibson et al. 1979; Pimlott 2005; Syrota 1987).

In vivo blocking (or displacement) experiments using target-selective drugs can be performed to prove that uptake of radioactivity in the tissue of interest is caused by a specific interaction of the injected probe with its target (i.e., is saturable, stereoselective, and specific). Such drugs can be antagonists or agonists for (subtypes of) the target receptor, enzyme inhibitors, or transport modulators. Co-injection of these nonradioactive drugs with the imaging probe should result in a strong reduction (or, in the case of transport modulators, a strong increase (Hendrikse et al. 1999; van Waarde et al. 2009)) of probe uptake in the tissue of interest if drugs and probe bind to the same target. The ratio of tissue uptake of radioactivity at baseline and after treatment of animals with a specific drug indicates the magnitude of the fraction of tissue radioactivity that reflects specific target binding. When nonradioactive target-selective drugs have little impact on uptake of radioactivity in the tissue of interest, the radiotracer fails in pharmacological tests and cannot be considered as a suitable candidate for PET imaging (Andersen et al. 2015; van Waarde et al. 1992b, 2008). However, when the drugs have a strong and significant impact on radioactivity levels in target tissue, the radiotracer passes the tests and can proceed to the next phase of probe development (Law 1993; van Waarde et al. 1992b, 1995, 1998). Specificity of probe association can be demonstrated by the fact that drugs selective for the proper target have a strong impact on probe binding in the tissue of interest, whereas drugs selective for a different target (subtype) do not affect probe binding at all. In some cases, genetically modified rodents in which the target has been knocked out can be used as an alternative to treatment of healthy animals with target-specific blockers (Eckelman 2003a, b). The specific interaction of the probe may be obscured, or artificial decreases of tracer binding may be generated by secondary effects of a competing drug unrelated to target binding. For instance, the drug may affect the clearance or the metabolism of the tracer. Therefore, plasma radioactivity and tracer metabolism should always be taken into account.

The kinetics of the tracer in the tissue of interest should match the half-life of the radionuclide and be appropriate for kinetic modeling. A tracer may fail in initial tests when its kinetics is too slow (or too fast) (Giron 2009). The kinetics of radiotracers that are very tightly (or irreversibly) bound during the scanning time may be highly dependent on blood flow, and their binding may not be sensitive to changes of target expression induced by disease or by an intervention (Eckelman et al. 2009). For PET probes which bind to a finite number of sites, the time to reach binding equilibrium should be long compared to the rate of washout of non-specifically bound tracer, but short relative to radionuclide decay (McCarthy et al. 2009).

Samples of arterial blood can be taken from animals after injection of a novel radiotracer, and the relative amounts of intact parent tracer and metabolites in these samples can be assessed with advanced chromatographic techniques, such as solid-phase extraction (SPE), high-performance liquid chromatography (HPLC), various forms of thin-layer chromatography (TLC, HPTLC, UPTLC), and [ultrahigh-performance] liquid chromatography-mass spectrometry ([UP]LC-MS) (Ma et al. 2003; Maziere et al. 1992). Moreover, samples of target tissue can be taken, homogenized in buffer, and the relative amounts of parent tracer and metabolites in tissue extracts can also be determined. Such measurements assess the in vivo stability of the tracer. Target tissue should contain mainly parent tracer and only a minor fraction of radioactive metabolites. When a major fraction of total radioactivity in target tissue reflects metabolites rather than intact parent tracer, the radiotracer fails in the stability test and cannot be considered as a suitable candidate for PET imaging.

The regional tissue distribution of the probe (e.g., its distribution within the brain or its uptake in various peripheral organs) and the absolute amount of tracer uptake in tissues of interest can be examined by PET imaging and by ex vivo measurement of radioactivity in tissue samples. This regional distribution should correspond to the known distribution of the target protein. When target expression is known to be heterogeneous (e.g., different in various organs or various brain regions), but probe radioactivity is homogeneously distributed, the radiotracer fails in the tissue distribution test and cannot be considered as a suitable candidate for PET imaging.

Dosimetry data acquired in biodistribution experiments are essential for translation of the probe to humans. Based on such data, the recommended dose of the tracer for human studies can be calculated. A tracer may fail in initial tests when it causes a very high radiation dose to some vital organs.

17.3.1 Specificity Testing in Practice

Step 1 Healthy rodents are treated either with solvent (without drugs) or with solvent containing a pharmacological dose of a target-selective drug. The animals are anesthetized, positioned in a PET camera for small animal imaging, and injected with a novel radiotracer. The kinetics of tracer uptake in the target organs is monitored with the PET camera for an extended period of time (depending on the half-life of the administered radionuclide, usually 0.5–2 h). In the case of PET studies in rats, many small (0.1 ml) samples of blood can be taken at different time intervals during the scan from a cannula placed in an artery (total volume drawn <15% of blood volume of animal, drawn blood replaced by warm saline). Radioactivity in these samples is then counted and used as input function for kinetic modeling of tracer uptake in the target organ. Differences between tracer uptake at baseline and after drug treatment and alterations in the shape of the time-activity curves in blood and target tissue are carefully monitored (Fig. 17.1). In terminal experiments, animals are euthanized after the scan and tissue samples are collected to study the distribution of radioactivity in organs outside the field of view of the PET camera (e.g., for dosimetry purposes), to validate the PET measurements, or to

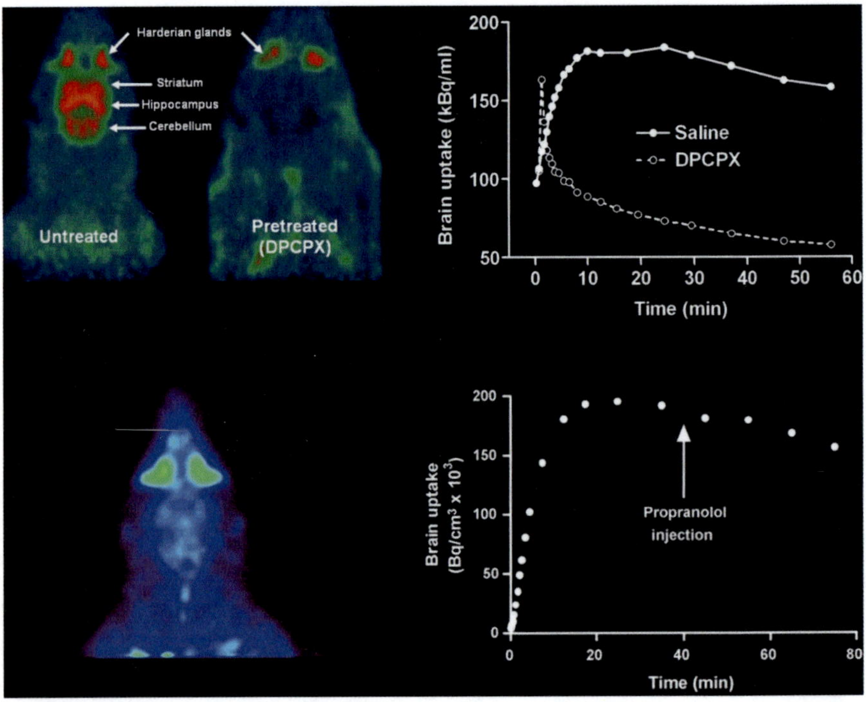

Fig. 17.1 MicroPET images made with a successful and a non-successful receptor ligand. Upper row: Data for the adenosine A1 receptor ligand ^{11}C-MPDX. Uptake of this ligand showed regional differences and was highest in the hippocampus, striatum, and cerebellum, as expected. After pretreatment of animals with a nonradioactive xanthine (*DPCPX*), brain uptake of the radioligand was strongly suppressed and regional differences were no longer visible. *Bottom row*: Data for the ß-adrenoceptor ligand ^{11}C-exaprolol. Uptake of this tracer was homogeneous throughout the brain and did not reflect the known distribution of ß-adrenoceptors. When a large dose of the beta-blocker propranolol was administered after injection of the radioligand, the kinetics and uptake of ^{11}C-exaprolol in rat brain were unaffected. Thus, ^{11}C-MPDX is suitable for visualization of adenosine A1 receptors, but ^{11}C-exaprolol cannot be used to visualize ß-adrenoceptors in the rodent brain (Data from Paul et al. (2011), van Waarde et al. (2008))

determine the expression of the target with independent tests (immunohistochemistry, autoradiography, Western blotting).

Milestone 1 If target-selective drugs (or target knockout) cause a statistically significant, dose-dependent and strong change of tracer uptake in target tissue at several time points during the scan, and if the distribution of the tracer reflects the known distribution of target expression, the radiotracer proceeds to the next phase of probe development. However, if target-selective drugs (or target knockout) have very little impact on tracer uptake, and/or the regional distribution of the tracer is homogeneous and not related to regional levels of target expression, the tracer fails in step 1.

17.3.2 Stability Testing in Practice

Step 2 For accurate quantification of target expression in living subjects with PET, information should be gathered on metabolic stability of the injected tracer. In some cases this information can already be acquired during step 1, but in other cases assessment of the metabolic stability of the tracer requires the use of a different group of animals for technical reasons (e.g., a large amount of blood or tissue is required for the metabolite analysis and such an additional large amount cannot be taken during the PET scan when blood sampling is already performed for kinetic modeling purposes and target tissue is required for immunohistochemistry, autoradiography, or Western blotting rather than metabolite assay). Rodents are treated either with solvent (without drugs) or with a solution containing a pharmacological dose of a target-selective drug. The animals are anesthetized and injected with a radiotracer. A few blood samples with large volumes (0.5–1 ml) are taken at different intervals after tracer injection (depending on the kinetics of tracer binding which is known from data acquired in step 1, total volume drawn <15 % of blood volume of animal, drawn blood replaced by warm saline). Animals are then terminated; samples of target tissue are taken and homogenized. Protein-free extracts of blood plasma and target tissue homogenates are prepared, and radioactive compounds in these extracts are separated using chromatographic techniques. The fraction of total radioactivity in blood plasma or target tissue reflecting intact parent compound is determined (Fig. 17.2).

Milestone 2 For proper interpretation of the imaging signal, it is essential that metabolite levels in target tissue are low. When radioactivity in target tissue reflects mainly the presence of intact parent tracer (even after an interval of 0.5–2 h) and only small amounts of metabolites are detected, the radiotracer will proceed to the next phase of probe development. The outcome of the metabolite assays in blood plasma will then be used to correct the input function of kinetic models for the presence of radioactive metabolites. However, when a large fraction of radioactivity (>25 %) in target tissue is found to reflect the presence of metabolites rather than injected parent tracer, the radiotracer fails in the metabolic stability test.

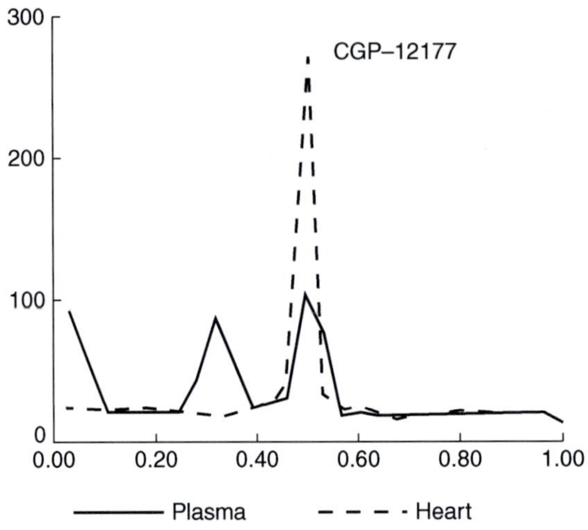

Fig. 17.2 Radiochromatograms of extracts of rat plasma and heart, made 80 min after injection of ^{3}H-CGP12177. Plasma (*solid line*) contains both parent tracer and metabolites at this time point, whereas myocardial tissue (*dotted line*) contains only intact parent tracer. The peak at Rf 0.50 represents unmodified ^{3}H-CGP12177, whereas the peaks at Rf values 0.05 and 0.26 represent radioactive metabolites. These data indicate that CGP12177 has the required metabolic stability for visualization of ß-adrenoceptors in the heart (Data from van Waarde et al. (1992a))

17.4 Proving Sensitivity of Probe Binding to Changes of Target Expression

Radiotracers which passed the tests of steps 1 and 2 are finally tested for their capability to detect changes of target expression as a consequence of disease or of some specific intervention. Animal models of disease and other intervention models (with known changes of target expression) are used for this purpose. The particular model that is chosen will depend on the target which the radiotracer should visualize. As was explained above, reproducibility of the PET measurements may have to be determined in a so-called "test-retest experiment" before a candidate radiotracer is tested in a disease or an intervention model, if the expected changes of target availability due to disease or to the specific intervention are small. Healthy rodents (rats or mice) are then scanned twice with the tracer candidate, under identical conditions, on two different occasions (e.g., with an interval of 1 week). The outcome of repeated estimations of target expression is compared. Good tracers show a test-retest reproducibility better than 10 %. Data from a test-retest experiment can be used for the planning of subsequent imaging studies in disease models (e.g., for the calculation of group sizes using a power analysis). An ideal radiotracer for PET imaging should be capable of detecting changes in target availability of 15 % or more.

Since the tracers which are developed in our institution are aimed at visualizing targets in neurodegenerative diseases, psychiatric disorders, cardiovascular disease, infections, inflammation and cancer, animal models of multiple sclerosis, activated microglia, encephalitis, peripheral inflammation, and cancer are frequently used in the last step of preclinical testing. We have chosen models associated with acceptable (minor to moderate) animal discomfort, which can yield important information regarding the in vivo behavior of a tracer candidate.

Questions that can be answered during step 3 of preclinical testing are the following:

1. Do changes of target expression result in altered probe binding in the tissue of interest?
2. Is the spatial distribution of changes of probe binding identical to the spatial distribution of changes of target expression?
3. Are the temporal patterns of changes of probe binding and changes of target expression similar?
4. What is the ratio of tracer uptake in diseased and normal tissue (e.g., inflamed and non-inflamed regions, tumor, and contralateral healthy areas)?
5. Is the probe specific for one particular kind of disease (e.g., does it preferentially accumulate in tumors and much less in inflammatory tissue; can the probe visualize a particular type of tumor)?
6. Can even small changes of target expression be detected? What is the detection limit of PET scans with the novel probe?
7. Are both the (negative) consequences of disease and the (positive) consequences of therapy detectable?

17.4.1 Testing of a Neuroinflammation Tracer

Most tracers for neurodegenerative diseases which are developed in our institution should visualize inflammatory processes in the central nervous system. Such tracers tend to show a very low uptake in the healthy brain, but their uptake should be strongly increased in inflamed brain regions. A PET scan of diseased animals can be made, and tracer uptake can be expressed in various ways: regional standardized uptake value (SUV), target-to-nontarget ratios of radioactivity (uptake in inflamed areas divided by uptake in non-inflamed areas), regional distribution volume determined by graphical analysis or kinetic modeling, and binding potential (estimated by kinetic modeling). These outcome parameters are chosen because they provide quantitative data on regional tracer uptake and they can later also be measured in humans (patients and healthy control subjects) with PET imaging. When the expected increase (or decrease) in diseased animals is observed and if the regional distribution of radioactivity corresponds to regional numbers of activated microglia (or loss of myelin), the tracer passes the disease model test (its uptake is then sensitive to pathophysiological changes of target availability). However, when tracer uptake in diseased animals is not significantly different from that observed in healthy controls, the tracer candidate fails.

Depending on the tracer target and the human disease for which the tracer was intended, one of the following neuroinflammation models was frequently chosen in our institution:

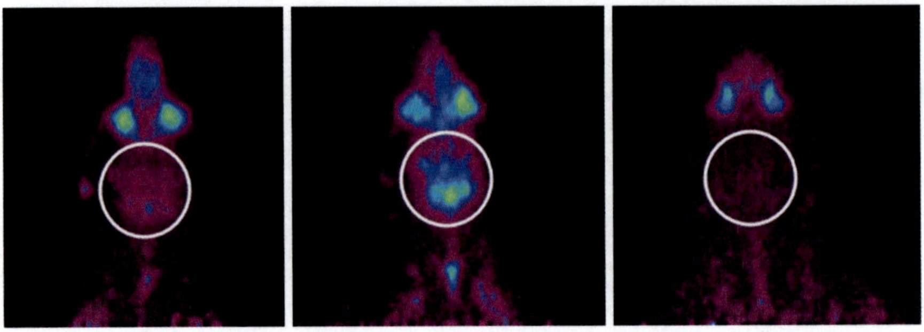

Fig. 17.3 MicroPET images of rats made with [^{11}C]DPA-713, a radiotracer for the translocator protein TSPO which is strongly overexpressed in activated microglia. The image at the *left* shows regional tracer uptake in the head-and-neck region of a healthy rat, the image at the center uptake in a rat with herpes simplex virus-induced encephalitis, and the image at the *right* uptake in an animal with encephalitis which had been pretreated with a nonradioactive ligand for TSPO (PK11195). *White circles* indicate the position of the brain. Tracer uptake in the healthy brain was negligible, as expected, but a strong increase was observed in inflamed brain areas. This increase could be blocked by pretreating animals with a specific ligand for TSPO. Thus, [^{11}C]DPA-713 is suitable for imaging of neuroinflammation (Data from Doorduin et al. (2009)

17.4.1.1 Viral Infection Model

Rats are intranasally inoculated with herpes simplex virus type-1 (HSV-1). The applied virus enters the brain via the olfactory nerve, resulting in neuroinflammation. We have used this model for at least 10 years in the evaluation of tracers for the inflammatory component of neurodegenerative diseases (e.g., tracers for the translocator protein (TSPO) (Antunes et al. 2012a; Buursma et al. 2005b; Doorduin et al. 2009, 2010, 2014; Paul et al. 2014; Vallez Garcia et al. 2015); see Fig. 17.3). The animals are intranasally inoculated with a solution of HSV-1 in saline using a micropipette, or they are sham-inoculated by applying saline without virus. Animals can remain either untreated or be treated with an anti-inflammatory drug (e.g., a NSAID or dexamethasone, to study the impact of drug treatment on neuroinflammation). The first signs of disease (irritated mouth and eyes) appear at day 5 after inoculation. Infected rats are scanned with a tracer candidate for PET imaging on day 6 or 7 after inoculation. The day of scanning depends on their disease symptoms. Infected rats will show irritated mouth and eyes, piloerection, hunched posture, and a sluggish response to stimuli on day 7. In some individuals, these symptoms already appear at day 6. Animals are scanned as soon as behavioral symptoms of encephalitis appear, and they are terminated after the scan. In this way, unnecessary suffering and a large variation in symptom severity are prevented. On the scanning day, the rats are anesthetized (isoflurane or sevoflurane) and cannulas are placed in a vein (for tracer injection) and a femoral artery (for rapid blood sampling). Some animals may be treated with a solution of a target-selective drug in saline, whereas other animals are treated only with saline. The anesthetized animals are positioned in a PET camera and injected with the novel radiotracer. The kinetics of tracer uptake in various brain regions is monitored with this camera for an extended period of time (usually 0.5–2 h, depending on the half-life of the administered radionuclide,

20.4 min for ^{11}C and 109.8 min for ^{18}F). During the PET scan, many small (0.1 ml) blood samples are drawn at different time intervals from the arterial cannula. Total blood volume withdrawn is <15% of the blood volume of the animal, and drawn blood is replaced by warm saline. Radioactivity in the samples (and in plasma acquired from these samples by centrifugation) is determined with a calibrated gamma counter and used as input function for kinetic modeling of regional tracer uptake. After the scan, animals are killed. Tissue samples are collected to study the distribution of radioactivity in organs outside the field of view of the PET camera (e.g., for calculation of dosimetry) and to determine regional expression levels of the target with independent tests (e.g., immunohistochemistry, autoradiography, Western blotting).

17.4.1.2 Intracerebroventricular Injection of Lipopolysaccharide (LPS)

Rats are anesthetized by intraperitoneal injection of a mixture of ketamine (25 mg/kg) and medetomidine (0.2 mg/kg) and are placed in a stereotaxic frame. Duratears Z eye cream is applied to prevent dehydration of the conjunctivae. Animals receive a mask for oxygenation and are placed on heating pads to maintain body temperature during surgery. A longitudinal incision is made along the medial line of the skull. The skin and fascia are pushed aside and the skull is exposed. A single hole is drilled at the proper coordinates, until the dura can be seen and opened. Using a Hamilton injection needle, 5–7 μL of sterile saline containing either bacterial lipopolysaccharide (LPS, *Escherichia coli* 020:B6 0.5 ug/uL) or nothing (sham-surgery controls) is injected. The injection takes 10 min. After an additional waiting time of 5 min, the syringe is withdrawn and the skin is closed. Saline is injected subcutaneously to avoid dehydration. Anti-sedan is used to wake up the animal. After stereotactic injection, lidocaine is applied on the head of the rat as an analgesic. Animals are scanned 2–3 days after LPS injection, when the neuroinflammation response is maximal. The scanning protocol is the same as described above for the viral infection model. The same neuroinflammation model can also be set up in mice (Dobos et al. 2012).

17.4.1.3 Stereotactic Injection of Lysolecithin

Rats are anesthetized with isoflurane and placed in a stereotaxic frame. Duratears Z eye cream is applied to prevent dehydration of the conjunctivae. After one longitudinal incision along the medial line of the skull, the skin and fascia are pushed aside and the skull is exposed. At the proper coordinates, a single hole is drilled, till the dura can be seen and opened. With a Hamilton injection needle, 1–2 ul of a 1–2% solution of lysolecithin in saline is deposited in the cerebellar peduncle. The needle is withdrawn and the skin is closed. On the day of stereotactic surgery and during the following 2 days, analgesia is applied to suppress pain (buprenorphine, 0.01–0.05 mg/kg, s.c.). Lysolecithin induces an inflammatory response resulting in local demyelination which peaks around 7 days, after which spontaneous remyelination occurs. This model has been used by us for the evaluation of tracers that should visualize demyelination in patients with multiple sclerosis (de Paula Faria et al. 2014).

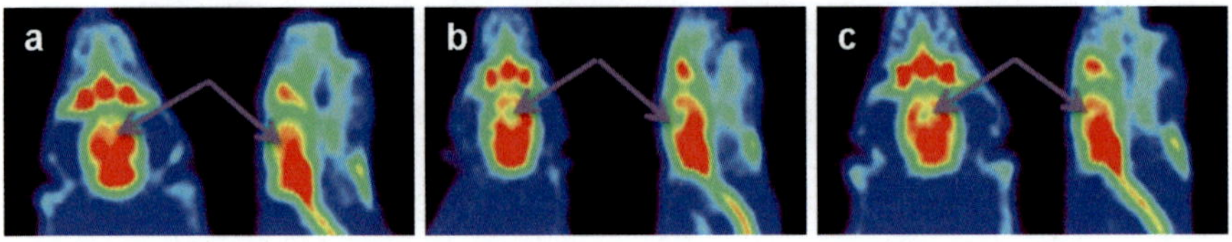

Fig. 17.4 MicroPET images of rats made with [^{11}C]MeDAS, a tracer which binds to myelin. *Arrows* point to the location of the lesion. Panel (**a**) Animals were injected with saline and scanned after 1 week. This sham lesion did not result in any loss of myelin or decrease of tracer uptake. Panel (**b**) Animals were injected with lysolecithin and scanned after 1 week. Strong demyelination was clearly visible at the lesion site. Panel (**c**) Animals were injected with lysolecithin and scanned after 4 weeks. Partial remyelination was accompanied by increased tracer uptake at the lesion site (compare panels **c** and **b**) (Data from de Paula Faria et al. 2014)

Animals are scanned 1 week after lysolecithin injection (to study the impact of demyelination on tracer uptake) or 4–6 weeks after lysolecithin injection (to evaluate whether the tracer can detect remyelination; see Fig. 17.4). The scanning protocol is the same as described above for the viral infection model.

Each of the mentioned inflammation models has specific advantages and disadvantages. The HSV-encephalitis model is suitable for the evaluation of tracers which should visualize the expression or function of viral proteins (Buursma et al. 2005b) and for evaluation of tracers which should target activated microglia or endangered neurons (Antunes et al. 2012a; Doorduin et al. 2009, 2010, 2014; Paul et al. 2014; Vallez Garcia et al. 2015). An advantage of the model is that it does not require any surgery or application of analgesics. A disadvantage of the model is that the disease symptoms can be variable (both in time course and extent). The LPS model is suitable for the evaluation of tracers which should target activated microglia, and the lysolecithin model for tracers which should visualize demyelination. Both models result in highly reproducible, local, and reversible lesions. Tracer uptake in the lesion and in contralateral healthy brain tissue can be directly compared; thus, the animal can serve as its own control. Longitudinal study designs can be applied to investigate the ability of the tracer candidate to detect temporal changes in target expression. However, for obvious reasons, these two models are not suitable for the evaluation of tracers that should visualize the expression or function of viral proteins, and both models are associated with an invasive surgical procedure and the application of analgesia.

17.4.2 Testing of a Tumor or Peripheral Inflammation Tracer

In oncologic research, it may be necessary to verify that a radiotracer can visualize rapidly dividing cells in tumors and accumulates selectively in tumor cells rather than in inflamed tissue. The tracer candidate is injected in animals which bear both a tumor and some form of peripheral inflammation. Uptake of the tracer in both types of tissue is directly compared, and the animal serves as its own control. A PET scan is made and tracer uptake is expressed in various ways: standardized uptake

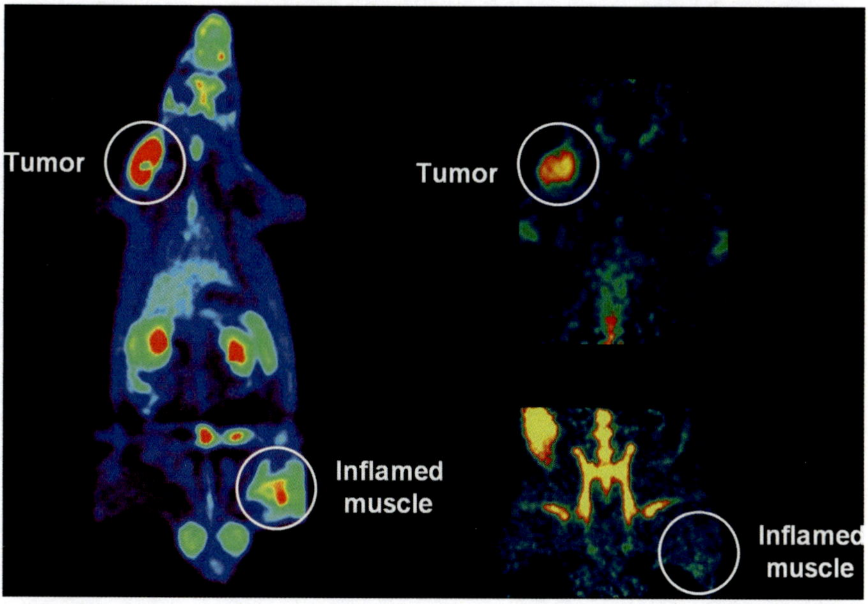

Fig. 17.5 MicroPET images of rats bearing both a tumor (in one shoulder) and a sterile inflammation (in one hind leg). The image at the *left* was made with the glucose analog ^{18}F-FDG, whereas the images at the *right* were acquired with the nucleoside 4′-[methyl-^{11}C]thiothymidine. *White circles* indicate the position of the tumor and the sterile inflammation. FDG accumulated both in tumor and inflammatory tissue, in contrast to thiothymidine, which accumulated only in the tumor (Data from Toyohara et al. (2012), van Waarde and Elsinga (2008))

values (SUV) in tumor, inflamed and healthy tissue, target-to-nontarget ratios of radioactivity, regional distribution volumes determined by graphical analysis or kinetic modeling, and binding potentials (estimated by kinetic modeling). When the tracer displays a high uptake in tumor tissue but a much lower uptake in inflammatory cells, the oncologic tracer candidate passes the test (it shows then both a high and a specific uptake in tumor tissue; see Fig. 17.5). However, when the tracer shows little accumulation in tumor tissue and the tumor is barely visualized, or if the tracer is strongly accumulated both in tumor and inflammatory tissue, the tracer candidate fails. Thus, a tracer may fail because of a low sensitivity, a low specificity, or a combination of low sensitivity and low specificity. The mentioned outcome parameters are chosen because they provide quantitative data on regional tracer uptake and they can later also be measured in humans (patients and healthy control subjects) with PET imaging.

A simplified version of the animal model is used to verify that an inflammation tracer can visualize inflammatory cells and accumulates selectively in these cells rather than in non-inflamed tissue. In this case, animals bear only a sterile inflammation and a tumor is lacking.

Depending on the tracer target (type of protein to which the tracer binds), one of the following animal models has been chosen:

17.4.2.1 Rat Glioma/Sterile Inflammation Model

Rats (normal Wistars) are subcutaneously inoculated with 2.5 million C6 cells (1:1 suspension of tumor cells in culture medium and Matrigel) in their right shoulder. A tumor appears in that position after a few days. The growth of this tumor is carefully monitored. When the tumor reaches a diameter of 1 cm (after an interval of 7–10 days), a sterile inflammation is created. Animals are then anesthetized with isoflurane and 0.1 ml of turpentine is intramuscularly injected in the thigh of their left hind leg. Within 24 h after this injection, they are scanned with the tracer candidate and terminated. Animal suffering is minimized by limiting the growth of the tumor and by reducing the interval between turpentine injection and PET scanning to a single day. On the scanning day, the rats are anesthetized (isoflurane or sevoflurane) and cannulas are placed in a vein (for tracer injection) and a femoral artery (for rapid blood sampling). Some animals may be treated with a solution of a target-selective drug, whereas other animals are treated only with vehicle. The anesthetized animals are positioned in a PET camera and injected with the novel radiotracer. The kinetics of tracer uptake in tumor and inflammatory tissue is monitored with this camera for an extended period of time (usually 0.5–2 h, depending on the half-life of the administered radionuclide, 20.4 min for ^{11}C and 109.8 min for ^{18}F). During the PET scan, many small (0.1 ml) blood samples are drawn at different time intervals from the arterial cannula. Total blood volume withdrawn is <15 % of the blood volume of the animal, and drawn blood is replaced by warm saline. Radioactivity in the samples (and in plasma acquired from these samples by centrifugation) is determined with a calibrated gamma counter and used as input function for kinetic modeling of regional tracer uptake. After the scan, animals are killed. Tissue samples are collected for various purposes (ex vivo counting of radioactivity, metabolite analysis, histological or histochemical examination). We have employed this animal model for more than 10 years in the evaluation of oncologic tracers (Antunes et al. 2012c, d; Toyohara et al. 2012; van Waarde et al. 2004b, 2006; van Waarde and Elsinga 2008). Although the animals are tumor-bearing and may develop a visible swelling of the hind leg, their behavior remains normal and their locomotion is unimpaired. Turpentine injection serves as an animal model of *acute* inflammation (granulocyte infiltration of inflamed tissue).

17.4.2.2 Xenograft Model of Inflammation

As an alternative to the turpentine injection described above, Wistar rats may be inoculated with various amounts of activated human peripheral blood mononuclear cells (1:1 mixture of hPBMC in PBS and Matrigel), 15 min before the PET scan with the novel radiotracer. This model is not associated with significant discomfort for the animals since the rats are anesthetized with isoflurane or sevoflurane before inoculation and all subsequent actions take place under deep, general anesthesia. The scanning procedure is identical to the one described above. The xenograft model serves as an animal model of *chronic* inflammation (since chronic inflammation is associated with infiltration of PBMC), but in contrast to a real chronic inflammation, this model is not associated with significant animal discomfort. We have employed this animal model for the evaluation of radiolabeled interleukins (Di Gialleonardo et al. 2012).

17.4.3 Testing the Capability of a Tracer to Visualize a Particular Type of Tumor

A final animal procedure aims to verify that an oncological radiotracer can visualize a particular type of tumor or a specific biomarker (e.g., drug target) on these tumor cells. The tracer candidate is injected in immune-deficient rats or mice bearing a human tumor xenograft, immune-competent rats bearing a rat tumor, or immune-competent mice bearing a murine tumor. The employed tumor models can either be heterotopic or orthotopic. Orthotopic models may be preferred since they better reflect the human situation (Bibby 2004; Hoffman 1994, 1999; Killion et al. 1998; Loi et al. 2011). Immune-competent animals are required when the radiotracer is developed for monitoring of cancer immunotherapy. Uptake of the tracer in the tumor and surrounding tissues is measured for an extended period of time (1–2 h) with a PET camera. The scanning procedure is similar to that described above, but a simplified procedure is used for mice. Since mice are too small for repeated arterial blood sampling and input function determination, tracer uptake in this species can only be expressed in the following ways: target-to-nontarget (e.g., tumor-to-muscle) ratio of radioactivity and standardized uptake value (SUV). These outcome parameters are chosen because they provide quantitative data on tracer uptake in tumor and healthy tissue, and they can later also be determined in humans (patients and healthy control subjects) with PET imaging. When the tracer displays a high target-to-nontarget ratio of radioactivity at certain intervals after injection (i.e., much greater than 1, preferably severalfold), the tracer candidate passes the tumor model test (it shows then both a high and a specific uptake in tumor tissue). However, when the tracer shows little accumulation in tumor tissue and the tumor is barely visualized, the tracer candidate fails.

Depending on the tracer target (type of protein to which the tracer binds) and the intended use of the tracer, a particular tumor model will be chosen. Mice or rats are subcutaneously inoculated with tumor cells (1:1 suspension of tumor cells in culture medium and Matrigel). A tumor appears at the site of inoculation after a few days to a few weeks, depending on the proliferation rate of the tumor cells. The growth of this tumor is carefully monitored. When the tumor reaches a size of 0.3–0.6 ml (for mice) or 0.5–1 ml (for rats), animals are scanned with the tracer candidate and terminated. Animal suffering is minimized by limiting the growth of the tumor. On the scanning day, the rodents are anesthetized (isoflurane or sevoflurane). Some animals may be treated with a solution of a target-selective drug, whereas others are treated only with the solvent. The anesthetized animals are positioned in a PET camera and injected with the novel radiotracer. The kinetics of tracer uptake in tumor and normal tissues is monitored with this camera for an extended period of time (usually 0.5–2 h, depending on the half-life of the administered radionuclide, 20.4 min for ^{11}C and 109.8 min for ^{18}F). After the scan, animals are killed. Tissue samples are collected for various purposes (ex vivo counting of radioactivity, metabolite analysis, histological or histochemical examination). We have employed tumor-bearing animals for more than 10 years in the evaluation of oncological tracers, both for PET and SPECT. Animal models of the following human tumors were successfully used: lung cancer (N417 (van Waarde et al. 2004a)), prostate cancer

(PC3 cells (Ananias et al. 2011; Carlucci et al. 2013, 2015; Yu et al. 2013)), melanoma (A375M cells (Rybczynska et al. 2013)), fibrosarcoma (HT1080 cells (Matusiak et al. 2015)), glioblastoma/astrocytoma (U373 cells (Buursma et al. 2005a)), and pancreatic carcinoid tumor (BON cells (Kuik et al. 2015; Neels et al. 2008)). Rat glioma (C6 (Antunes et al. 2012b; Rybczynska et al. 2009; van Waarde et al. 2007)), murine colon carcinoma (CT26 (Antunes et al. 2010)), and murine lung cancer (TC-1) models were also employed.

17.4.4 Conclusion

Milestone 3 If model-associated changes of tracer uptake reflect known changes of target expression (both in terms of time course and regional distribution) and if even small changes of target expression can be detected with PET, the radiotracer passes the sensitivity test and can be considered as a suitable candidate for future application in humans. However, when the disease or the intervention changes the expression of the target but such changes are not detected with PET or are detected with poor sensitivity (a large change of target expression resulting only in a barely detectable change of uptake of the PET probe), the radiotracer fails in step 3.

17.5 Caveats and Disclaimer

1. Radiolabeled receptor ligands, enzyme, transporter, or channel inhibitors should have a sufficiently high specific radioactivity at the time of injection, in order to detect specific binding of the probe to the small number of sites in the tissue of interest (Hume et al. 1998; Hume and Myers 2002; Jagoda et al. 2004; Kung and Kung 2005; Lancelot and Zimmer 2010).
2. The injected radiotracer should have a high chemical and radiochemical purity, since impurities in the tracer solution may interfere with in vivo binding of the probe. Nonradioactive precursor material in the tracer solution may compete with the radioligand for binding to its intended target.
3. Known species differences (e.g., between rodents and humans) should be considered in order to decide which animal species is most appropriate for tracer evaluation. Sex differences should also be taken into account. Particularly differences of metabolism can have a strong impact on radiotracer kinetics. General guidelines cannot be given, as each PET probe is unique (de Jong and Maina 2010; Hicks et al. 2006; Pakzad et al. 2005).
4. Target-selective drugs which are used in blocking experiments should bind to the same site and have similar physicochemical characteristics as the radiotracer candidate, but be chemically different from the substance under test. When "cold compound" (i.e., nonradioactive material that is chemically identical to the tracer molecule) is used for blocking purposes, blocker and probe may both bind to multiple cellular components and target selectivity of the PET probe cannot be proven (Chopra et al. 2011).

5. Target-selective drugs may not only block their intended targets but may also alter blood flow in the tissue of interest, change tracer transport and metabolism, and affect the activity of drug efflux pumps. In order to assess the potential involvement of such confounding factors, blood samples can be drawn during a PET scan and the time-dependent uptake of the probe can be subjected to pharmacokinetic analysis (Eckelman 2012).
6. Even if a tracer has the proper lipophilicity for passage of the blood-brain barrier, it may not enter the brain to a significant extent when it is a substrate for P-glycoprotein or any of the other efflux transporters. Thus, a good radioligand should not be a substrate for these transporters, unless one intends to use it for quantification of transporter activity (Ametamey et al. 2008; Giron 2009; Honer et al. 2014; Pike 2009).
7. In contrast to PET scanning in humans, small animal imaging requires immobilization of the animal which is usually achieved by the use of anesthesia. The impact of the applied anesthesia on tracer pharmacokinetics should therefore be considered (Ametamey et al. 2008; de Jong and Maina 2010; Giron 2009; Lancelot and Zimmer 2010). Tracers that are efficiently trapped (e.g., FDG) may be injected into awake rodents. Animals are then only anesthetized after tracer uptake has been completed and a steady state has been reached in target tissue, so that tracer distribution can be assessed by a late, static scan. This approach is only feasible when information on tracer kinetics is not required.

Disclaimer The procedures described above constitute the general approach for validation of a novel radiotracer. However, the milestones on the way should not be interpreted as absolute go/no-go moments. If a tracer fails in one test but passes all others, and if the point of failure concerns an issue which could be present in rodents but be absent in humans (e.g., rapid metabolism), a limited pilot study in primates can still be carried out in order to avoid the premature discarding of a valuable radiopharmaceutical. Such a decision may particularly be made if no other tracers for the target are available.

References

Aboagye EO, Luthra SK, Brady F, Poole K, Anderson H, Jones T, Boobis A, Burtles SS, Price P. Cancer Research UK procedures in manufacture and toxicology of radiotracers intended for pre-phase I positron emission tomography studies in cancer patients. Br J Cancer. 2002;86:1052–6.

Alexoff DL, Vaska P, Marsteller D, Gerasimov T, Li J, Logan J, Fowler JS, Taintor NB, Thanos PK, Volkow ND. Reproducibility of 11C-raclopride binding in the rat brain measured with the microPET R4: effects of scatter correction and tracer specific activity. J Nucl Med. 2003;44:815–22.

Ametamey SM, Honer M, Schubiger PA. Molecular imaging with PET. Chem Rev. 2008;108:1501–16.

Ananias HJ, Yu Z, Dierckx RA, van der Wiele C, Helfrich W, Wang F, Yan Y, Chen X, de Jong I, Elsinga PH. (99m)technetium-HYNIC(tricine/TPPTS)-Aca-bombesin(7-14) as a targeted imaging agent with microSPECT in a PC-3 prostate cancer xenograft model. Mol Pharm. 2011;8:1165–73.

Andersen VL, Hansen HD, Herth MM, Dyssegaard A, Knudsen GM, Kristensen JL. (11)C-labeling and preliminary evaluation of pimavanserin as a 5-HT2A receptor PET-radioligand. Bioorg Med Chem Lett. 2015;25:1053–6.

Antunes IF, Haisma HJ, Elsinga PH, Dierckx RA, de Vries EF. Synthesis and evaluation of [(18) F]-FEAnGA as a PET tracer for beta-glucuronidase activity. Chem: Bioconjug; 2010.

Antunes IF, Doorduin J, Haisma HJ, Elsinga PH, van Waarde A, Willemsen AT, Dierckx RA, de Vries EF. 18F-FEAnGA for PET of beta-glucuronidase activity in neuroinflammation. J Nucl Med. 2012a;53:451–8.

Antunes IF, Haisma HJ, Elsinga PH, Di Gialleonardo V, van Waarde A, Willemsen AT, Dierckx RA, de Vries EF. Induction of beta-glucuronidase release by cytostatic agents in small tumors. Mol Pharm. 2012b;9:3277–85.

Antunes IF, Haisma HJ, Elsinga PH, Sijbesma JW, van Waarde A, Willemsen AT, Dierckx RA, de Vries EF. In vivo evaluation of [18F]FEAnGA-Me: a PET tracer for imaging beta-glucuronidase (beta-GUS) activity in a tumor/inflammation rodent model. Nucl Med Biol. 2012c;39:854–63.

Antunes IF, Haisma HJ, Elsinga PH, van Waarde A, Willemsen AT, Dierckx RA, de Vries EF. In vivo evaluation of 1-O-(4-(2-fluoroethyl-carbamoyloxymethyl)-2-nitrophenyl)-O-beta-D-glucopyronurona te: a positron emission tomographic tracer for imaging beta-glucuronidase activity in a tumor/inflammation rodent model. Mol Imaging. 2012d;11:77–87.

Aronson JK. Biomarkers and surrogate endpoints. Br J Clin Pharmacol. 2005;59:491–4.

Backer MV, Backer JM. Imaging key biomarkers of tumor angiogenesis. Theranostics. 2012;2:502–15.

Bibby MC. Orthotopic models of cancer for preclinical drug evaluation: advantages and disadvantages. Eur J Cancer. 2004;40:852–7.

Biomarker Definitions Working Group. Biomarkers and surrogate endpoints: preferred definitions and conceptual framework. Clin Pharmacol Ther. 2001;69:89–95.

Brooks DJ, Pavese N. Imaging biomarkers in Parkinson's disease. Prog Neurobiol. 2011;95:614–28.

Buursma AR, Beerens AM, de Vries EF, van Waarde A, Rots MG, Hospers GA, Vaalburg W, Haisma HJ. The human norepinephrine transporter in combination with 11C-m-hydroxyephedrine as a reporter gene/reporter probe for PET of gene therapy. J Nucl Med. 2005a;46:2068–75.

Buursma AR, de Vries EF, Garssen J, Kegler D, van Waarde A, Schirm J, Hospers GA, Mulder NH, Vaalburg W, Klein HC. [18F]FHPG positron emission tomography for detection of herpes simplex virus (HSV) in experimental HSV encephalitis. J Virol. 2005b;79:7721–7.

Carlucci G, Ananias HJ, Yu Z, Hoving HD, Helfrich W, Dierckx RA, Liu S, de Jong I, Elsinga PH. Preclinical evaluation of a novel (1)(1)(1)In-labeled bombesin homodimer for improved imaging of GRPR-positive prostate cancer. Mol Pharm. 2013;10:1716–24.

Carlucci G, Kuipers A, Ananias HJ, de Paula Faria D, Dierckx RA, Helfrich W, Rink R, Moll GN, de Jong I, Elsinga PH. GRPR-selective PET imaging of prostate cancer using [(18) F]-lanthionine-bombesin analogs. Peptides. 2015;67:45–54.

Chopra A, Shan L, Eckelman WC, Leung K, Menkens AE. Important parameters to consider for the characterization of PET and SPECT imaging probes. Nucl Med Biol. 2011;38:1079–84.

Dandekar M, Tseng JR, Gambhir SS. Reproducibility of 18F-FDG microPET studies in mouse tumor xenografts. J Nucl Med. 2007;48:602–7.

de Jong M, Maina T. Of mice and humans: are they the same? – Implications in cancer translational research. J Nucl Med. 2010;51:501–4.

de Paula Faria D, de Vries EF, Sijbesma JW, Buchpiguel CA, Dierckx RA, Copray SC. PET imaging of glucose metabolism, neuroinflammation and demyelination in the lysolecithin rat model for multiple sclerosis. Mult Scler. 2014;20:1443–52.

Di Gialleonardo V, Signore A, Willemsen AT, Sijbesma JW, Dierckx RA, de Vries EF. Pharmacokinetic modelling of N-(4-[(18)F]fluorobenzoyl)interleukin-2 binding to activated lymphocytes in an xenograft model of inflammation. Eur J Nucl Med Mol Imaging. 2012;39:1551–60.

Dishino DD, Welch MJ, Kilbourn MR, Raichle ME. Relationship between lipophilicity and brain extraction of C-11-labeled radiopharmaceuticals. J Nucl Med. 1983;24:1030–8.

Dobos N, de Vries EF, Kema IP, Patas K, Prins M, Nijholt IM, Dierckx RA, Korf J, den Boer JA, Luiten PG, Eisel UL. The role of indoleamine 2,3-dioxygenase in a mouse model of neuroinflammation-induced depression. J Alzheimers Dis. 2012;28:905–15.

Doorduin J, Klein HC, Dierckx RA, James M, Kassiou M, de Vries EF. [11C]-DPA-713 and [18F]-DPA-714 as new PET tracers for TSPO: a comparison with [11C]-(R)-PK11195 in a rat model of herpes encephalitis. Mol Imaging Biol. 2009;11:386–98.

Doorduin J, Klein HC, de Jong JR, Dierckx RA, de Vries EF. Evaluation of [11C]-DAA1106 for imaging and quantification of neuroinflammation in a rat model of herpes encephalitis. Nucl Med Biol. 2010;37:9–15.

Doorduin J, de Vries EF, Dierckx RA, Klein HC. P-glycoprotein activity in the blood-brain barrier is affected by virus-induced neuroinflammation and antipsychotic treatment. Neuropharmacology. 2014;85:548–53.

Doze P, Elsinga PH, de Vries EF, van Waarde A, Vaalburg W. Mutagenic activity of a fluorinated analog of the beta-adrenoceptor ligand carazolol in the Ames test. Nucl Med Biol. 2000a;27:315–9.

Doze P, van Waarde A, Elsinga PH, Hendrikse NH, Vaalburg W. Enhanced cerebral uptake of receptor ligands by modulation of P-glycoprotein function in the blood-brain barrier. Synapse. 2000b;36:66–74.

Duffy SW, Treasure FP. Potential surrogate endpoints in cancer research – some considerations and examples. Pharm Stat. 2011;10:34–9.

Eckelman WC. The testing of putative receptor binding radiotracers in vivo. In: Diksic M, Reba RC, editors. Radiopharmaceuticals and brain pathology studied with PET and SPECT. Boca Raton: CRC Press; 1991. p. 41–68.

Eckelman WC. The application of receptor theory to receptor-binding and enzyme-binding oncologic radiopharmaceuticals. Nucl Med Biol. 1994;21:759–69.

Eckelman WC. Sensitivity of new radiopharmaceuticals. Nucl Med Biol. 1998;25:169–73.

Eckelman WC. The use of gene-manipulated mice in the validation of receptor binding radiotracer. Nucl Med Biol. 2003a;30:851–60.

Eckelman WC. The use of PET and knockout mice in the drug discovery process. Drug Discov Today. 2003b;8:404–10.

Eckelman WC. Targeted molecular imaging: target significance and probe validation. JACC Cardiovasc Imaging. 2012;5:616–8.

Eckelman WC, Mathis CA. Targeting proteins in vivo: in vitro guidelines. Nucl Med Biol. 2006;33:161–4.

Eckelman WC, Reba RC, Kelloff GJ. Targeted imaging: an important biomarker for understanding disease progression in the era of personalized medicine. Drug Discov Today. 2008;13:748–59.

Eckelman WC, Kilbourn MR, Mathis CA. Specific to nonspecific binding in radiopharmaceutical studies: it's not so simple as it seems! Nucl Med Biol. 2009;36:235–7.

Fischman AJ, Alpert NM, Rubin RH. Pharmacokinetic imaging: a noninvasive method for determining drug distribution and action. Clin Pharmacokinet. 2002;41:581–602.

Gibson RE, Eckelman WC, Rzeszotarski WJ, Jiang VW, Mazaitis A, Paik C, Komai T, Reba RC. Radiotracer localization by ligand-receptor interactions. In: Colombetti LG, editor. Principles of radiopharmacology, vol. 2. West Palm Beach: CRC Press; 1979. p. 17–40.

Giron MC. Radiopharmaceutical pharmacokinetics in animals: critical considerations. Q J Nucl Med Mol Imaging. 2009;53:359–64.

Giron MC, Portolan S, Bin A, Mazzi U, Cutler CS. Cytochrome P450 and radiopharmaceutical metabolism. Q J Nucl Med Mol Imaging. 2008;52:254–66.

Hendrikse NH, de Vries EG, Eriks-Fluks L, van der Graaf WT, Hospers GA, Willemsen AT, Vaalburg W, Franssen EJ. A new in vivo method to study P-glycoprotein transport in tumors and the blood-brain barrier. Cancer Res. 1999;59:2411–6.

Hicks RJ, Dorow D, Roselt P. PET tracer development – a tale of mice and men. Cancer Imaging. 2006;6:S102–6.

Hoffman RM. Orthotopic is orthodox: why are orthotopic-transplant metastatic models different from all other models? J Cell Biochem. 1994;56:1–3.

Hoffman RM. Orthotopic metastatic mouse models for anticancer drug discovery and evaluation: a bridge to the clinic. Invest New Drugs. 1999;17:343–59.

Honer M, Gobbi L, Martarello L, Comley RA. Radioligand development for molecular imaging of the central nervous system with positron emission tomography. Drug Discov Today. 2014;19:1936–44.

Hume SP, Myers R. Dedicated small animal scanners: a new tool for drug development? Curr Pharm Des. 2002;8:1497–511.

Hume SP, Gunn RN, Jones T. Pharmacological constraints associated with positron emission tomographic scanning of small laboratory animals. Eur J Nucl Med. 1998;25:173–6.

Ingvar M, Eriksson L, Rogers GA, Stone-Elander S, Widen L. Rapid feasibility studies of tracers for positron emission tomography: high-resolution PET in small animals with kinetic analysis. J Cereb Blood Flow Metab. 1991;11:926–31.

Ishiwata K, Kawamura K, Yanai K, Hendrikse NH. In vivo evaluation of P-glycoprotein modulation of 8 PET radioligands used clinically. J Nucl Med. 2007;48:81–7.

Jacobson O, Chen X. Interrogating tumor metabolism and tumor microenvironments using molecular positron emission tomography imaging. Theranostic approaches to improve therapeutics. Pharmacol Rev. 2013;65:1214–56.

Jagoda EM, Vaquero JJ, Seidel J, Green MV, Eckelman WC. Experiment assessment of mass effects in the rat: implications for small animal PET imaging. Nucl Med Biol. 2004;31:771–9.

Killion JJ, Radinsky R, Fidler IJ. Orthotopic models are necessary to predict therapy of transplantable tumors in mice. Cancer Metastasis Rev. 1998;17:279–84.

Kramer-Marek G, Capala J. Can PET imaging facilitate optimization of cancer therapies? Curr Pharm Des. 2012;18:2657–69.

Kroll T, Elmenhorst D, Weisshaupt A, Beer S, Bauer A. Reproducibility of non-invasive A1 adenosine receptor quantification in the rat brain using [(18)F]CPFPX and positron emission tomography. Mol Imaging Biol. 2014;16:699–709.

Kuik WJ, Kema IP, Brouwers AH, Zijlma R, Neumann KD, Dierckx RA, DiMagno SG, Elsinga PH. In vivo biodistribution of no-carrier-added 6-18F-fluoro-3,4-dihydroxy-L-phenylalanine (18F-DOPA), produced by a new nucleophilic substitution approach, compared with carrier-added 18F-DOPA, prepared by conventional electrophilic substitution. J Nucl Med. 2015;56:106–12.

Kung MP, Kung HF. Mass effect of injected dose in small rodent imaging by SPECT and PET. Nucl Med Biol. 2005;32:673–8.

Lamoureux M, Thorn S, Dumouchel T, Renaud JM, Klein R, Mason S, Lortie M, DaSilva JN, Beanlands RS, De Kemp RA. Uniformity and repeatability of normal resting myocardial blood flow in rats using [13N]-ammonia and small animal PET. Nucl Med Commun. 2012;33:917–25.

Lancelot S, Zimmer L. Small-animal positron emission tomography as a tool for neuropharmacology. Trends Pharmacol Sci. 2010;31:411–7.

Laruelle M, Slifstein M, Huang Y. Relationships between radiotracer properties and image quality in molecular imaging of the brain with positron emission tomography. Mol Imaging Biol. 2003;5:363–75.

Laven M, Markides K, Langstrom B. Analysis of microsomal metabolic stability using high-flow-rate extraction coupled to capillary liquid chromatography-mass spectrometry. J Chromatogr B Analyt Technol Biomed Life Sci. 2004;806:119–26.

Law MP. Demonstration of the suitability of CGP 12177 for in vivo studies of beta-adrenoceptors. Br J Pharmacol. 1993;109:1101–9.

Levin VA. Relationship of octanol/water partition coefficient and molecular weight to rat brain capillary permeability. J Med Chem. 1980;23:682–4.

Loi M, Di PD, Becherini P, Zorzoli A, Perri P, Carosio R, Cilli M, Ribatti D, Brignole C, Pagnan G, Ponzoni M, Pastorino F. The use of the orthotopic model to validate antivascular therapies for cancer. Int J Dev Biol. 2011;55:547–55.

Ma Y, Lang L, Kiesewetter DO, Jagoda E, Sassaman MB, Der M, Eckelman WC. Liquid chromatography-tandem mass spectrometry identification of metabolites of two 5-HT1A antagonists, N-[2-[4-(2-methoxylphenyl)piperazino]ethyl]-N-(2-pyridyl) trans- and cis-4-fluorocyclohexanecarboxamide, produced by human and rat hepatocytes. J Chromatogr B Biomed Sci Appl. 2001;755:47–56.

Ma Y, Kiesewetter DO, Jagoda EM, Huang BX, Eckelman WC. Identification of metabolites of fluorine-18-labeled M2 muscarinic receptor agonist, 3-(3-[(3-fluoropropyl)thio]-1,2,5-thiadiazol-4-yl)-1,2,5,6-tetrahydro-1-methylpyr idine, produced by human and rat hepatocytes. J Chromatogr B Analyt Technol Biomed Life Sci. 2002a;766:319–29.

Ma Y, Lang L, Kiesewetter DO, Eckelman WC. Liquid chromatography-tandem mass spectrometry identification of metabolites of three phenylcarboxyl derivatives of the 5-HT(1A) antagonist, N-(2-(4-(2-methoxyphenyl)-1-piperazinyl)ethyl)-N-(2-pyridyl) trans-4-fluorocyclohexanecarboxamide (FCWAY), produced by human and rat hepatocytes. J Chromatogr B Analyt Technol Biomed Life Sci. 2002b;780:99–110.

Ma Y, Kiesewetter D, Lang L, Eckelman WC. Application of LC-MS to the analysis of new radiopharmaceuticals. Mol Imaging Biol. 2003;5:397–403.

Marzin D. Preclinical evaluation of radiopharmaceutical: toxicological prerequisites. Nucl Med Biol. 1998;25:733–6.

Matusiak N, Castelli R, Tuin AW, Overkleeft HS, Wisastra R, Dekker FJ, Prely LM, Bischoff RP, van Waarde A, Dierckx RA, Elsinga PH. A dual inhibitor of matrix metalloproteinases and a disintegrin and metalloproteinases, [(1)(8)F]FB-ML5, as a molecular probe for non-invasive MMP/ADAM-targeted imaging. Bioorg Med Chem. 2015;23:192–202.

Maziere B, Cantineau R, Coenen HH. PET radiopharmaceutical metabolism – plasma metabolite analysis. In: Stöcklin G, Pike VW, editors. Radiopharmaceuticals for positron emission tomography: methodological aspects. Dordrecht: Kluwer Academic Publishers; 1992. p. 151–78.

McCarthy DJ, Halldin C, Andersson JD, Pierson ME. Discovery of novel positron emission tomography tracers. Annu Rep Med Chem. 2009;44:501–13.

Moerlein SM, Laufer P, Stocklin G. Effect of lipophilicity on the in vivo localization of radiolabelled spiperone analogues. Int J Nucl Med Biol. 1985;12:353–6.

Moerlein SM, Weisman RA, Beck D, Li AP, Welch MJ. Metabolism in vitro of radioiodinated N-isopropyl-p-iodoamphetamine by isolated hepatocytes. Nucl Med Biol. 1993;20:49–56.

Neels OC, Koopmans KP, Jager PL, Vercauteren L, van Waarde A, Doorduin J, Timmer-Bosscha H, Brouwers AH, de Vries EG, Dierckx RA, Kema IP, Elsinga PH. Manipulation of [11C]-5-hydroxytryptophan and 6-[18F]fluoro-3,4-dihydroxy-L-phenylalanine accumulation in neuroendocrine tumor cells. Cancer Res. 2008;68:7183–90.

Nordberg A. Molecular imaging in Alzheimer's disease: new perspectives on biomarkers for early diagnosis and drug development. Alzheimers Res Ther. 2011;3:34.

Pakzad F, Ell PJ, Carrio I. Molecular imaging in animal models of disease – every little detail counts! Eur J Nucl Med Mol Imaging. 2005;32:899–900.

Palumbo B, Buresta T, Nuvoli S, Spanu A, Schillaci O, Fravolini ML, Palumbo I. SPECT and PET serve as molecular imaging techniques and in vivo biomarkers for brain metastases. Int J Mol Sci. 2014;15:9878–93.

Passchier J, van Waarde A, Doze P, Elsinga PH, Vaalburg W. Influence of P-glycoprotein on brain uptake of [18F]MPPF in rats. Eur J Pharmacol. 2000;407:273–80.

Patel S, Gibson R. In vivo site-directed radiotracers: a mini-review. Nucl Med Biol. 2008;35:805–15.

Paul S, Khanapur S, Rybczynska AA, Kwizera C, Sijbesma JW, Ishiwata K, Willemsen AT, Elsinga PH, Dierckx RA, van Waarde A. Small-animal PET study of adenosine A(1) receptors in rat brain: blocking receptors and raising extracellular adenosine. J Nucl Med. 2011;52:1293–300.

Paul S, Khanapur S, Boersma W, Sijbesma JW, Ishiwata K, Elsinga PH, Meerlo P, Doorduin J, Dierckx RA, van Waarde A. Cerebral adenosine A(1) receptors are upregulated in rodent encephalitis. Neuroimage. 2014;92:83–9.

Pike VW. PET radiotracers: crossing the blood-brain barrier and surviving metabolism. Trends Pharmacol Sci. 2009;30:431–40.

Pimlott SL. Radiotracer development in psychiatry. Nucl Med Commun. 2005;26:183–8.
Pomper MG, Lee JS. Small animal imaging in drug development. Curr Pharm Des. 2005;11:3247–72.
Puntmann VO. How-to guide on biomarkers: biomarker definitions, validation and applications with examples from cardiovascular disease. Postgrad Med J. 2009;85:538–45.
Richter WS. Imaging biomarkers as surrogate endpoints for drug development. Eur J Nucl Med Mol Imaging. 2006;33 Suppl 1:6–10.
Rybczynska AA, Elsinga PH, Sijbesma JW, Ishiwata K, de Jong JR, de Vries EF, Dierckx RA, van Waarde A. Steroid hormones affect binding of the sigma ligand 11C-SA4503 in tumour cells and tumour-bearing rats. Eur J Nucl Med Mol Imaging. 2009;36:1167–75.
Rybczynska AA, de Bruyn M, Ramakrishnan NK, de Jong JR, Elsinga PH, Helfrich W, Dierckx RA, van Waarde A. In vivo responses of human A375M melanoma to a sigma ligand: 18F-FDG PET imaging. J Nucl Med. 2013;54:1613–20.
Silberstein EB. Preclinical evaluation of radiopharmaceutical toxicology: prerequisites. Nucl Med Biol. 2000;27:101.
Strimbu K, Tavel JA. What are biomarkers? Curr Opin HIV AIDS. 2010;5:463–6.
Syrota A. Investigation of myocardial receptors by PET in heart diseases. In: Heiss WD, editor. Clinical efficacy of positron emission tomography. Dordrecht: Martinus Nijhoff; 1987. p. 253–63.
Thackeray JT, Renaud JM, Kordos M, Klein R, dekemp RA, Beanlands RS, DaSilva JN. Test-retest repeatability of quantitative cardiac 11C-meta-hydroxyephedrine measurements in rats by small animal positron emission tomography. Nucl Med Biol. 2013;40:676–81.
Toyohara J, Elsinga PH, Ishiwata K, Sijbesma JW, Dierckx RA, van Waarde A. Evaluation of 4'-[methyl-11C]thiothymidine in a rodent tumor and inflammation model. J Nucl Med. 2012;53:488–94.
Tseng JR, Dandekar M, Subbarayan M, Cheng Z, Park JM, Louie S, Gambhir SS. Reproducibility of 3'-deoxy-3'-18F-fluorothymidine MicroPET studies in tumor xenografts in mice. J Nucl Med. 2005;46:1851–7.
Vallez Garcia D, de Vries EF, Toyohara J, Ishiwata K, Hatano K, Dierckx RA, Doorduin J. Evaluation of [C]CB184 for imaging and quantification of TSPO overexpression in a rat model of herpes encephalitis. Eur J Nucl Med Mol Imaging. 2015;42(7):1106–18.
van Waarde A, Elsinga PH. Proliferation markers for the differential diagnosis of tumor and inflammation. Curr Pharm Des. 2008;14:3326–39.
van Waarde A, Meeder JG, Blanksma PK, Bouwer J, Visser GM, Elsinga PH, Paans AMJ, Vaalburg W, Lie KI. Suitability of CGP12177 and CGP26505 for quantitative imaging of β adrenoceptors. Nucl Med Biol. 1992a;19:711–8.
van Waarde A, Meeder JG, Blanksma PK, Brodde OE, Visser GM, Elsinga PH, Paans AM, Vaalburg W, Lie KI. Uptake of radioligands by rat heart and lung in vivo: CGP 12177 does and CGP 26505 does not reflect binding to beta-adrenoceptors. Eur J Pharmacol. 1992b;222:107–12.
van Waarde A, Elsinga PH, Brodde OE, Visser GM, Vaalburg W. Myocardial and pulmonary uptake of S-1'-[18F]fluorocarazolol in intact rats reflects radioligand binding to beta-adrenoceptors. Eur J Pharmacol. 1995;272:159–68.
van Waarde A, Elsinga PH, Doze P, Heldoorn M, Jaeggi KA, Vaalburg W. A novel beta-adrenoceptor ligand for positron emission tomography: evaluation in experimental animals. Eur J Pharmacol. 1998;343:289–96.
van Waarde A, Buursma AR, Hospers GA, Kawamura K, Kobayashi T, Ishii K, Oda K, Ishiwata K, Vaalburg W, Elsinga PH. Tumor imaging with 2 sigma-receptor ligands, 18F-FE-SA5845 and 11C-SA4503: a feasibility study. J Nucl Med. 2004a;45:1939–45.
van Waarde A, Cobben DC, Suurmeijer AJ, Maas B, Vaalburg W, de Vries EF, Jager PL, Hoekstra HJ, Elsinga PH. Selectivity of 18F-FLT and 18F-FDG for differentiating tumor from inflammation in a rodent model. J Nucl Med. 2004b;45:695–700.
van Waarde A, Vaalburg W, Doze P, Bosker FJ, Elsinga PH. PET imaging of beta-adrenoceptors in human brain: a realistic goal or a mirage? Curr Pharm Des. 2004c;10:1519–36.

van Waarde A, Jager PL, Ishiwata K, Dierckx RA, Elsinga PH. Comparison of sigma-ligands and metabolic PET tracers for differentiating tumor from inflammation. J Nucl Med. 2006;47:150–4.

van Waarde A, Shiba K, de Jong JR, Ishiwata K, Dierckx RA, Elsinga PH. Rapid reduction of sigma1-receptor binding and 18F-FDG uptake in rat gliomas after in vivo treatment with doxorubicin. J Nucl Med. 2007;48:1320–6.

van Waarde A, Doorduin J, de Jong JR, Dierckx RA, Elsinga PH. Synthesis and preliminary evaluation of (S)-[11C]-exaprolol, a novel beta-adrenoceptor ligand for PET. Neurochem Int. 2008;52:729–33.

van Waarde A, Ramakrishnan NK, Rybczynska AA, Elsinga PH, Berardi F, de Jong JR, Kwizera C, Perrone R, Cantore M, Sijbesma JW, Dierckx RA, Colabufo NA. Synthesis and preclinical evaluation of novel PET probes for P-glycoprotein function and expression. J Med Chem. 2009;52:4524–32.

Vanderheyden JL. The use of imaging in preclinical drug development. Q J Nucl Med Mol Imaging. 2009;53:374–81.

Waterhouse RN. Determination of lipophilicity and its use as a predictor of blood-brain barrier penetration of molecular imaging agents. Mol Imaging Biol. 2003;5:376–89.

Wong DF, Pomper MG. Predicting the success of a radiopharmaceutical for in vivo imaging of central nervous system neuroreceptor systems. Mol Imaging Biol. 2003;5:350–62.

Wu C, Li F, Niu G, Chen X. PET imaging of inflammation biomarkers. Theranostics. 2013;3:448–66.

Yu Z, Carlucci G, Ananias HJ, Dierckx RA, Liu S, Helfrich W, Wang F, de Jong I, Elsinga PH. Evaluation of a technetium-99m labeled bombesin homodimer for GRPR imaging in prostate cancer. Amino Acids. 2013;44:543–53.

Zootechnical Issues in Small Animal Imaging

18

Jürgen W.A. Sijbesma, Janine Doorduin, and Aren van Waarde

Abstract

This chapter is focused on animal handling during rodent imaging. Particularly in studies of peripheral organs, the nutritional status of an animal may affect the imaging results. Anesthetics can also have a strong impact on scan data, for example, in drug research or studies of the brain. Physiological parameters like body temperature, heart rate, ventilation frequency, and oxygenation of the blood should always be carefully monitored and be kept close to their normal values or be standardized as much as possible when data from different animals are compared. Most PET and SPECT studies have employed the intravenous route for tracer administration. Several other routes are possible although these are probably not as widely applicable. For many studies, the combination of functional (PET, SPECT, fMRI) and anatomic (CT, US, MRI) imaging offers significant advantages, particularly if functional and anatomic data can be acquired simultaneously.

18.1 Introduction

This chapter is focused on important issues of animal handling in rodent imaging. Researchers should be aware of the fact that zootechnical procedures (i.e., animal housing, care, and nutrition) have a strong impact on the final outcome of a scanning protocol. Since our own expertise is related mainly to small animal PET (positron emission tomography) and SPECT (single photon emission computed tomography)

J.W.A. Sijbesma • J. Doorduin • A. van Waarde (✉)
Department of Nuclear Medicine and Molecular Imaging, University of Groningen,
University Medical Center Groningen, Hanzeplein 1, Groningen 9713GZ, The Netherlands
e-mail: a.van.waarde@umcg.nl

A.W.J.M. Glaudemans et al. (eds.), *Quality in Nuclear Medicine*,
DOI 10.1007/978-3-319-33531-5_18

imaging, emphasis will be placed on these modalities. For similar reasons, the subject matter of the chapter has been limited to the handling of rats and mice. Ferrets, pigs, and nonhuman primates can be used in the preclinical evaluation of nuclear medicine tracers, but a discussion of the handling of these species is outside the scope of this review.

Mice are commonly used in radiotracer development, as this rodent species offers several advantages. Mice are cheap, their biology is well known, and inbred strains and transgenic mouse models of human diseases are readily available. However, since the dimensions of an adult mouse (body weight about 20 g) are small compared to the linear resolution of a PET or SPECT camera (≥1 and 0.3 mm, respectively), small anatomical details in the brain, thorax, or abdomen cannot be distinguished. Moreover, the blood volume of a mouse is small (about 1.5 ml), which limits the possibilities of repeated blood sampling. For this reason, mice are not very suitable for studies which require pharmacokinetic modeling.

Rats offer most of the advantages of mice, although less transgenic models have been developed in this species. The larger dimensions of rats as compared to mice allow the quantification of tracer uptake in individual brain regions rather than the entire brain, and visualization of relevant anatomical details. Since the blood volume of an adult rat is considerable (about 25 ml for an animal of 300 g), repeated blood sampling is possible in this species. Data of such samples can be used for pharmacokinetic modeling.

18.2 Nutritional Status of the Scanned Animal

Diet composition, food intake, or duration of fasting before the onset of the scan may affect the outcome of rodent imaging. An early biodistribution study reported that glucose ([^{18}F]-FDG) uptake in rat heart, testis, and brown fat are strongly affected by the nutritional status of the animal. In myocardium and brown adipose tissue, tracer uptake was reduced two to threefold after 24 h of fasting, in contrast to the situation in testis, where a small increase was noted (Paul et al. 1987).

Fasting (20 h) of tumor-bearing mice resulted in a strong decline of the levels of blood glucose both in awake and anesthetized animals (ketamine/xylazine or pentobarbital). This decline was accompanied by an almost fourfold increase in tumor glucose ([^{18}F]-FDG) uptake and a significantly improved tumor-to-background contrast in PET images (Lee et al. 2005). In severe combined immunodeficient (SCID) mice bearing a human A431 epidermal carcinoma or U251 glioblastoma, fasting (8–12 h) or warming the animals during the scan significantly reduced [^{18}F]-FDG uptake in brown fat and strongly improved tumor visualization (Fueger et al. 2006). In contrast to [^{18}F]-FDG uptake in peripheral organs (tumor, muscle, and heart), glucose metabolism in the brain of male Black 6 mice (C57BL/6) was not significantly affected by fasting (Wong et al. 2011).

The biodistribution of other metabolic PET tracers (e.g., amino acids) is also affected by nutritional status. An early PET study reported that the uptake of [^{13}N]-glutamate in rat pancreas is significantly higher when animals are subjected to overnight fasting rather than allowed free access to pellet food (Kubota et al. 1983).

Composition of the diet (either standard or high-energy) was shown to affect tumor [^{18}F]-FDG uptake and cell proliferation in mice bearing MC38 colon carcinomas. A high-energy diet induced hyperinsulinemia, activated insulin receptors in tumor cells, and increased tumor uptake of [^{18}F]-FDG. These negative effects of the high-energy diet could be blocked by treating mice with metformin, a drug which reduces hepatic gluconeogenesis and insulin levels in the circulation (Mashhedi et al. 2011).

Uptake of inflammatory markers ([^{18}F]-galacto-RGD, [^{18}F]-FDG) in murine atherosclerotic lesions is related to the lipid/cholesterol content of the diet and reduced after lipid-lowering interventions (Saraste et al. 2012; Silvola et al. 2011).

These limited data indicate that a short period of fasting may be useful in scanning protocols aimed at visualization of the peripheral tumors, the atherosclerotic lesions, the pancreas, or the heart. However, fasting seems to offer no significant advantages in studies of the brain.

18.3 Anesthesia: A Necessary Evil?

Rodents are usually anesthetized during a scan, in order to prevent them from moving during the imaging procedure. However, anesthetics limit the capability of an animal to maintain homeostasis. Anesthesia affects several physiological parameters, such as myocardial function and blood flow (Cavazzuti et al. 1987; Croteau et al. 2004; Gjedde et al. 1980; Hansen et al. 1988; Hendrich et al. 2001; LaManna et al. 1986; Lenz et al. 1998, 1999; Maekawa et al. 1986; Saija et al. 1989; Todd et al. 1996; Zanelli et al. 1975), blood volume in tissue (Todd et al. 1996; Zanelli et al. 1975), gastrointestinal motion (Yamashita et al. 2011), and inflammatory responses (Chiang et al. 2008; Fortis et al. 2012). Anesthesia is associated with alterations of cerebral energy metabolism (Cavazzuti et al. 1987; Crosby et al. 1982; Dam et al. 1990; Eintrei et al. 1999; Hodes et al. 1985; Lenz et al. 1998, 1999; Maekawa et al. 1986; Ori et al. 1986; Saija et al. 1989; Sokoloff et al. 1977) and neurotransmission (Ford et al. 1986; Shahani et al. 2002). For these reasons, PET findings in anesthetized rodents may not be a proper representation of the physiology of the conscious animal.

Experimental animals can be trained to stay quiet during a PET or MRI scan and be accustomed to a restraining device (Becerra et al. 2011; Chen et al. 2010; Ferris et al. 2006; Hosoi et al. 2005; Itoh et al. 2009; King et al. 2005; Lahti et al. 1998; Lee et al. 2005; Mizuma et al. 2010; Momosaki et al. 2004). Using such a device, the side effects of anesthetics can be avoided since the scanned subject remains conscious. However, physical restraint will always cause some stress, even in trained rodents. PET data of conscious animals kept in a restrainer can therefore not be considered as an exact replica of processes in the undisturbed situation.

Restraint stress can be avoided by using a portable imaging device such as the *RatCap* (Schulz et al. 2011) or a system which corrects for motion such as the *AwakeSPECT* (Baba et al. 2013). Using such devices, imaging data can be acquired from unrestrained animals. However, because of the weight and/or the physical dimensions of the devices, the scanned animals are not stress-free.

Although the impact of anesthetics on scan data is probably great, their exact consequences are frequently unknown. Because of the lack of a true control or an absolute gold standard, evaluation of the impact of anesthetics is difficult. Three different approaches have been used to assess this impact:

(i) Animals are scanned using an identical procedure but different anesthetics (Alstrup et al. 2011; Casteels et al. 2010; Croteau et al. 2004; Elfving et al. 2003; Flores et al. 2008; Fuchs et al. 2013; Kersemans et al. 2011; Matsumura et al. 2003; Yu et al. 2009). This approach may reveal differences between anesthetic drugs, but it cannot indicate which anesthetic procedure results in the smallest disturbance of the normal tissue homeostasis.
(ii) Awake and anesthetized animals are scanned with the same tracer (Chen et al. 2010; Hosoi et al. 2005; Itoh et al. 2009; Lee et al. 2005; McCormick et al. 2011; Mizuma et al. 2010; Momosaki et al. 2004; Yamashita et al. 2011). Using this approach, observed differences between the study groups may be due both to the anesthetic and to restraint stress in the group which is awake.
(iii) Awake rodents are injected with radiotracer and allowed free movement in their home cages or in an open-field arena. After a prolonged interval, when the regional distribution of the tracer has approached a steady state, the animals are anesthetized and a PET scan is made (Fueger et al. 2006; Matsumura et al. 2003; Patel et al. 2008; Radonjic et al. 2013; Schiffer et al. 2007; Shih et al. 2008; Toyama et al. 2004). A great advantage of this approach is that data from the scan represent distribution of the tracer in the conscious state. However, the kinetics of tracer uptake during that state are unknown, and for this reason, tracer-kinetic modeling is not possible. In some cases, tracer distribution volumes can be calculated from a delayed scan using a simulated input function based on validated assumptions (Tantawy et al. 2011).

Anesthesia procedures for rodent imaging have been the subject of several excellent reviews (Alstrup et al. 2013; Gargiulo et al. 2012a, b; Hanusch et al. 2007; Hildebrandt et al. 2008; Tremoleda et al. 2012). Some known effects of anesthetics are discussed below.

18.3.1 Impact of Anesthetics on Glucose Metabolism

In the ground-breaking paper of Louis Sokoloff concerning measurement of the metabolic rate of glucose with [^{14}C]-deoxyglucose and ex vivo autoradiography, striking regional differences of metabolism were observed in the brain of conscious rats, the highest levels occurring in gray matter of certain cortical areas, e.g., auditory cortex, and the lowest levels in white matter regions. Thiopental anesthesia markedly reduced glucose metabolic rate, particularly in gray matter, and metabolic rate became more uniform throughout the brain (Sokoloff et al. 1977).

In subsequent years, the [^{14}C]-deoxyglucose method has been applied to study the impact of different anesthetics on cerebral glucose metabolism in rodents. Barbiturates such as phenobarbital (Hodes et al. 1985) or pentobarbital (Saija et al. 1989); inhalation anesthetics such as isoflurane (Lenz et al. 1998, 1999; Maekawa et al. 1986; Ori et al. 1986), sevoflurane (Lenz et al. 1998), or desflurane (Lenz et al. 1999); and propofol, a modulator of GABA receptor-mediated signal transduction (Dam et al. 1990), were found to cause widespread, dose-dependent reductions of glucose metabolism particularly in gray matter areas of the brain. However, ketamine anesthesia resulted in a unique metabolic response, with striking increases of glucose consumption in limbic areas (cingulate gyrus, hippocampus, striatum, extrapyramidal motor system, olfactory tubercle, corpus callosum) and decreases of energy metabolism in somatosensory and auditory systems (Cavazzuti et al. 1987; Crosby et al. 1982; Eintrei et al. 1999; Saija et al. 1989). Ketamine-induced increases of glucose metabolism in limbic areas were blocked after coadministration of diazepam (Eintrei et al. 1999).

Effects of anesthesia on glucose metabolism in rodent tissues have also been studied with PET and 2-deoxy-2-[^{18}F] fluoro-D-glucose ([^{18}F]-FDG). The imaging findings were in accordance with previously reported data from ex vivo autoradiography. In a study comparing six different anesthetics (ketamine, ketamine/xylazine, chloral hydrate, pentobarbital, propofol, isoflurane), all anesthetics – with the exception of ketamine – were found to reduce glucose metabolism in rat brain (Matsumura et al. 2003). Reductions of brain metabolism by anesthetics were a general finding in [^{18}F]-FDG-PET studies, both of mice (Toyama et al. 2004) and rats (Fig. 18.1), but glucose uptake in the myocardium and in implanted tumors was found to be affected by the type of anesthetic, some anesthetics (e.g., isoflurane) causing an increase (Toyama et al. 2004) and others (e.g., ketamine/xylazine, pentobarbital) causing a decline (Lee et al. 2005; Toyama et al. 2004). These differences may be related to the fact that ketamine/xylazine, in contrast to isoflurane or sevoflurane, strongly increases levels of nonradioactive glucose in the blood, which competes with [^{18}F]-FDG for uptake in target tissues (Flores et al. 2008; Fueger et al. 2006; Woo et al. 2008; Yu et al. 2009).

Thus, the regional distribution and intensity of glucose metabolism, both in the brain and in peripheral organs, are strongly dependent on animal handling, particularly the duration or depth of anesthesia and the type of anesthetic. Vital parameters (levels of glucose and oxygen in the blood, body temperature, ventilation frequency, and heart rate) should be carefully monitored during PET studies of anesthetized rodents and be maintained at identical levels in all study groups.

18.3.2 Impact of Anesthetics on Neurotransmission

18.3.2.1 Dopaminergic System

Since the neurotransmitter dopamine plays an important role in motor function, addiction, and reward, dopaminergic neurotransmission is frequently studied in biomedical research. Changes of dopaminergic neurotransmission are implied in Parkinson's disease and schizophrenia, and dopamine receptor antagonists are widely employed as antipsychotic drugs. Several findings in experimental animals have indicated that anesthesia may affect the dopaminergic system.

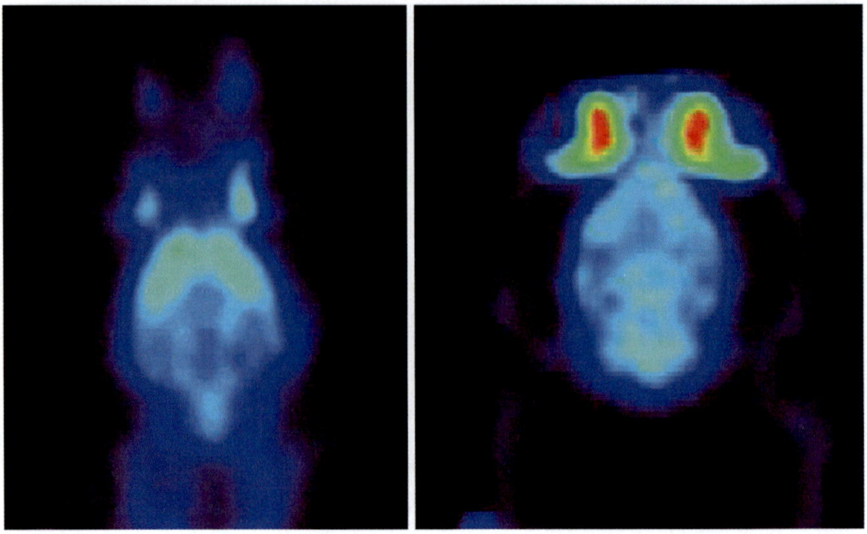

Fig. 18.1 Impact of anesthesia on glucose metabolism in the rat brain. *Left image*: [^{18}F]-FDG injected intraperitoneally in a conscious rat which was then allowed to explore a novel environment for 45 min. After this period, the animal was anesthetized with isoflurane and a 20 min static scan was made. *Right image*: [^{18}F]-FDG injected intravenously in an animal which was under anesthesia with pentobarbital. In the conscious animal, striking regional differences of tracer uptake were noted, with particularly high uptake in the forebrain. In the anesthetized animal, glucose uptake was reduced, and although the difference between gray matter and white matter remained visible, regional differences were largely abolished (Unpublished data of A.van Waarde)

Target-to-nontarget ratios of the dopamine reuptake tracer [^{125}I]-PE2I were decreased after anesthetizing rats with ketamine/xylazine or isoflurane, but unaltered after anesthesia with zoletile mixture or halothane (Elfving et al. 2003). The specific binding fraction and the kinetics of [^{11}C]-cocaine in the brain were different when rats were anesthetized with α-chloralose or isoflurane, suggesting differences of dopamine transporter availability (Du et al. 2009). The binding potential of the dopamine transporter ligand [^{123}I]-ioflupane in awake mice was about 50 % of that which was observed in mice which were anesthetized with isoflurane (Baba et al. 2013).

Binding potential (k_3/k_4) values of the dopamine D1 receptor tracer [^{11}C]-SCH23390 were significantly increased (by 36–46 %) when rats were anesthetized with chloral hydrate or ketamine and significantly decreased (by 41 %) after anesthesia with pentobarbital (Momosaki et al. 2004). These findings may be related to blood flow changes, since chloral hydrate and ketamine increase and pentobarbital decreases perfusion of the brain (Alstrup et al. 2013). Another possible (but unproven) mechanism is that anesthetics modify the affinity of D1 receptors for radioligand binding.

Binding potential values (distribution volume ratios minus one) of the dopamine D2/D3 ligand [^{11}C]-raclopride in rats anesthetized with isoflurane were twice as high as in animals anesthetized with fentanyl-fluanisone-midazolam (Alstrup et al. 2011). Binding of the dopamine D2/D3 agonist [^{11}C]-(+)-PHNO in rat brain was also increased when animals were anesthetized with isoflurane, and the reduction of [^{11}C]-(+)-PHNO binding by amphetamine was greater in isoflurane-anesthetized animals than in awake rats (McCormick et al. 2011). However, the striatal binding of [^{11}C]-raclopride in animals anesthetized with ketamine/xylazine was not significantly different from that observed in freely moving rodents, and drug challenges (methamphetamine, gamma-vinyl-GABA) affected [^{11}C]-raclopride binding similarly in both study groups (Patel et al. 2008). In contrast to the increases reported for [^{11}C]-raclopride and [^{11}C]-(+)-PHNO, binding potential (BP_{ND}) values of the dopamine D2 receptor ligand [^{18}F]-fallypride in rat striatum were found to be 30 % lower in isoflurane-anesthetized animals compared to awake controls (Tantawy et al. 2011).

Many literature findings indicate that anesthetics alter dopamine transporter activity (Shahani et al. 2002) and trafficking (Byas-Smith et al. 2004; Votaw et al. 2003, 2004), extracellular dopamine concentration (Adachi et al. 2005; Votaw et al. 2003), and metabolism of dopamine to 3,4-dihydroxyphenylacetic acid (Adachi et al. 2005; Ford et al. 1986). Via such mechanisms, anesthetics affect the outcome of PET and SPECT studies of the dopaminergic system.

18.3.2.2 Serotonergic System

PET and SPECT imaging of other neurotransmitter systems is also influenced by anesthesia. Using a constant infusion protocol and arterial blood sampling, Tokugawa et al. monitored tissue-to-plasma ratios of the serotonin 5-HT$_{1A}$ receptor ligand [^{18}F]-FPWAY in awake and isoflurane-anesthetized rats. Stable ratios were reached within 30 min after the start of tracer infusion. Ratios in lateral hippocampus and cerebellum of anesthetized animals were found to be greater (by 32–63 %) than in awake rats. This difference was explained by the assumption that levels of extracellular serotonin are reduced under isoflurane anesthesia (Tokugawa et al. 2007). In an earlier study, target-to-background ratios of the serotonin transporter ligand [^{3}H]-*(S)*-citalopram were found to be increased by isoflurane or halothane and decreased by ketamine/xylazine, whereas ratios of the serotonin 5-HT$_2$ ligand [^{18}F]-altanserin were unaffected (Elfving et al. 2003). It is not known whether all of these changes are related to altered concentrations of extracellular serotonin.

18.3.2.3 Cholinergic System

Using a bolus plus constant infusion protocol, American authors studied the in vivo binding of the muscarinic cholinoceptor ligand N-[^{18}F]-fluoroethyl-piperidinyl benzilate ([^{18}F]-FEPB) in rats (Kilbourn et al. 2007). Both isoflurane and pentobarbital caused a strong (65–90 %) increase of tracer distribution volume in receptor-rich regions of the brain (striatum, cortex, hippocampus). Pretreatment of animals with an acetylcholinesterase inhibitor (phenserine) caused a strong increase of tracer binding (70 %) in awake rats, but not in animals anesthetized with isoflurane or pentobarbital. The mechanisms underlying these phenomena are not understood, but it is evident that anesthesia can affect the outcome of PET studies with cholinergic tracers and may even obscure the result of pharmacological challenges.

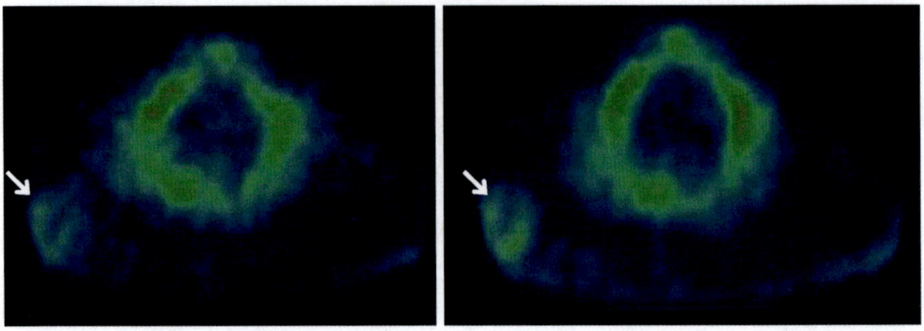

Fig. 18.2 Impact of anesthesia on sigma-1 receptor imaging in a tumor. A rat with a C6 glioma implanted subcutaneously in its right shoulder was scanned twice with [^{11}C]-SA4503. *Left image*: animal shortly anesthetized (< 20 min before start of the scan). *Right image*: animal anesthetized for 3 h with pentobarbital. *Arrows* indicate the position of the tumor. Tumor uptake of the radioligand is significantly increased after prolonged anesthesia (Data from Rybczynska et al. 2009)

18.3.2.4 Other Aspects of Neurotransmission

Using in vivo saturation experiments with increasing masses of *(R)*-rolipram and [^{11}C]-*(R)*-rolipram as tracer, Itoh et al. determined the B_{max} and K_d of phospodiesterase-4 in the brain of conscious and isoflurane-anesthetized rats. Significantly higher values (by 29 % and 59 %, respectively) were observed in conscious as opposed to anesthetized animals (Itoh et al. 2009).

The binding of a sigma-1 receptor ligand, particularly to sigma-1 receptors in peripheral tumors, is significantly and time dependently increased when animals are anesthetized with pentobarbital (Rybczynska et al. 2009). Pentobarbital interferes with steroid metabolism, resulting in reduced levels of progesterone and a decreased competition of this endogenous antagonist with the radioligand for binding to the sigma-1 receptor protein (Fig. 18.2). In contrast to the increases induced by pentobarbital, the radioligand binding to sigma-1 receptors is significantly decreased when animals are anesthetized with racemic ketamine (van Waarde et al. 2004). The *(R)*-enantiomer of ketamine has significant affinity for sigma-1 receptors.

In contrast to findings reported for other neuroreceptors, no significant changes in cerebral uptake of the cannabinoid CB1 receptor ligand [^{18}F]-MK-9470 were noted in rats anesthetized with pentobarbital or isoflurane as compared to freely moving animals, neither with in vivo techniques (parametric PET images, statistical parametric mapping) nor with ex vivo autoradiography, although relative tracer uptake in the cortex seemed to be slightly (9–13 %) decreased and relative uptake in cerebellum was slighty (13–14 %) increased (Casteels et al. 2010).

18.3.2.5 Use Anesthetics with Care

In conclusion, anesthetics can have species-specific and dose-dependent effects on the binding properties of neuroreceptors, transporters, and enzymes. Some anesthetics may even interfere directly with the target receptor. Consideration of the possible undesired effects of anesthesia is necessary when an imaging study is planned, and the applied anesthetic should be carefully chosen, depending on the study target. Vital parameters should be monitored, and the scanning conditions should be standardized as much as possible during PET studies of the brain.

18.3.3 Monitoring of Physiological Parameters in Anesthetized Rodents

An anesthetized animal is limited in its capability to maintain homeostasis. This limitation becomes more severe when the experimental procedure is more invasive, when the animal is anesthetized longer (Tremoleda et al. 2012) or when drugs are administered which potentiate the effect of anesthetics, such as adenosine A1 receptor agonists (Paul et al. 2014).

Negative side effects of anesthetics are depressions of the respiratory, cardiovascular, and thermoregulatiory systems. For this reason, these systems should be monitored during animal experiments (Tremoleda et al. 2012; Zutphen et al. 2001). Monitoring of the clinical and physiological parameters of an anesthetized animal is required since it allows the investigator to maintain the animal in a steady state, e.g., by adjusting the depth of anesthesia or the settings of an artificial respirator, the animal can be kept in a constant condition (Tremoleda et al. 2012; Zutphen et al. 2001).

Any monitoring procedure starts with checking the condition of the animal before the experiment (Tremoleda et al. 2012). If undesired or unexpected abnormalities in the clinical or physiological parameters are noted during the subsequent experimental procedures, data from the affected animal should be excluded from the final study report.

18.3.3.1 Respiratory System

Poor exchange of O_2 and CO_2 or administration of excessive concentrations of anesthetics can cause hypoxia and eventually lead to respiratory arrest. Monitoring of the animal's breathing frequency and ventilatory motion besides regular inspection for the symptoms of cyanosis can inform the investigator that the animal is developing hypoxia (Tremoleda et al. 2012; Zutphen et al. 2001). Continuous monitoring is possible by using a capnograph which measures CO_2 concentration in the exhaled air. The gold standard for measurement of respiratory function is blood gas analysis (Tremoleda et al. 2012; Zutphen et al. 2001).

18.3.3.2 Cardiovascular System

The cardiovascular system can be monitored by examining heart rate, stroke volume, and capillary refill time (Tremoleda et al. 2012; Zutphen et al. 2001). More advanced techniques are the use of an electrocardiograph (ECG) to monitor the electrical activity of the heart, a pulse oximeter to measure the myocardial pulse and oxygenation level of the arterial blood, and pressure transducers to record changes of blood pressure (Tremoleda et al. 2012; Zutphen et al. 2001).

Some imaging modalities offer the possibility of respiratory and cardiovascular gating. Gating is used to avoid image artifacts due to cardiac and/or respiratory

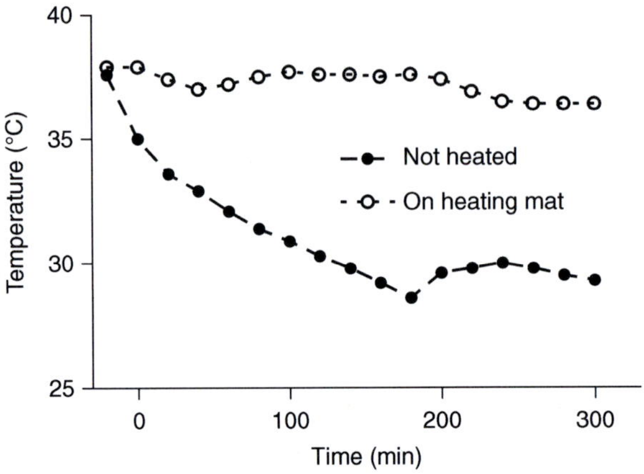

Fig. 18.3 Impact of anesthesia on rodent thermoregulation. An adult rat (body weight 300–350 g) which is anesthetized with pentobarbital (and is kept in this condition with small additional intraperitoneal injections of the drug) is not in a steady state. Body temperature of the animal drops dramatically. The increase of body temperature at 3 h is caused by shivering. When the same rat is anesthetized but artificially warmed, using a heating mat and an electronic temperature controller, the normal tissue homeostasis can be approached much more closely. Rectal temperatures are plotted

movement or to get information about the cardiac and/or the respiratory cycle (Szymanski et al. 2012; Tahari et al. 2014). Gating software can also be employed to monitor the respiratory and cardiovascular systems of a scanned animal.

18.3.3.3 Thermoregulatory System

Rodents have a high skin-surface-to-body-weight ratio and a high metabolic rate, which makes them vulnerable to hypothermia and also to hyperthermia when they are artificially heated. For body temperature monitoring, the core temperature of the animal can be measured with a rectal probe and an electronic thermometer (Tremoleda et al. 2012; Zutphen et al. 2001).

For continuous monitoring and maintenance of body temperature close to the physiological value, commercially available controllers can be used (Fig. 18.3). These consist of a temperature probe, an adjustable electronic thermostat, and some source of heat (heating pad, infrared lamp, or circulating water system).

For a more detailed overview of monitoring possibilities and their physiological background, the reader is advised to consult textbooks about laboratory animal science.

18.4 Tracer Administration

18.4.1 Possible Routes of Tracer Administration

A crucial action in small animal PET/SPECT imaging is the administration or delivery of the radiotracer to the animal. It is important to consider possible routes of administration and their pros and cons during the planning phase. The route of choice will depend on the animal species, sex, experimental design (longitudinal versus single study), pharmacokinetics of the radiotracer, and practical feasibility. This section of our chapter describes the most common administration methods based on the expertise in our institution and on literature data. Administration methods can be divided in four groups.

18.4.1.1 Transdermal Route

Transdermal means "through the skin." Although this administration method is technically easy, it is not often used in PET/SPECT imaging. The chemical structure of the radiotracer can prevent its penetration through the skin. Moreover, the transdermal application method can result in a slow delivery of the tracer with unknown kinetics. This causes difficulties for quantification of tracer uptake in the target organ. However, if the labeled compound is quickly absorbed through the skin, this route of application may be suitable for imaging purposes, e.g., the monitoring of transdermal drug delivery (Petroni et al. 2011).

18.4.1.2 Enteral Route

Enteral ("through the intestines") refers to oral administration via the food or drinking water or rectal administration. The method is technically easy and results in low discomfort for the animals, but a few things should be taken into account. The chemical structure of the radiotracer can change when it is mixed with food or water and passes the stomach and gut. Addition of the tracer can have a negative effect on the taste of the animal's diet. This last complication can be avoided by using intragastric gavage (Sarparanta et al. 2011; Yamashita et al. 2011) in anesthetized or conscious animals, although this is associated with some risk of damaging the esophagus. Another option is using a carrier like a silicon capsule or silicon particles for tracer administration (Sarparanta et al. 2011; Shingaki et al. 2012). Since the enteral administration of a radiotracer results in a rather slow entry of radioactivity in the circulation, this route is less suitable for isotopes with short half lives such as ^{15}O, ^{13}N, and ^{11}C.

18.4.1.3 Administration Through the Respiratory System

Radioactively labeled gasses such as [^{15}O]-oxygen, carbon dioxide, or carbon monoxide can be administered through the respiratory system, i.e., by inhalation. This method is technically challenging. Animals must be anesthetized and be connected to a closed ventilation system by the use of a trachea tube or tracheotomy (Watabe et al. 2013; Yee et al. 2006). The method also requires additional equipment to control the influx and efflux of gas from the animal's lungs. This includes an artificial ventilator, additional connecting tubes, and electronic equipment for ventilation monitoring (Watabe et al. 2013; Yee et al. 2006).

The pulmonary deposition of drug aerosols and nanoparticles has been studied, using PET and SPECT. Such studies require an even greater technical effort because the administered aerosols need to meet specific requirements of particle diameter since the pulmonary disposition is directly related to particle size (Asgharian et al. 2003; Kuehl et al. 2012; Palko et al. 2010). Thus, an additional aerosol generator, pump, flow meter, filters, and tubing are required (Asgharian et al. 2003; Kuehl et al. 2012). For the administration of nanoparticles, a flat-tipped syringe placed in the trachea or bronchial gavage may suffice, but with the risk of damaging the esophagus (Palko et al. 2010).

18.4.1.4 Parenteral Routes

Parenteral indicates the use of an administration route other than transdermal, enteral, or through the respiratory system (Palko et al. 2010). Radiotracers for PET and SPECT are frequently injected. Standard injection methods are (Zutphen et al. 2001):

- Intracutaneous (i.c.): injection in the skin
- Subcutaneous (s.c.): injection under the skin
- Intramuscular (i.m.): injection in the muscle
- Intraperitoneal (i.p.): injection in the abdominal cavity
- Intravenous (i.v.): injection in a vein

Since intracutaneous, subcutaneous, and intramuscular injections have the same disadvantages as the transdermal administration route, intraperitoneal and intravenous injections are commonly applied.

Intraperitoneal Administration

Injection in the abdominal cavity is relatively easy. A skilled person can do this within seconds with relatively little preparation. Another advantage of this technique is that injections can be done both in anesthetized and awake rodents. Although the method is technically not very challenging, the success rate is lower than expected. Even after taking all the necessary precautions (holding the animal and needle in the proper way), in 15 % of the injections (Vines et al. 2011), the radiotracer ended up in the intestines where it got trapped, resulting in a useless scan. Another disadvantage of intraperitoneal tracer injections is that the technique results in a rather slow entry of the radiotracer in the circulation (Wong et al. 2011; Yoder et al. 2011). In practice this means that i.p. injections may only be suitable for microPET scans with metabolic tracers such as [^{18}F]-FDG. For the same reason, i.p. injections are not appropriate for dynamic scanning protocols or for studies involving pharmacokinetic modeling (Nanni et al. 2007; Vines et al. 2011; Wong et al. 2011; Yoder et al. 2011).

Intravenous Injection

The most frequently used method for radiotracer delivery is intravenous injection. Since the tracer is directly administered into the circulation, this technique results in rapid pharmacokinetics and is suitable for dynamic scanning protocols (Nanni et al. 2007; Vines et al. 2011). The method can be applied both in awake and in anesthetized animals. Tracer injection can be done manually (for bolus injections) or with an infusion pump (for bolus injections and/or slow infusions). Intravenous injection is technically more challenging than intraperitoneal tracer administration. It is an invasive method which requires preparations (e.g., the insertion of a cannula) and considerable care before, during, and after the procedure.

When animals are anesthetized with a substance causing vasoconstriction (Nanni et al. 2007; Vines et al. 2011), small veins are hard to find. Vasoconstriction can partly be prevented by heating the tissue around the target vein right after the animal has been anesthetized, using warm water or an infrared lamp. The injection can cause hemorrhages. Bleeding can be prevented by putting pressure on the target vein after injection. Repeated injections or puncturing can cause tissue damage, fibrosis (Vines et al. 2011), and even complete degradation of the vein. It is advised to practice the method in order to gain experience and reduce the chances of failure and discomfort before starting small animal imaging experiments.

18.4.2 Selection of a Blood Vessel for Tracer Administration

The answer to the question which vein should be employed as an injection pathway depends on many variables. Rats and mice have a very long tail with two lateral veins which can be used for manual or pump-controlled radiotracer injections. Because of the length of this tail, tail veins can be repeatedly used for multiple injections without running the risk of venous degradation. The length of the tail makes it also possible to inject the animal when it is lying in the scanner as the injection site is usually outside the field of view and far from any target organ.

In our institution we use a 29G $x^1/_2$ (0.33 × 12 mm) insulin needle for injections in a preheated mouse tail and a 26G $x^3/_4$ (0.64 × 19 mm) butterfly for injections in a preheated rat tail. Although tail veins are easily accessible, this injection pathway has some disadvantages. Tails cool rapidly, and tail veins are therefore very sensitive to vasoconstriction, especially when anesthetized animals are housed in a cold room. Several studies have shown that even after correct intravenous injection, extravasation of the radiotracer may occur in the upper part of the tail, resulting in a slow release of part of the injected dose from a depot and difficulties in quantitative analysis of the PET data (Groman et al. 2004; Nanni et al. 2007; Vines et al. 2011).

A suitable alternative for the technically challenging tail vein injection is an injection of the radiotracer in the retro-orbital venous sinus (Nanni et al. 2007; Schoell et al. 2009; Steel et al. 2008). Although some expertise is required, several publications indicate that retro-orbital injections are easy, can be rapidly performed, and result in rapid drug delivery to target organs (Nanni et al. 2007; Schoell et al. 2009). The technique is reproducible and can be repeated without any serious complications (Nanni et al. 2007).

However, it is difficult to use this injection route when the animal is lying inside a PET or SPECT camera. Retro-orbital injections are thus not very suitable for dynamic scanning protocols. Moreover, the volume which can be injected is more limited than in tail vein injections; therefore, the injected tracer should have a high specific radioactivity (Nanni et al. 2007; Steel et al. 2008). Finally, it is advised to not use this technique for studies of the brain. Elevated levels of radioactivity at the injection site can result in spillover to regions of interest within the brain and can negatively affect the brain data (Greeuw et al. 2013).

A method which has been widely used in our institution is tracer injection through the penile vein. This method has a success rate of 95 % for rats. The high rate of success is related to the absence of vasoconstriction under normal conditions. Because the penis of a rat or mouse is hidden in a sheath and is kept close to the abdomen, the organ is maintained at body temperature. Pulling the penis out of its sheath causes obstruction of the blood flow in this organ. The penile vein swells, and the tracer can be injected in rats with a 27G $x^3/_4$ (0.4 × 19 mm) needle. The success rate in mice is even higher than 95 %. The penis of a mouse contains a dense capillary microcirculation which is comparable with the retro-orbital area. Injection with a 29G $x^1/_2$ (0.33 × 12 mm) insulin needle just under the skin is enough to deliver the radiotracer into the blood stream. The technique is easy to learn and is suitable for pump infusion (Kononov et al. 1994).

Only in rare cases, penile vein injections fail. Injection failures cause an interstitial swelling which is clearly visible. Animals with such swellings can be excluded from the data analysis. Even when the tracer gets trapped under the skin or in erectile tissue, radioactivity will be slowly released into the blood because of the presence of a dense cluster of blood vessels, especially when the penis is put back in its sheath.

Besides these advantages, penile vein injections have also some disadvantages. For obvious reasons, the method can only be used in male rodents. When repeated injections are required, the penis may develop fibrotic scar tissue which lowers the success rate.

For rats, a catheter in the vena femoralis is a very safe pathway for delivery of the radiotracer. This technique can be combined with a catheter in the arteria femoralis for arterial blood sampling or blood pressure measurements. Although we have employed femoral cannulas only in terminal experiments and anesthetized rodents, it is possible to use such catheters in conscious, freely moving rats (Hall et al. 1984; Peternel et al. 2010).

The ideal position for a vena femoralis catheter is in the deeper part of the groin next to the femoral artery and saphenous nerve (Hall et al. 1984; Jespersen et al. 2012; Peternel et al. 2010). The vein can be easily reached by making a small incision on the ventral side of the animal, 1 or 2 cm from the median (Fig. 18.4). After fixation of the vein, a small hole can be made with a bended 25G $x^5/_8$ (0.5 × 16 mm) needle. Subsequently, a fine bore polythene tube (0.40 mm inner diameter, 0.80 mm outer diameter) can be inserted into the vein and be pushed up almost to the upper part of the inferior vena cava. The whole procedure takes 10–15 min. Because the vena femoralis is a large blood vessel, it is possible to draw some blood as a confirmation that the catheter is in the right position (Hall et al. 1984; Jespersen et al. 2012; Peternel et al. 2010). Because the catheter is close to the upper part of the inferior vena cava, the injected radiotracer reaches the heart almost immediately. From there, it is distributed to the

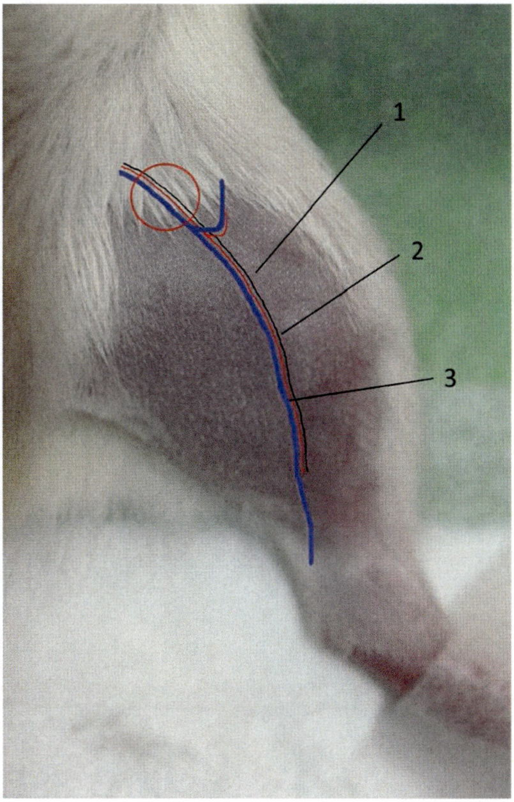

Fig. 18.4 Anatomy of the hind leg of a rat, showing the position of the saphenous nerve (*1*), the femoral artery (*2*), and the femoral vein (*3*). The *circle* shows the insertion side for the polythene tube

rest of the body. Femoral vein catheters can be used both for manual injections and pump infusion protocols.

18.5 Combining Different Imaging Modalities

Since PET and SPECT provide specific biochemical but not anatomic information, these nuclear imaging techniques are frequently combined with other imaging modalities (CT or MRI) which can visualize anatomical details. The images of the different modalities are then fused (Jan et al. 2005; Pascau et al. 2012), and in the joined images, the position of radiotracer accumulation can be clearly identified. Structural information from CT or MRI images can also be used to derive a transmission map for object-specific attenuation correction. Hybrid scanners combining PET, SPECT, and CT (Sanchez et al. 2013), PET and MRI (Herzog et al. 2010; Herzog 2012; Judenhofer et al. 2008; Maramraju et al. 2011; Raylman et al. 2007), or fluorescence tomography, SPECT, and CT (Solomon et al. 2013) have been developed, allowing co-registration of radionuclide, optical, and anatomical data with minimized movement of the subject.

A conventional small animal CT scan results in radiation doses ranging from 70 to 400 mGy (Taschereau et al. 2006). Doses of a few Gy can already have significant biological effects (e.g., reduction of tumor growth, damage to rapidly dividing tissues), whereas doses between 6.5 and 7 Gy are lethal to mice. With conventional equipment, repeated CT scanning is possible, but the total number of scans in a single animal is definitely limited. Recent advances in rodent CT scanners (low-dose detector hardware) have resulted in very significant (up to 90%) reductions in radiation dose, making microCT suitable for longitudinal study protocols (Osborne et al. 2012).

18.5.1 SPECT/CT

MicroSPECT/CT (using ^{99m}Tc-labeled human albumin nanoparticles) has been successfully applied to study the pattern of lymphatic flow from heterotopic abdominal cardiac grafts in mice. Mediastinal lymph nodes were identified as the draining nodes (Brown et al. 2011). Monitoring of stem cell trafficking (Gildehaus et al. 2011) or of viral spread along a lymphatic network (Raty et al. 2007) in the living organism was another application of this form of multimodal imaging. The use of microSPECT/CT rather than microSPECT has been proven to result in a more accurate quantification of heterogeneous intratumoral tracer uptake in human pancreatic cancer xenografts (Carlson et al. 2006) and sarcomas (Umeda et al. 2012). SPECT/CT has proven useful for the localization of pulmonary (Hayakawa et al. 2013) and abdominal (Huhtala et al. 2010; Nayak et al. 2013; Pool et al. 2012) lesions in mouse models of human cancer and atherosclerotic plaques in mouse aorta (Li et al. 2010). Moreover, SPECT/CT has been used for assessment of age-dependent changes of pulmonary function (ventilation/perfusion) in mice (Jobse et al. 2012) and of particle-size-dependent deposition of aerosols in mouse and rat lungs (Kuehl et al. 2012). Focused ultrasound-induced increases of blood-brain barrier permeability in rats (Lin et al. 2009; Yang et al. 2011) and hypoperfusion in a rodent model of stroke (Seo et al. 2007) could also be assessed with this technique.

18.5.2 SPECT/MRI

MicroSPECT/MRI has been applied to identify the location of atherosclerotic plaques in large blood vessels (Li et al. 2010) and orthotopic pleural mesothelioma in the mouse abdomen (Nayak et al. 2013).

18.5.3 SPECT/US

Ultrasound-derived partial volume correction resulted in improved quantification of myocardial segmental perfusion with 99mTc-tetrofosmin in rats (Goethals et al. 2012).

18.5.4 PET/CT

Combination of PET and CT has proven useful for the localization of abdominal lesions in experimental animals, e.g., pancreatic (Fendrich et al. 2011; Flores et al. 2009) and prostate (Garrison et al. 2007) tumors, and for identifying inflammation in murine atherosclerotic plaques (Nahrendorf et al. 2008, 2009. The use of microPET/CT rather than microPET resulted in a more accurate quantification of infarct size in mouse models of myocardial infarction (Gargiulo et al. 2012c; Greco et al. 2012) and of [^{18}F]-FDG uptake in an orthotopic model of glioblastoma multiforme after radiotherapy (Park et al. 2011) and in thymic lymphoma after chemotherapy (Walter et al. 2010). Iodinated contrast media can be used in small animal PET/CT in order to improve tumor delineation and diagnostic performance (Lasnon et al. 2013). Small animal PET/CT has been applied to assess bone damage in ovariectomized rats (Li et al. 2011) and adrenergic activation of interscapular brown adipose tissue in mice (Mirbolooki et al. 2014), using [^{18}F]-fluoride and [^{18}F]-FDG as radiotracers. Copper metabolism in the liver of an animal model of Wilson's disease could also be studied using this technique (Peng et al. 2012).

18.5.5 PET/MRI

Simultaneous small animal PET and MRI has been successfully applied for the study of cardiac metabolism and function in mice (Buscher et al. 2010) and rheumatoid arthritis in rats (Zhang et al. 2013). A recent animal study has indicated that FDG-PET and contrast-enhanced MRI may play complementary roles in the imaging of certain types of carcinomas characterized by poor FDG uptake and abundant cancer-associated stroma, as FDG-PET alone is not sufficient to estimate the total tumor burden for radiotherapy planning (Farace et al. 2012).

In conclusion, combination of PET or SPECT imaging with data from other modalities (CT, MRI, and ultrasound) may offer significant advantages. The precise anatomical location of tracer uptake (e.g., in segments of the heart, atherosclerotic plaques, lymph nodes, brown fat, abdominal organs, and small tumor metastases) can be determined. Data from CT or MRI also allow more accurate correction for partial volume effects besides attenuation and scatter of the emitted gamma radiation. Although multimodality imaging may result in longer scanning protocols (and thus may be more challenging from the perspective of animal care and maintenance of homeostasis), the resulting increase of information will definitely have added value. With multimodality scanners, comprehensive data sets can be collected on multiple physiological events, e.g., regional blood flow, glucose metabolism and drug-receptor interaction, or regional brain stimulation and neurotransmitter synthesis.

Disclaimer This chapter could only discuss some important aspects of animal handling related to our own field of expertise. Species other than mice or rats (e.g., guinea pigs, ferrets, Göttingen minipigs, cynomolgus monkeys, and baboons) are used by many institutions in the preclinical evaluation of PET tracers. For information about such species, the reader should consult the specialized literature.

References

Adachi YU, Yamada S, Satomoto M, Higuchi H, Watanabe K, Kazama T. Isoflurane anesthesia induces biphasic effect on dopamine release in the rat striatum. Brain Res Bull. 2005;67:176–81.

Alstrup AK, Smith DF. Anaesthesia for positron emission tomography scanning of animal brains. Lab Anim. 2013;47:12–8.

Alstrup AK, Simonsen M, Landau AM. Type of anesthesia influences positron emission tomography measurements of dopamine D2/D3 receptor binding in the rat brain. Scand J Lab Anim Sci. 2011;38:195–200.

Alstrup AK, Landau AM, Holden JE, Jakobsen S, Schacht AC, Audrain H, Wegener G, Hansen AK, Gjedde A, Doudet DJ. Effects of anesthesia and species on the uptake or binding of radioligands in vivo in the Göttingen minipig. Biomed Res Int. 2013;2013:808713.

Asgharian B, Kelly JT, Tewksbury EW. Respiratory deposition and inhalability of monodisperse aerosols in Long-Evans rats. Toxicol Sci. 2003;71:104–11.

Baba JS, Endres CJ, Foss CA, Nimmagadda S, Jung H, Goddard JS, Lee S, McKisson J, Smith MF, Stolin AV, Weisenberger AG, Pomper MG. Molecular imaging of conscious, unrestrained mice with AwakeSPECT. J Nucl Med. 2013;54:969–76.

Becerra L, Chang PC, Bishop J, Borsook D. CNS activation maps in awake rats exposed to thermal stimuli to the dorsum of the hindpaw. Neuroimage. 2011;54:1355–66.

Brown K, Badar A, Sunassee K, Fernandes MA, Shariff H, Jurcevic S, Blower PJ, Sacks SH, Mullen GE, Wong W. SPECT/CT lymphoscintigraphy of heterotopic cardiac grafts reveals novel sites of lymphatic drainage and T cell priming. Am J Transplant. 2011;11:225–34.

Buscher K, Judenhofer MS, Kuhlmann MT, Hermann S, Wehrl HF, Schäfers KP, Schäfers M, Pichler BJ, Stegger L. Isochronous assessment of cardiac metabolism and function in mice using hybrid PET/MRI. J Nucl Med. 2010;51:1277–84.

Byas-Smith MG, Li J, Szlam F, Eaton DC, Votaw JR, Denson DD. Isoflurane induces dopamine transporter trafficking into the cell cytoplasm. Synapse. 2004;53:68–73.

Carlson SK, Classic KL, Hadac EM, Bender CE, Kemp BJ, Lowe VJ, Hoskin TL, Russell SJ. In vivo quantitation of intratumoral radioisotope uptake using micro-single photon emission computed tomography/computed tomography. Mol Imaging Biol. 2006;8:324–32.

Casteels C, Bormans G, Van Laere K. The effect of anaesthesia on [18F]MK-9470 binding to the type 1 cannabinoid receptor in the rat brain. Eur J Nucl Med Mol Imaging. 2010;37:1164–73.

Cavazzuti M, Porro CA, Biral GP, Benassi C, Barbieri GC. Ketamine effects on local cerebral blood flow and metabolism in the rat. J Cereb Blood Flow Metab. 1987;7:806–11.

Chen YY, Shih YY, Lo YC, Lu PL, Tsang S, Jaw FS, Liu RS. MicroPET imaging of noxious thermal stimuli in the conscious rat brain. Somatosens Mot Res. 2010;27:69–81.

Chiang N, Schwab JM, Fredman G, Kasuga K, Gelman S, Serhan CN. Anesthetics impact the resolution of inflammation. PLoS One. 2008;3:e1879.

Crosby G, Crane AM, Sokoloff L. Local changes in cerebral glucose utilization during ketamine anesthesia. Anesthesiology. 1982;56:437–43.

Croteau E, Benard F, Bentourkia M, Rousseau J, Paquette M, Lecomte R. Quantitative myocardial perfusion and coronary reserve in rats with 13N-ammonia and small animal PET: impact of anesthesia and pharmacologic stress agents. J Nucl Med. 2004;45:1924–30.

Dam M, Ori C, Pizzolato G, Ricchieri GL, Pellegrini A, Giron GP, Battistin L. The effects of propofol anesthesia on local cerebral glucose utilization in the rat. Anesthesiology. 1990;73:499–505.

Du C, Tully M, Volkow ND, Schiffer WK, Yu M, Luo Z, Koretsky AP, Benveniste H. Differential effects of anesthetics on cocaine's pharmacokinetic and pharmacodynamic effects in brain. Eur J Neurosci. 2009;30:1565–75.

Eintrei C, Sokoloff L, Smith CB. Effects of diazepam and ketamine administered individually or in combination on regional rates of glucose utilization in rat brain. Br J Anaesth. 1999;82:596–602.

Elfving B, Bjornholm B, Knudsen GM. Interference of anaesthetics with radioligand binding in neuroreceptor studies. Eur J Nucl Med Mol Imaging. 2003;30:912–5.

Farace P, Conti G, Merigo F, Tambalo S, Marzola P, Sbarbati A, Quarta C, D'Ambrosio D, Chondrogiannis S, Nanni C, Rubello D. Potential role of combined FDG PET/CT and contrast enhancement MRI in a rectal carcinoma model with nodal metastases characterized by a poor FDG-avidity. Eur J Radiol. 2012;81:658–62.

Fendrich V, Schneider R, Maitra A, Jacobsen ID, Opfermann T, Bartsch DK. Detection of precursor lesions of pancreatic adenocarcinoma in PET-CT in a genetically engineered mouse model of pancreatic cancer. Neoplasia. 2011;13:180–6.

Ferris CF, Febo M, Luo F, Schmidt K, Brevard M, Harder JA, Kulkarni P, Messenger T, King JA. Functional magnetic resonance imaging in conscious animals: a new tool in behavioural neuroscience research. J Neuroendocrinol. 2006;18:307–18.

Flores JE, McFarland LM, Vanderbilt A, Ogasawara AK, Williams SP. The effects of anesthetic agent and carrier gas on blood glucose and tissue uptake in mice undergoing dynamic FDG-PET imaging: sevoflurane and isoflurane compared in air and in oxygen. Mol Imaging Biol. 2008;10:192–200.

Flores LG, Bertolini S, Yeh HH, Young D, Mukhopadhyay U, Pal A, Ying Y, Volgin A, Shavrin A, Soghomonyan S, Tong W, Bornmann W, Alauddin MM, Logsdon C, Gelovani JG. Detection of pancreatic carcinomas by imaging lactose-binding protein expression in peritumoral pancreas using [18F]fluoroethyl-deoxylactose PET/CT. PLoS One. 2009;4:e7977.

Ford AP, Marsden CA. Influence of anaesthetics on rat striatal dopamine metabolism in vivo. Brain Res. 1986;379:162–6.

Fortis S, Spieth PM, Lu WY, Parotto M, Haitsma JJ, Slutsky AS, Zhong N, Mazer CD, Zhang H. Effects of anesthetic regimes on inflammatory responses in a rat model of acute lung injury. Intensive Care Med. 2012;38:1548–55.

Fuchs K, Kukuk D, Mahling M, Quintanilla-Martinez L, Reischl G, Reutershan J, Lang F, Rocken M, Pichler BJ, Kneilling M. Impact of anesthetics on 3'-[18F]fluoro-3'-deoxythymidine ([18F]FLT) uptake in animal models of cancer and inflammation. Mol Imaging. 2013;12:277–87.

Fueger BJ, Czernin J, Hildebrandt I, Tran C, Halpern BS, Stout D, Phelps ME, Weber WA. Impact of animal handling on the results of 18F-FDG PET studies in mice. J Nucl Med. 2006;47:999–1006.

Gargiulo S, Greco A, Gramanzini M, Esposito S, Affuso A, Brunetti A, Vesce G. Mice anesthesia, analgesia, and care, Part I: anesthetic considerations in preclinical research. ILARJ. 2012a;53:E55–69.

Gargiulo S, Greco A, Gramanzini M, Esposito S, Affuso A, Brunetti A, Vesce G. Mice anesthesia, analgesia, and care, Part II: anesthetic considerations in preclinical imaging studies. ILARJ. 2012b;53:E70–81.

Gargiulo S, Greco A, Gramanzini M, Petretta MP, Ferro A, Larobina M, Panico M, Brunetti A, Cuocolo A. PET/CT imaging in mouse models of myocardial ischemia. J Biomed Biotechnol. 2012c;2012:541872.

Garrison JC, Rold TL, Sieckman GL, Figueroa SD, Volkert WA, Jurisson SS, Hoffman TJ. In vivo evaluation and small-animal PET/CT of a prostate cancer mouse model using 64Cu bombesin analogs: side-by-side comparison of the CB-TE2A and DOTA chelation systems. J Nucl Med. 2007;48:1327–37.

Gildehaus FJ, Haasters F, Drosse I, Wagner E, Zach C, Mutschler W, Cumming P, Bartenstein P, Schieker M. Impact of indium-111 oxine labelling on viability of human mesenchymal stem cells in vitro, and 3D cell-tracking using SPECT/CT in vivo. Mol Imaging Biol. 2011;13:1204–14.

Gjedde A, Rasmussen M. Pentobarbital anesthesia reduces blood-brain glucose transfer in the rat. J Neurochem. 1980;35:1382–7.

Goethals LR, De GF, Vanhove C, Roosens B, Devos H, Lahoutte T. Improved quantification in pinhole gated myocardial perfusion SPECT using micro-CT and ultrasound information. Contrast Media Mol Imaging. 2012;7:167–74.

Greco A, Petretta MP, Larobina M, Gargiulo S, Panico M, Nekolla SG, Esposito G, Petretta M, Brunetti A, Cuocolo A. Reproducibility and accuracy of non-invasive measurement of infarct size in mice with high-resolution PET/CT. J Nucl Cardiol. 2012;19:492–9.

Greeuw I, Bergstra R. Retro-orbitale injectie van radioactieve stoffen bij gebruik in een PET scanner. Biotechniek. 2013;5:9–14.

Groman EV, Reinhardt CP. Method to quantify tail vein injection technique in small animals. Contemp Top Lab Anim Sci. 2004;43:35–8.

Hall RI, Ross LH, Bozovic M, Grant JP. A simple method of obtaining repeated venous blood samples from the conscious rat. J Surg Res. 1984;36:92–5.

Hansen TD, Warner DS, Todd MM, Vust LJ, Trawick DC. Distribution of cerebral blood flow during halothane versus isoflurane anesthesia in rats. Anesthesiology. 1988;69:332–7.

Hanusch C, Hoeger S, Beck GC. Anaesthesia of small rodents during magnetic resonance imaging. Methods. 2007;43:68–78.

Hayakawa T, Mutoh M, Imai T, Tsuta K, Yanaka A, Fujii H, Yoshimoto M. SPECT/CT of lung nodules using 111In-DOTA-c(RGDfK) in a mouse lung carcinogenesis model. Ann Nucl Med. 2013;27:640–7.

Hendrich KS, Kochanek PM, Melick JA, Schiding JK, Statler KD, Williams DS, Marion DW, Ho C. Cerebral perfusion during anesthesia with fentanyl, isoflurane, or pentobarbital in normal rats studied by arterial spin-labeled MRI. Magn Reson Med. 2001;46:202–6.

Herzog H. PET/MRI: challenges, solutions and perspectives. Z Med Phys. 2012;22:281–98.

Herzog H, Pietrzyk U, Shah NJ, Ziemons K. The current state, challenges and perspectives of MR-PET. Neuroimage. 2010;49:2072–82.

Hildebrandt IJ, Su H, Weber WA. Anesthesia and other considerations for in vivo imaging of small animals. ILARJ. 2008;49:17–26.

Hodes JE, Soncrant TT, Larson DM, Carlson SG, Rapoport SI. Selective changes in local cerebral glucose utilization induced by phenobarbital in the rat. Anesthesiology. 1985;63:633–9.

Hosoi R, Matsumura A, Mizokawa S, Tanaka M, Nakamura F, Kobayashi K, Watanabe Y, Inoue O. MicroPET detection of enhanced 18F-FDG utilization by PKA inhibitor in awake rat brain. Brain Res. 2005;1039:199–202.

Huhtala T, Laakkonen P, Sallinen H, Yla-Herttuala S, Narvanen A. In vivo SPECT/CT imaging of human orthotopic ovarian carcinoma xenografts with 111In-labeled monoclonal antibodies. Nucl Med Biol. 2010;37:957–64.

Itoh T, Abe K, Zoghbi SS, Inoue O, Hong J, Imaizumi M, Pike VW, Innis RB, Fujita M. PET measurement of the in vivo affinity of 11C-(R)-rolipram and the density of its target, phosphodiesterase-4, in the brains of conscious and anesthetized rats. J Nucl Med. 2009;50:749–56.

Jan ML, Chuang KS, Chen GW, Ni YC, Chen S, Chang CH, Wu J, Lee TW, Fu YK. A three-dimensional registration method for automated fusion of micro PET-CT-SPECT whole-body images. IEEE Trans Med Imaging. 2005;24:886–93.

Jespersen B, Knupp L, Northcott CA. Femoral arterial and venous catheterization for blood sampling, drug administration and conscious blood pressure and heart rate measurements. J Vis Exp. 2012;59:(pii: 3496).

Jobse BN, Rhem RG, McCurry CA, Wang IQ, Labiris NR. Imaging lung function in mice using SPECT/CT and per-voxel analysis. PLoS One. 2012;7:e42187.

Judenhofer MS, Wehrl HF, Newport DF, Catana C, Siegel SB, Becker M, Thielscher A, Kneilling M, Lichy MP, Eichner M, Klingel K, Reischl G, Widmaier S, Rocken M, Nutt RE, Machulla HJ, Uludag K, Cherry SR, Claussen CD, Pichler BJ. Simultaneous PET-MRI: a new approach for functional and morphological imaging. Nat Med. 2008;14:459–65.

Kersemans V, Cornelissen B, Hueting R, Tredwell M, Hussien K, Allen PD, Falzone N, Hill SA, Dilworth JR, Gouverneur V, Muschel RJ, Smart SC. Hypoxia imaging using PET and SPECT: the effects of anesthetic and carrier gas on [64Cu]-ATSM, [99mTc]-HL91 and [18F]-FMISO tumor hypoxia accumulation. PLoS One. 2011;6:e25911.

Kilbourn MR, Ma B, Butch ER, Quesada C, Sherman PS. Anesthesia increases in vivo N-([18F] fluoroethyl)piperidinyl benzilate binding to the muscarinic cholinergic receptor. Nucl Med Biol. 2007;34:479–82.

King JA, Garelick TS, Brevard ME, Chen W, Messenger TL, Duong TQ, Ferris CF. Procedure for minimizing stress for fMRI studies in conscious rats. J Neurosci Methods. 2005;148:154–60.

Kononov A, Browne EZ, Alexander F, Porvasnik S. Continuous rat intravenous infusion. Microsurgery. 1994;15:443–5.

Kubota K, Fukuda H, Yamada K, Endo S, Ito M, Abe Y, Yamaguchi T, Fujiwara T, Sato T, Yamaura H. Experimental pancreas imaging study with 13N-glutamate using positron computer tomography. Eur J Nucl Med. 1983;8:528–30.

Kuehl PJ, Anderson TL, Candelaria G, Gershman B, Harlin K, Hesterman JY, Holmes T, Hoppin J, Lackas C, Norenberg JP, Yu H, McDonald JD. Regional particle size dependent deposition of inhaled aerosols in rats and mice. Inhal Toxicol. 2012;24:27–35.

Lahti KM, Ferris CF, Li F, Sotak CH, King JA. Imaging brain activity in conscious animals using functional MRI. J Neurosci Methods. 1998;82:75–83.

LaManna JC, Harik SI. Regional studies of blood-brain barrier transport of glucose and leucine in awake and anesthetized rats. J Cereb Blood Flow Metab. 1986;6:717–23.

Lasnon C, Quak E, Briand M, Gu Z, Louis MH, Aide N. Contrast-enhanced small-animal PET/CT in cancer research: strong improvement of diagnostic accuracy without significant alteration of quantitative accuracy and NEMA NU 4-2008 image quality parameters. EJNMMI Res. 2013;3:5.

Lee KH, Ko BH, Paik JY, Jung KH, Choe YS, Choi Y, Kim BT. Effects of anesthetic agents and fasting duration on 18F-FDG biodistribution and insulin levels in tumor-bearing mice. J Nucl Med. 2005;46:1531–6.

Lenz C, Rebel A, Van AK, Kuschinsky W, Waschke KF. Local cerebral blood flow, local cerebral glucose utilization, and flow-metabolism coupling during sevoflurane versus isoflurane anesthesia in rats. Anesthesiology. 1998;89:1480–8.

Lenz C, Frietsch T, Futterer C, Rebel A, Van AK, Kuschinsky W, Waschke KF. Local coupling of cerebral blood flow to cerebral glucose metabolism during inhalational anesthesia in rats: desflurane versus isoflurane. Anesthesiology. 1999;91:1720–3.

Li D, Patel AR, Klibanov AL, Kramer CM, Ruiz M, Kang BY, Mehta JL, Beller GA, Glover DK, Meyer CH. Molecular imaging of atherosclerotic plaques targeted to oxidized LDL receptor LOX-1 by SPECT/CT and magnetic resonance. Circ Cardiovasc Imaging. 2010;3:464–72.

Li ZC, Jiang SD, Yan J, Jiang LS, Dai LY. Small-animal PET/CT assessment of bone microdamage in ovariectomized rats. J Nucl Med. 2011;52:769–75.

Lin KJ, Liu HL, Hsu PH, Chung YH, Huang WC, Chen JC, Wey SP, Yen TC, Hsiao IT. Quantitative micro-SPECT/CT for detecting focused ultrasound-induced blood-brain barrier opening in the rat. Nucl Med Biol. 2009;36:853–61.

Maekawa T, Tommasino C, Shapiro HM, Keifer-Goodman J, Kohlenberger RW. Local cerebral blood flow and glucose utilization during isoflurane anesthesia in the rat. Anesthesiology. 1986;65:144–51.

Maramraju SH, Smith SD, Junnarkar SS, Schulz D, Stoll S, Ravindranath B, Purschke ML, Rescia S, Southekal S, Pratte JF, Vaska P, Woody CL, Schlyer DJ. Small animal simultaneous PET/MRI: initial experiences in a 9.4 T microMRI. Phys Med Biol. 2011;56:2459–80.

Mashhedi H, Blouin MJ, Zakikhani M, David S, Zhao Y, Bazile M, Birman E, Algire C, Aliaga A, Bedell BJ, Pollak M. Metformin abolishes increased tumor [18F]-2-fluoro-2-deoxy-D-glucose uptake associated with a high energy diet. Cell Cycle. 2011;10:2770–8.

Matsumura A, Mizokawa S, Tanaka M, Wada Y, Nozaki S, Nakamura F, Shiomi S, Ochi H, Watanabe Y. Assessment of microPET performance in analyzing the rat brain under different types of anesthesia: comparison between quantitative data obtained with microPET and ex vivo autoradiography. Neuroimage. 2003;20:2040–50.

McCormick PN, Ginovart N, Wilson AA. Isoflurane anaesthesia differentially affects the amphetamine sensitivity of agonist and antagonist D2/D3 positron emission tomography radiotracers: implications for in vivo imaging of dopamine release. Mol Imaging Biol. 2011;13:737–46.

Mirbolooki MR, Upadhyay SK, Constantinescu CC, Pan ML, Mukherjee J. Adrenergic pathway activation enhances brown adipose tissue metabolism: a [18F]FDG PET/CT study in mice. Nucl Med Biol. 2014;41:10–6.

Mizuma H, Shukuri M, Hayashi T, Watanabe Y, Onoe H. Establishment of in vivo brain imaging method in conscious mice. J Nucl Med. 2010;51:1068–75.

Momosaki S, Hatano K, Kawasumi Y, Kato T, Hosoi R, Kobayashi K, Inoue O, Ito K. Rat-PET study without anesthesia: anesthetics modify the dopamine D1 receptor binding in rat brain. Synapse. 2004;54:207–13.

Nahrendorf M, Zhang H, Hembrador S, Panizzi P, Sosnovik DE, Aikawa E, Libby P, Swirski FK, Weissleder R. Nanoparticle PET-CT imaging of macrophages in inflammatory atherosclerosis. Circulation. 2008;117:379–87.

Nahrendorf M, Keliher E, Panizzi P, Zhang H, Hembrador S, Figueiredo JL, Aikawa E, Kelly K, Libby P, Weissleder R. [18F]-4V for PET-CT imaging of VCAM-1 expression in atherosclerosis. JACC Cardiovasc Imaging. 2009;2:1213–22.

Nanni C, Pettinato C, Ambrosini V, Spinelli A, Trespidi S, Rubello D, Al-Nahhas A, Franchi R, Alavi A, Fanti S. Retro-orbital injection is an effective route for radiopharmaceutical administration in mice during small-animal PET studies. Nucl Med Commun. 2007;28:547–53.

Nayak TK, Bernardo M, Milenic DE, Choyke PL, Brechbiel MW. Orthotopic pleural mesothelioma in mice: SPECT/CT and MR imaging with HER1- and HER2-targeted radiolabeled antibodies. Radiology. 2013;267:173–82.

Ori C, Dam M, Pizzolato G, Battistin L, Giron G. Effects of isoflurane anesthesia on local cerebral glucose utilization in the rat. Anesthesiology. 1986;65:152–6.

Osborne DR, Yan S, Stuckey A, Pryer L, Richey T, Wall JS. Characterization of X-ray dose in murine animals using microCT, a New Low-Dose detector and nanoDot dosimeters. PLoS One. 2012;7:e49936.

Palko HA, Fung JY, Louie AY. Positron emission tomography: a novel technique for investigating the biodistribution and transport of nanoparticles. Inhal Toxicol. 2010;22:657–88.

Park SS, Chunta JL, Robertson JM, Martinez AA, Oliver Wong CY, Amin M, Wilson GD, Marples B. MicroPET/CT imaging of an orthotopic model of human glioblastoma multiforme and evaluation of pulsed low-dose irradiation. Int J Radiat Oncol Biol Phys. 2011;80:885–92.

Pascau J, Vaquero JJ, Chamorro-Servent J, Rodriguez-Ruano A, Desco M. A method for small-animal PET/CT alignment calibration. Phys Med Biol. 2012;57:N199–207.

Patel VD, Lee DE, Alexoff DL, Dewey SL, Schiffer WK. Imaging dopamine release with positron emission tomography (PET) and [11C]-raclopride in freely moving animals. Neuroimage. 2008;41:1051–66.

Paul R, Kiuru A, Soderstrom KO, Tuominen J, Johansson R, Haaparanta M, Roeda D, Solin O. Organ and tumor distribution of [18F]-2-fluoro-2-deoxy-D-glucose in fasting and non-fasting rats. Life Sci. 1987;40:1609–16.

Paul S, Khanapur S, Sijbesma JW, Ishiwata K, Elsinga PH, Meerlo P, Dierckx RA, Van Waarde A. Use of [11C]-MPDX and PET to study adenosine A1 receptor occupancy by nonradioactive agonists and antagonists. JNuclMed. 2014;55:315–20.

Peng F, Lutsenko S, Sun X, Muzik O. Imaging copper metabolism imbalance in Atp7b (-/-) knock-out mouse model of Wilson's disease with PET-CT and orally administered [64Cu]Cl2. Mol Imaging Biol. 2012;14:600–7.

Peternel L, Skrajnar S, Cerne M. A comparative study of four permanent cannulation procedures in rats. J Pharmacol Toxicol Methods. 2010;61:20–6.

Petroni D, Menichetti L, Sorace O, Poli M, Vanasia M, Salvadori PA. [11C]diclofenac sodium: synthesis and PET assessment of transdermal penetration. Nucl Med Biol. 2011;38:181–9.

Pool SE, ten Hagen TL, Koelewijn S, de J M, Koning GA. Multimodality imaging of somatostatin receptor-positive tumors with nuclear and bioluminescence imaging. Mol Imaging. 2012;11:27–32.

Radonjic M, Cappaert NL, de Vries EF, de Esch CE, Kuper FC, van Waarde A, Dierckx RA, Wadman WJ, Wolterbeek AP, Stierum RH, de Groot DM. Delay and impairment in brain development and function in rat offspring after maternal exposure to methylmercury. Toxicol Sci. 2013;133:112–24.

Raty JK, Liimatainen T, Huhtala T, Kaikkonen MU, Airenne KJ, Hakumaki JM, Narvanen A, Yla-Herttuala S. SPECT/CT imaging of baculovirus biodistribution in rat. Gene Ther. 2007;14:930–8.

Raylman RR, Majewski S, Velan SS, Lemieux S, Kross B, Popov V, Smith MF, Weisenberger AG. Simultaneous acquisition of magnetic resonance spectroscopy (MRS) data and positron emission tomography (PET) images with a prototype MR-compatible, small animal PET imager. J Magn Reson. 2007;186:305–10.

Rybczynska AA, Elsinga PH, Sijbesma JW, Ishiwata K, de Jong JR, de Vries EF, Dierckx RA, van Waarde A. Steroid hormones affect binding of the sigma ligand [11C]-SA4503 in tumour cells and tumour-bearing rats. Eur J Nucl Med Mol Imaging. 2009;36:1167–75.

Saija A, Princi P, De PR, Costa G. Modifications of the permeability of the blood-brain barrier and local cerebral metabolism in pentobarbital- and ketamine-anaesthetized rats. Neuropharmacology. 1989;28:997–1002.

Sanchez F, Orero A, Soriano A, Correcher C, Conde P, Gonzalez A, Hernandez L, Moliner L, Rodriguez-Alvarez MJ, Vidal LF, Benlloch JM, Chapman SE, Leevy WM. ALBIRA: a small animal PETSPECTCT imaging system. Med Phys. 2013;40:051906.

Saraste A, Laitinen I, Weidl E, Wildgruber M, Weber AW, Nekolla SG, Holzlwimmer G, Esposito I, Walch A, Leppanen P, Lisinen I, Luppa PB, Yla-Herttuala S, Wester HJ, Knuuti J, Schwaiger M. Diet intervention reduces uptake of alphavbeta3 integrin-targeted PET tracer [18F]-galacto-RGD in mouse atherosclerotic plaques. J Nucl Cardiol. 2012;19:775–84.

Sarparanta M, Makila E, Heikkila T, Salonen J, Kukk E, Lehto VP, Santos HA, Hirvonen J, Airaksinen AJ. ^{18}F-labeled modified porous silicon particles for investigation of drug delivery carrier distribution in vivo with positron emission tomography. MolPharm. 2011;8:1799–806.

Schiffer WK, Mirrione MM, Dewey SL. Optimizing experimental protocols for quantitative behavioral imaging with [18F]-FDG in rodents. J Nucl Med. 2007;48:277–87.

Schoell AR, Heyde BR, Weir DE, Chiang PC, Hu Y, Tung DK. Euthanasia method for mice in rapid time-course pulmonary pharmacokinetic studies. J Am Assoc Lab Anim Sci. 2009;48:506–11.

Schulz D, Southekal S, Junnarkar SS, Pratte JF, Purschke ML, Stoll SP, Ravindranath B, Maramraju SH, Krishnamoorthy S, Henn FA, O'Connor P, Woody CL, Schlyer DJ, Vaska P. Simultaneous assessment of rodent behavior and neurochemistry using a miniature positron emission tomograph. Nat Methods. 2011;8:347–52.

Seo Y, Gao DW, Hasegawa BH, Dae MW, Franc BL. Rodent brain imaging with SPECT/CT. Med Phys. 2007;34:1217–20.

Shahani SK, Lingamaneni R, Hemmings HC. General anesthetic actions on norepinephrine, dopamine, and gamma-aminobutyric acid transporters in stably transfected cells. Anesth Analg. 2002;95:893–9, table.

Shih YY, Chiang YC, Chen JC, Huang CH, Chen YY, Liu RS, Chang C, Jaw FS. Brain nociceptive imaging in rats using [18F]-fluorodeoxyglucose small-animal positron emission tomography. Neuroscience. 2008;155:1221–6.

Shingaki T, Takashima T, Wada Y, Tanaka M, Kataoka M, Ishii A, Shigihara Y, Sugiyama Y, Yamashita S, Watanabe Y. Imaging of gastrointestinal absorption and biodistribution of an orally administered probe using positron emission tomography in humans. Clin Pharmacol Ther. 2012;91:653–9.

Silvola JM, Saraste A, Laitinen I, Savisto N, Laine VJ, Heinonen SE, Yla-Herttuala S, Saukko P, Nuutila P, Roivainen A, Knuuti J. Effects of age, diet, and type 2 diabetes on the development and FDG uptake of atherosclerotic plaques. JACC Cardiovasc Imaging. 2011;4:1294–301.

Sokoloff L, Reivich M, Kennedy C, Des Rosiers MH, Patlak CS, Pettigrew KD, Sakurada O, Shinohara M. The [14C]deoxyglucose method for the measurement of local cerebral glucose utilization: theory, procedure, and normal values in the conscious and anesthetized albino rat. J Neurochem. 1977;28:897–916.

Solomon M, Nothdruft RE, Akers W, Edwards WB, Liang K, Xu B, Suddlow GP, Deghani H, Tai YC, Eggebrecht AT, Achilefu S, Culver JP. Multimodal fluorescence-mediated tomography and SPECT/CT for small-animal imaging. J Nucl Med. 2013;54:639–46.

Steel CD, Stephens AL, Hahto SM, Singletary SJ, Ciavarra RP. Comparison of the lateral tail vein and the retro-orbital venous sinus as routes of intravenous drug delivery in a transgenic mouse model. Lab Anim (NY). 2008;37:26–32.

Szymanski MK, Kruizinga S, Tio RA, Willemsen AT, Schäfers MA, Stegger L, Dierckx RA, Hillege HL, Slart RH. Use of gated [13N]-NH3 micro-PET to examine left ventricular function in rats. Nucl Med Biol. 2012;39:724–9.

Tahari AK, Lodge MA, Wahl RL. Respiratory-gated PET/CT versus delayed images for the quantitative evaluation of lower pulmonary and hepatic lesions. J Med Imaging Radiat Oncol. 2014;58:277–82.

Tantawy MN, Peterson TE, Jones CK, Johnson K, Rook JM, Conn PJ, Baldwin RM, Ansari MS, Kessler RM. Impact of isoflurane anesthesia on D2 receptor occupancy by [18F]fallypride measured by microPET with a modified Logan plot. Synapse. 2011;65:1173–80.

Taschereau R, Chow PL, Chatziioannou AF. Monte Carlo simulations of dose from microCT imaging procedures in a realistic mouse phantom. Med Phys. 2006;33:216–24.

Todd MM, Weeks J. Comparative effects of propofol, pentobarbital, and isoflurane on cerebral blood flow and blood volume. J Neurosurg Anesthesiol. 1996;8:296–303.

Tokugawa J, Ravasi L, Nakayama T, Lang L, Schmidt KC, Seidel J, Green MV, Sokoloff L, Eckelman WC. Distribution of the 5-HT1A receptor antagonist [18F]FPWAY in blood and brain of the rat with and without isoflurane anesthesia. Eur J Nucl Med Mol Imaging. 2007;34:259–66.

Toyama H, Ichise M, Liow JS, Vines DC, Seneca NM, Modell KJ, Seidel J, Green MV, Innis RB. Evaluation of anesthesia effects on [18F]FDG uptake in mouse brain and heart using small animal PET. Nucl Med Biol. 2004;31:251–6.

Tremoleda JL, Kerton A, Gsell W. Anaesthesia and physiological monitoring during in vivo imaging of laboratory rodents: considerations on experimental outcomes and animal welfare. EJNMMI Res. 2012;2:44.

Umeda IO, Tani K, Tsuda K, Kobayashi M, Ogata M, Kimura S, Yoshimoto M, Kojima S, Moribe K, Yamamoto K, Moriyama N, Fujii H. High resolution SPECT imaging for visualization of intratumoral heterogeneity using a SPECT/CT scanner dedicated for small animal imaging. Ann Nucl Med. 2012;26:67–76.

van Waarde A, Buursma AR, Hospers GA, Kawamura K, Kobayashi T, Ishii K, Oda K, Ishiwata K, Vaalburg W, Elsinga PH. Tumor imaging with 2 sigma-receptor ligands, [18F]-FE-SA5845 and [11C]-SA4503: a feasibility study. J Nucl Med. 2004;45:1939–45.

Vines DC, Green DE, Kudo G, Keller H. Evaluation of mouse tail-vein injections both qualitatively and quantitatively on small-animal PET tail scans. J Nucl Med Technol. 2011;39:264–70.

Votaw J, Byas-Smith M, Hua J, Voll R, Martarello L, Levey AI, Bowman FD, Goodman M. Interaction of isoflurane with the dopamine transporter. Anesthesiology. 2003;98:404–11.

Votaw JR, Byas-Smith MG, Voll R, Halkar R, Goodman MM. Isoflurane alters the amount of dopamine transporter expressed on the plasma membrane in humans. Anesthesiology. 2004;101:1128–35.

Walter MA, Hildebrandt IJ, Hacke K, Kesner AL, Kelly O, Lawson GW, Phelps ME, Czernin J, Weber WA, Schiestl RH. Small-animal PET/CT for monitoring the development and response to chemotherapy of thymic lymphoma in Trp53-/- mice. J Nucl Med. 2010;51:1285–92.

Watabe T, Shimosegawa E, Watabe H, Kanai Y, Hanaoka K, Ueguchi T, Isohashi K, Kato H, Tatsumi M, Hatazawa J. Quantitative evaluation of cerebral blood flow and oxygen metabolism in normal anesthetized rats: [15O]-labeled gas inhalation PET with MRI Fusion. J Nucl Med. 2013;54:283–90.

Wong KP, Sha W, Zhang X, Huang SC. Effects of administration route, dietary condition, and blood glucose level on kinetics and uptake of [18F]-FDG in mice. J Nucl Med. 2011;52:800–7.

Woo SK, Lee TS, Kim KM, Kim JY, Jung JH, Kang JH, Cheon GJ, Choi CW, Lim SM. Anesthesia condition for [18F]-FDG imaging of lung metastasis tumors using small animal PET. Nucl Med Biol. 2008;35:143–50.

Yamashita S, Takashima T, Kataoka M, Oh H, Sakuma S, Takahashi M, Suzuki N, Hayashinaka E, Wada Y, Cui Y, Watanabe Y. PET imaging of the gastrointestinal absorption of orally administered drugs in conscious and anesthetized rats. J Nucl Med. 2011;52:249–56.

Yang FY, Wang HE, Lin GL, Teng MC, Lin HH, Wong TT, Liu RS. Micro-SPECT/CT-based pharmacokinetic analysis of [99mTc]-diethylenetriaminepentaacetic acid in rats with blood-brain barrier disruption induced by focused ultrasound. J Nucl Med. 2011;52:478–84.

Yee SH, Lee K, Jerabek PA, Fox PT. Quantitative measurement of oxygen metabolic rate in the rat brain using microPET imaging of briefly inhaled [15O]-labelled oxygen gas. Nucl Med Commun. 2006;27:573–81.

Yoder KK, Mock BH, Zheng QH, McCarthy BP, Riley AA, Hutchins GD. Assessment of i.p. injection of [18F]fallypride for behavioral neuroimaging in rats. J Neurosci Methods. 2011;196:70–5.

Yu M, Guaraldi MT, Bozek J, Kagan M, Azure M, Radeke H, Cdebaca M, Robinson SP. Effects of food intake and anesthetic on cardiac imaging and uptake of BMS747158-02 in comparison with FDG. J Nucl Cardiol. 2009;16:763–8.

Zanelli GD, Lucas PB, Fowler JF. The effect of anaesthetics on blood perfusion in transplanted mouse tumours. Br J Cancer. 1975;32:380–90.

Zhang WT DUXK, Huo TL, Wei ZM, Hao CX, An B. Combination of [18F]-fluorodeoxyglucose positron emission tomography/computed tomography and magnetic resonance imaging is an optimal way to evaluate rheumatoid arthritis in rats dynamically. Chin Med J (Engl). 2013;126:3732–8.

Zutphen LFM, Baumans V, Beynen AC. Principles of laboratory animal science, Revised Edition edn. Amsterdam: Elsevier; 2001.

Part V

Management Instruments

Teamwork, Leadership, and Continuous Improvement

19

Wouter A. Keijser

Abstract

In this chapter, we describe the enhanced TeamSTEPPS® curriculum as fundament to creating a "culture of continuous improvement" in nuclear medicine. This evidence-based and modular teamwork system is deployed in concordance with a novel medical leadership development program. It provides a comprehensive and practical approach to improve performance and patient safety within nuclear medicine departments, hence across numerous multidisciplinary patient journeys that are influenced by effective (nuclear) medical imaging. The stepped approach of implementing and sustaining a shift towards a just and blame-free culture of multidisciplinary teamwork is described.

19.1 A Case for Teamwork and Leadership in Nuclear Medicine

Internal and external triggers of a nuclear medicine department influence the importance of investing in teamwork and leadership.

First of all, over the past 15 years, important healthcare issues increasingly gained attention, predominantly quality of care, patient safety, and cost-effectiveness. In 1999, the Institute of Medicine (IOM) published the report *To Err is Human: Building a Safer Health System*, which brought new public awareness of safety and quality issues in healthcare (Kohn 2000). This report as well as numerous other

W.A. Keijser, MD
University of Twente, Enschede, The Netherlands

Management and Organizational Behavior; Faculty of Behavioural,
Management and Social Sciences, Health Information Management SL, Barcelona, Spain
e-mail: Wouter@Keijser.com

A.W.J.M. Glaudemans et al. (eds.), *Quality in Nuclear Medicine*,
DOI 10.1007/978-3-319-33531-5_19

reports and scientific publications describe that one of the critical aspects of patient safety is the ability of healthcare professionals to perform effectively as teams. Healthcare can be seen as a result, the "product," of intensive collaboration of many involved: doctors, nurses, pharmacists, and other allied health professionals. In the clinical pathways followed by patients, optimal healthcare outcomes are linked to the level of continuous coordination, communication, and mutual support between a wide variety of professionals (Bridges 2011). Besides increased consciousness of patient safety, also external economic constraints, a fast evolution of technological and medical developments and innovation, a constant need for service optimization as well as staff shortages enforce nuclear medicine and other medical imaging specialties to have teamwork and leadership as primary considerations (UK Government 2014).

Secondly, several characteristics of the practice of nuclear medicine urge for outstanding teamwork and leadership. In a broad perspective, multidisciplinary teamwork in nuclear medicine should lead to excellence in the following key areas (EANM 2006):

- Quality of service provision (to patients and to referrers)
- Effectiveness (clinical as well as cost-effectiveness)
- Safety
- Employee satisfaction
- Innovation

Optimal outcomes in nuclear medicine range from developing scan protocols, individual planning of imaging and producing isotopes, to conducting and analyzing the final imaging examinations. Despite all these various activities, key performance indicators (e.g., justification of examination requests, including protocols, radiation protection, image acquisition, reporting, management, and service improvement) ask for a constant attention (The Royal College 2012). All this requires an intensive and constant merging of expertise from and close collaboration between various disciplines.

Optimal teamwork in delivering these elements of clinical imaging services is crucial. In day-to-day medical practice, nuclear medicine departments function as complex organizations with an "inner" and an "outer" world reality. Servicing imaging requests from external physicians, working with patients, and collaborating, intradepartmental as well as interdepartmental. Within the department, the foremost prerequisite for such complex and highly protocolled workflow is a close collaboration between several disciplines ranging from technologists, physicists, managers, radiographers, pharmacists, nurses, administrators, nuclear medicine physicians to safety experts and working based on a team-oriented approach. Here, a fragmented approach like "you make the isotope and I'll do the imaging" or "you scan them and I'll read them" can be detrimental to team effectiveness and service quality (Rohren 2012). As nuclear medicine departments function as "high reliability organizations," lack of teamwork can even bring about danger to safety of patients and team members (Baker 2006).

The practice of nuclear medicine goes beyond the boundaries of "isotope production units and camera rooms," as it entails also interdepartmental collaboration between many other specialties. Nuclear medicine departments very often provide services to and collaborate with a variety of other healthcare specialties. This requires optimal teamwork overarching individual departments. In clinical pathways stretched out within the network of specialties pharmacists, oncologists, surgeons, nuclear medicine physicians, pathologists, clinical physicists, clinical pharmacists, technologists, medical physicists, and many more can play a role (Beach et al. 2012; Kitajima 2005; Rohren 2012). Also, nuclear medicine departments often have regular clinical commitments to some specialist areas such as endocrinology, cardiology, oncology, pediatrics, neurology, nephrology, and orthopedics. For example, enhanced management of complex malignancies in cancer care involves frequent participation in multidisciplinary team meetings and departments that provide radionuclide therapy sustain close communication with endocrinology (e.g., treatment of thyroid disease). Furthermore, because interdepartmental collaboration can be associated with potential conflicting interests, also competencies in successfully resolving challenging multidisciplinary issues and even preventing looming conflicts are necessary.

Moreover, in nuclear medicine, research reports reveal that investing in multidisciplinary teamwork in nuclear medicine can result in optimization of workflow, patient as well as employee experience and safety (Tuttle 2004; Greaves 2013). Also in healthcare professionals, human nature fuels collaborative attitudes, as it was recently shown that clinical imaging professionals have a strong intrinsic need for "looking in each others' kitchen" in order to function optimally as a team (Rohren 2012). In other words, the performance of a nuclear medicine department entails all staff to understand each other's role and to communicate effectively. Additionally, the team should foster features like reflectivity, objectivity, sharing common goals, efficiency, patient perspective, and a shared, autonomous responsibility. In the decision-making process, each professional has a responsibility to contribute their skills and to acknowledge the goals of the department.

19.1.1 Evidence Based Teamwork

In healthcare, a growing body of evidence shows that the following key areas are highly influenced by optimization of teamwork (Borill 2001):

- Healthcare teams that function effectively provide higher-quality patient care.
- Members of teams that work well together have relatively low stress levels.
- A diverse range of professional groups working together is associated with higher levels of innovation in patient care.

Moreover, it is becoming widely recognized that individuals within healthcare teams should feel safe to share their concerns and mistakes in an environment where all staff feel supported. Teams fostering a just and blame-free climate and organizations that elicit intensive employee involvement in decision-making are more disposed to a culture of continuous learning and improvement. In other words, a blame culture is more likely to occur in healthcare organizations that rely predominantly on hierarchical, compliance-based functional management systems (Khatri 2009; The Royal College 2012).

Tightly related to teamwork and collaboration, leadership is a key aspect in high performing teams. Individual, managerial, and medical leadership and according competencies are fundamental for team effectiveness and employee satisfaction. Although leadership outside healthcare has been studied and described extensively in social and management sciences, medical leadership is an emerging theme in the healthcare quality arena (Dickson 2014).

19.2 Governing Teamwork and Leadership

There are several guiding principles in establishing and managing excellence in healthcare.

Clinical governance is a systematic approach for sustainably improving quality of patient care within a health system. Clinical governance consists of the following elements: clinical effectiveness, risk management effectiveness, patient experience, communication effectiveness, resources effectiveness, strategic effectiveness, and learning effectiveness. Implementation of clinical governance is facilitated through five key strategies:

1. System awareness
2. Teamwork
3. Communication
4. Ownership
5. Leadership (Degeling 2004)

Related to the nuclear medicine practice, the International Atomic Energy Agency has described "nuclear security culture" with characteristics in line with those of clinical governance (IAEA 2008). The IAEA implementing handbook provides the following principles for guiding decisions and behavior: motivation, leadership, commitment and responsibility, professionalism and competence, and learning and improvement.

Other national and international quality management and accreditation systems provide comprehensive aids to healthcare safety and quality, e.g., the Joint Commission International (JCI 2014) or the Dutch safety management system (VMS 2014). According to the European Foundation for Quality Management, teamwork and leadership are fundamental enablers as well as result in excellent organizations (EFQM 2014). The EFQM provides an "Excellence Model" model for managing sustainable excellence, also adaptable in nuclear medicine. Excellent organizations achieve and sustain outstanding results by valuing its staff and creating a culture of sharing mutual goals and promoting fairness and equality. In the

EFQM model, "leadership" is seen as a common attribute, not restricted to CEOs or bosses but to anyone that contributes to the organizations' quality and its (change) processes. Furthermore, the EFQM Excellence Model identifies performance indicators relevant to the "people's" teamwork:

- Involvement and engagement
- Target setting, competency, and performance management
- Leadership performance
- Training and career development
- Internal communications

The strategies and key performance indicators used in these models support an optimal managerial overview and control in managing organizations. However, many healthcare organizations do not show excellence in team climate and a just and blame-free culture. Also, medical leadership has only recently emerged in (continuing) medical education. Therefore, implementing the use of well-endorsed quality models also prompt practical questions like, "How do we create and sustain to a culture of excellence, of continuous improvement?" Like in other industries, healthcare's "ground zero" for sustainable change in healthcare lies in its professionals, the so-called "human" factor (Baker 2006). This also goes for clinical imaging services: its teams and members are most vital to excellent service delivery for patients and referrers.

19.3 Team Strategies and Tools to Enhance Performance and Patient Safety

In response to the IOM report, the Agency for Healthcare Research and Quality (AHRQ) and the Department of Defense (DoD) in the USA have been supporting research and development activities related to team performance in healthcare (Kohn 2000). In 2006, after about 2 years of field testing and adaptations, AHRQ and DoD released the initial 1.0 version of the TeamSTEPPS curriculum as the national standard for team training in healthcare (TeamSTEPPS 2.0 as of September 2015). TeamSTEPPS™, which stands for Team Strategies and Tools to Enhance Performance and Patient Safety, is based on 25-plus years of research on team performance (Clancy 2007). TeamSTEPPS is a toolkit that teaches four core components of teamwork that have been validated in the present literature: leadership, communication, mutual support, and situation monitoring (Salas et al. 2005). TeamSTEPPS is a teamwork system aimed at optimizing patient outcomes by improving communication and teamwork skills among healthcare professionals. Its content is based on a selection of state-of-the-art and well-proven strategies in healthcare quality and innovation, e.g., LEAN, crew resource management, and clinical microsystems (Godfrey et al. 2004). By combining them and rigorously testing them, TeamSTEPPS has optimized the availability of these "best of breeds" into a comprehensive, evidence-based, and practical curriculum.

19.3.1 Unique Curriculum

Foremost, the TeamSTEPPS system is a comprehensive set of ready-to-use materials to successfully integrate teamwork principles into any healthcare system (TeamSTEPPS 2014). The materials contain comprehensive curricula and instructional guides, including short case studies and videos illustrating teamwork opportunities and successes. Additional materials focus on change management, coaching, measurement, and implementation.

Compared with the numerous training and teaching programs available (commercial as well as noncommercial) a combination of three important characteristics makes TeamSTEPPS stand out:

1. Evidence based
   Founded in rigorous review of the literature (Baker 2003) and being researched and tested over a significant period of time, TeamSTEPPS can endure the often critical view of healthcare personnel that must be engaged in using the system.
2. Cost-efficient
   Delivering the program is done on site and is facilitated by people within the team or department (coach-the-coach principle), preventing high costs of external trainers or training facilities.
3. Tailored
   The curriculum was designed as a flexible toolkit for healthcare facilities and providers. Deployment implies connecting customizable with existing programs in a custom-made manner, in line with specific needs of local teams or departments.

19.3.2 Bringing It to the Team

The program is delivered to staff based on train-the-trainer and coach-the-coach principles. A "master trainer," previously trained in delivering the TeamSTEPPS program and knowledgeable about TeamSTEPPS acts as lead trainer. He/she is experienced in the application of tools and strategies to improve patient safety and the delivery of safe and efficient care and in turn trains and coaches staff in targeted work units, department, or facility level.

Master trainers preferably are also capable to in-depth perform site assessments (see below), determining critical performance gaps and potential implementation barriers. They also can coordinate implementing TeamSTEPPS initiatives across a number of units simultaneously and can provide process consultation to management. Their level of expertise and background varies; many local master trainers are chosen because of their preexisting role in patient safety or team training. Although statistics are unavailable to the author, based on practice-based evidence, it is estimated that the majority of these trainers have a nursing background. Some experienced master trainers provide additional (leadership) coaching to executive management and physicians and can provide valuable consultation on the organizations' strategic levels.

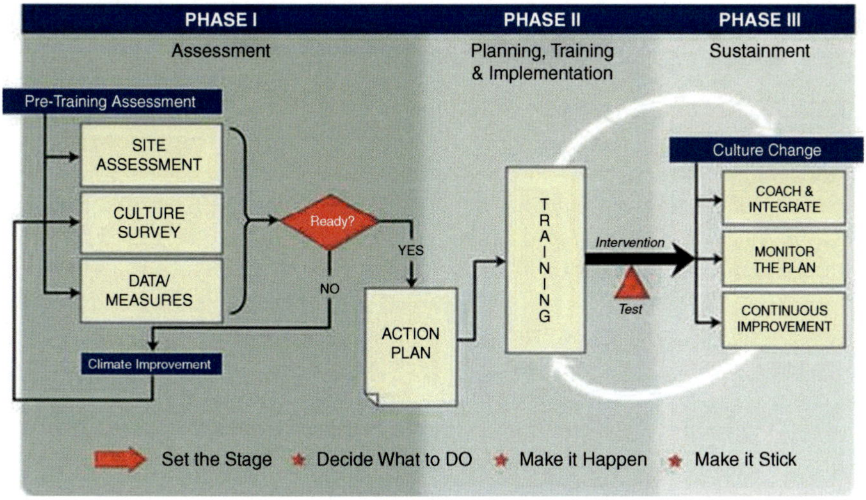

Fig. 19.1 Three-step TeamSTEPPS implementation (with permission of AHRQ)

Apart from the lead TeamSTEPPS master trainer, implementation entails the establishment of a group of internal team coaches. These individuals are selected based on their willingness and "profile" in the team. Their role is to act as informal coaches within the team providing role modeling and feedback, specifically referring to content discussed during team sessions. In collaboration with trainers, coaches can also be involved in the preparation and execution of the team training sessions. Preferably this internal corps of coaches and trainers reflects the department or team by a well-balanced number of nonphysicians as well as physicians in these roles.

19.3.3 Implementation Strategies

In many cases, local implementation of a TeamSTEPPS program resembles a cultural shift or transformation as teams change their ways of working combined with habits. Therefore, it is not surprising to recognize the work on change management by John Kotter et al., as TeamSTEPPS implementation follows the ten steps of change, as described in the well-known iceberg fable (Kotter 2006). Initially a steering committee or "change team" is formed, specifically with representation of all disciplines and active participation of physicians. The latter entails engaging physicians and others: a process that is not seldom seen as one of the greater challenges during implementation.[1] In a stepped approach, implementation typically occurs in three consecutive phases (Fig. 19.1). Each phase incorporates subsequent actions of setting the stage

[1] Informal exchange of experiences among master trainers during plenary discussion at the 2014 National TeamSTEPPS Conference (Minneapolis/St Pauls, Minnesota, USA) (Keijser 2014).

(assessment of "couleur locale" and needs), deciding what to do (tailoring the program), making it happen (training and coaching), and making it stick (sustaining).

19.3.3.1 Phase 1: Site Assessment

Preceding actual team sessions, the change team determines performance gaps and considers focus for change by coordinating a site assessment. Study of various data like performance data, measurements, and input from staff members (e.g., semistructured interviews) fuel into preparation of an implementation plan. This also includes a critical consideration of potential barriers and success factors, sometimes revolving in actions to improve preconditions, e.g., improving "buy-in" of team members. In this process, confronting teams with the results of their (online and anonymous) team climate measurement revealing often operates as an icebreaker – not to say crowbar – in creating a team climate of more openness.

The TeamSTEPPS curriculum contains several measurement tools for investigating pre-intervention status and monitoring progression in team performance, following the Kirkpatrick's levels for evaluating training programs (Kirkpatrick 1994). These include, e.g., course evaluation form, teamwork attitudes questionnaire, learning benchmarks, team performance observation tool, and teamwork perceptions questionnaire. Systematic measurement on critical teamwork domains like team structure, leadership, situation monitoring, mutual support, and communication provide a valid reflection of team performance (Baker 2008). Regular measurement of domains can be bolstered with more individual competency assessments, e.g., for (medical) leadership competency development (see further).

19.3.3.2 Phase 2: Planning, Training, and Implementation

Per team or unit, a change plan is completed: an improvement bundle of interventions, tailored to specific team characteristics and needs, and focusing on specific and measurable change. Detailed preparation comprises active knowledge of plan-do-study-act strategies, which can be brought in by a lead trainer. To apply these strategies, the team or unit uses various TeamSTEPPS worksheets and additional tools. In the process, teams are challenged to combine "hard" and "soft" aspects: merging of process redesigning in association with improvement of team skills and attitudes (see Fig. 19.2). In fact teams receive the task to collectively answer the question: *After we (re)define our work plans* [the 'hard' part], *which skills and attitudes* [the 'soft' part] *do we need to collectively adhere to these new plans? Especially during stressful situations?* Identification of specific needs for training revolves into a tailored course of multidisciplinary team sessions. The content of these sessions is based on the fundamental TeamSTEPPS training modules, comprising four core competency areas (see Table 19.1). Finally, all team members take part in a series of team sessions to train new work plans, skills, and attitudes. Team training sessions are a mixture of theoretic classroom information exchange and discussions and of interactive discussion and scenario-based roll play. Sessions are short (to a maximum of 1.5 h), with an optimum of 12–15 participants, without exception multidisciplinary and are held near or on the unit in order to enhance commitment and minimize no-shows.

As phase 2 progresses, discussions on attitude and behavior as well as skills, often result in higher levels of (renewed) trust within the team. Crucial for succes is

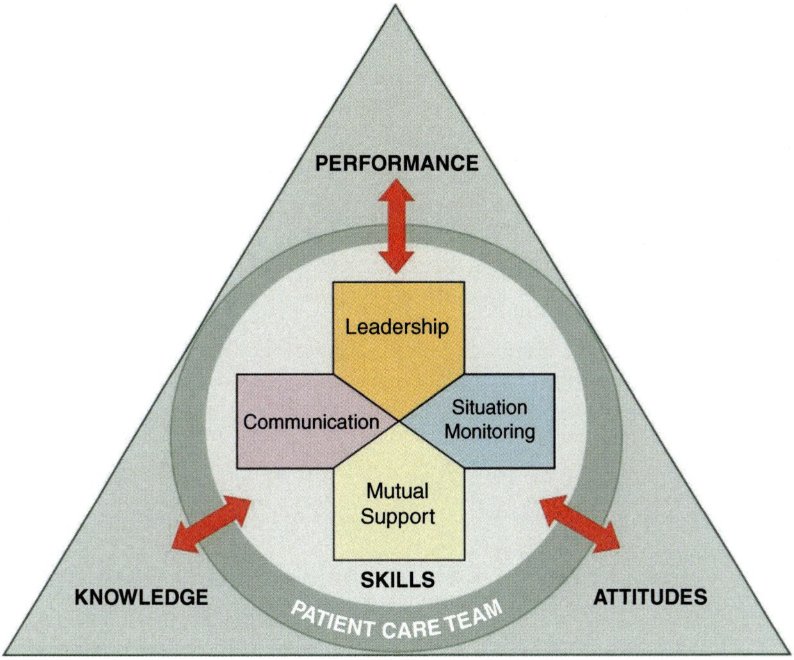

Fig. 19.2 TeamSTEPPS "Triangle" (with permission of AHRQ)

positive endoresement of departmental management and operational manager. Experiences has shown that in vase of their lack of involvement or support, implementation must be regarded as waste of resources.

19.3.3.3 Phase 3: Sustainment

In a final phase, the unit or department develops and executes a sustainability strategy also underpinning the cultural shift that coincides with sessions and other implementation efforts. Team knowledge, skills, and attitudes that have been trained and outcomes of improvement activities achieved during the second phase are essential to team development process. However, as TeamSTEPPS in essence is not to be used as an "ending project," certain activities are to be continued over time to maintain the teams' high performance. Also here lies an important responsibility of the departments or organizationals management.

New team culture can deteriorate rapidly by a variety of simple incidents or just lack of time and attention towards keeping the culture afloat. Effective teams should invest in their development on continuous bases. With the busy pace in healthcare and its professionals being uttermost dedicated, team members themselves and foremost their leadership and management should beware of deteriorating processes. Like teams, also formal and informal team leaders need time to develop their skills. Refresher sessions for teams as well as for leaders ware part of a sustainability plan.

As teams normally change over time, team members move from and new members enroll to the team. Excellent performing teams are very capable of depicting

Table 19.1 Teamwork competencies

Team competency I: Team leadership
Direct and coordinate activities of team members, assess team performance, assign tasks and responsibilities, develop team knowledge and skills, motivate team members, plan and organize, and create and maintain a positive team climate. Team leaders and team members learn to balance roles, responsibilities, and activities and proactively on relevant changes in the team environment
Examples of team training topics: briefing, debriefing, and huddling
Team competency II: Situation and mutual performance monitoring
(Re)establishing and learning to work according to a shared mental model, a "mutual framework of thinking, doing, and behaving." The team engages in describing common understandings of its environment and specific situations and applying appropriate strategies to monitor own and teammates' performance continuously and act accurately on potential disruptions
Examples of team training topics: role-play in mutual monitoring
Team competency III: Mutual support ("backup behavior")
Anticipating on other team members' needs and balancing workload among members to achieve balance over time (e.g., shifts) to keep a continuity in excellent safety and quality in team performance
Examples of team training topics: feedback, conflict management
Team competency IV: Communication
Training of efficiently sharing information and consultation between team members and other teams. All team members should foster situational awareness and communication skills, resulting in mutual respect among the team, regardless of each others' roles. As day-to-day workload can bring about stressful situation, the team engages also in training of conflict management and handling situation of nonprofessional behavior and other difficult situations between team members
Examples of team training topics: SBAR, professional behavior

the characteristics of its members, certainly in terms of knowledge, skills, and attitude. Subsequently, human resource units that work in close collaboration with teams can play an important role in remaining a high level of stability in teams across the organization (Khatri 2009).

A culture of continuous improvement contains not merely "soft" parts like the right skills and attitudes of team members and team leaders (see: Table 19.2). Teams and departments should also continuously focus on creating tangible change, improvement, and innovation on aggregated levels. Quality systems as described in other chapters of this book support execution of sustainment activities over time on a management and control level. Keeping knowledge, skills, and attitudes in teams and leadership competencies at excellent levels entails constant monitoring on micro-, meso-, and macrolevel in the organization, including measuring "hard" as well as "soft" characteristics of teams and leaders.

19.4 Team Priming and Leadership

Under supervision of its founders (AHRQ/DoD) and after a trailing period, the Dutch version of TeamSTEPPS (in Dutch: TeamSHOPP) was launched early 2012 in the Netherlands and ever since attained attention by several Dutch

Table 19.2 Behavior fosters better compliance with security regulations (IAEA 2008)

Leadership behavior
1. Expectations
2. Use of authority
3. Decision-making
4. Management oversight
5. Involvement of staff
6. Effective communications
7. Improving performance
8. Motivation
Personnel behavior
1. Professional conduct
2. Personal accountability
3. Adherence to procedures
4. Teamwork and cooperation
5. Vigilance

healthcare institutions (Keijser 2013). Translation into Dutch included some cultural adaptations and during the 2-year trail period, the TeamSTEPPS concept was regarded feasible in the Dutch healthcare setting. However, implementation experiences revealed a need for two additional adaptations of the original curriculum.

19.4.1 Priming

Firstly during sense-making sessions when assessing departments and teams in the preparatory phase, it became clear that internal conflicts often occur within multidisciplinary teams. Also, these conflicts frequently had hard-boiled over periods of years before, influencing communication and attitude of numerous team members. Further investigation of these hidden problems shed more light on distinct aspects of problems and their origin. Occasionally problems seemed to reflect common hierarchical challenges, typically between physicians and nonphysicians. Sometimes the department's history disclosed ineffective managerial conduct varying from having established a relatively repressive "blame" culture within the teams to a non-productive 'laiser faire' management climate.

These findings led to the conception of "mono-disciplinary priming" as a precondition for implementation of multidisciplinary team interventions (Keijser 2014). Such priming consists of team-based reflection on a team climate inventory of each monodisciplinary segment of the department or team, followed by adequate improvement efforts based on these baseline measurements. Often these additional efforts include sense-making discussions between peers (monodisciplinary), with a thawing effect on preexisting assumptions and attitudes to "the others" and vice versa. These priming efforts upfront can prevent TeamSTEPPS implementation for failure by increasing:

- Buy-in of all disciplines at team sessions
- Engagement of physicians
- Mutual trust between disciplines and between team members

These effects accelerate future adherence to the content of multidisciplinary team sessions focusing on team skills and behavior, like feedback and other communication skills. Additionally, priming efforts in the monodisciplinary teams and units of the department also help create a learning atmosphere among peers working in the same discipline, hence from the same perspective, which is fundamental to a culture of continuous improvement.

19.4.2 Medical Team Leadership

A second concern raised during early TeamSTEPPS implementation efforts. In the Netherlands was the engagement of physicians prior to and during team sessions as well as their medical leadership competencies. Skepticism among nonphysicians, no-show of doctors during team sessions, and troublesome planning of medical staff shifts contributed to an often suboptimal or even nonexistent role of physicians in team work improvements or innovation efforts. Subsequently this only fueled general presumptions about physician's attitudes towards team and teamwork initiatives. Intervening by undesirable "top-down" managerial leadership (e.g., mandating team efforts as mandatory, closure of operating rooms during team sessions, etc.) was only partially successful.

Engagement of doctors has been recognized as a crucial success factor in healthcare quality but remains a challenge for many (Clark 2012). This is the case in team initiatives in the Netherlands as well as in the USA.[2] Strategies to engage physicians in (continuous) quality improvement have been documented and are subject to research (Reinertsen 2007; Klugman2014). Also, physician engagement has been related to their leadership competencies (Denis 2013). Medical (team) leadership competencies are relatively new topics in the field of medical education (Blumenthal 2012). Also, only few countries have comprehensive medical leadership programs in place (Dickson 2014).

To enhance physician's empowerment in teamwork initiatives, the Dutch version of TeamSTEPPS recently was successfully implemented in concordance with a comprehensive medical leadership competency development program (Klein Ikkink 2013). This involves a four-stage approach:

1. Individual 360° assessment consisting of:
   (a) Inventory of personal orientation based on assessment of constructive and (passive and aggressive) defensive styles (see Fig. 19.3)
   (b) Inventory of emotional intelligence and mindfulness
   (c) Inventory of individual team leadership competencies
   (d) Inventory of reflective skills
2. Short-term intensive individual coaching by experienced medical leadership coach (also a physician)
3. Peer-to-peer coaching

[2] See footnote 1.

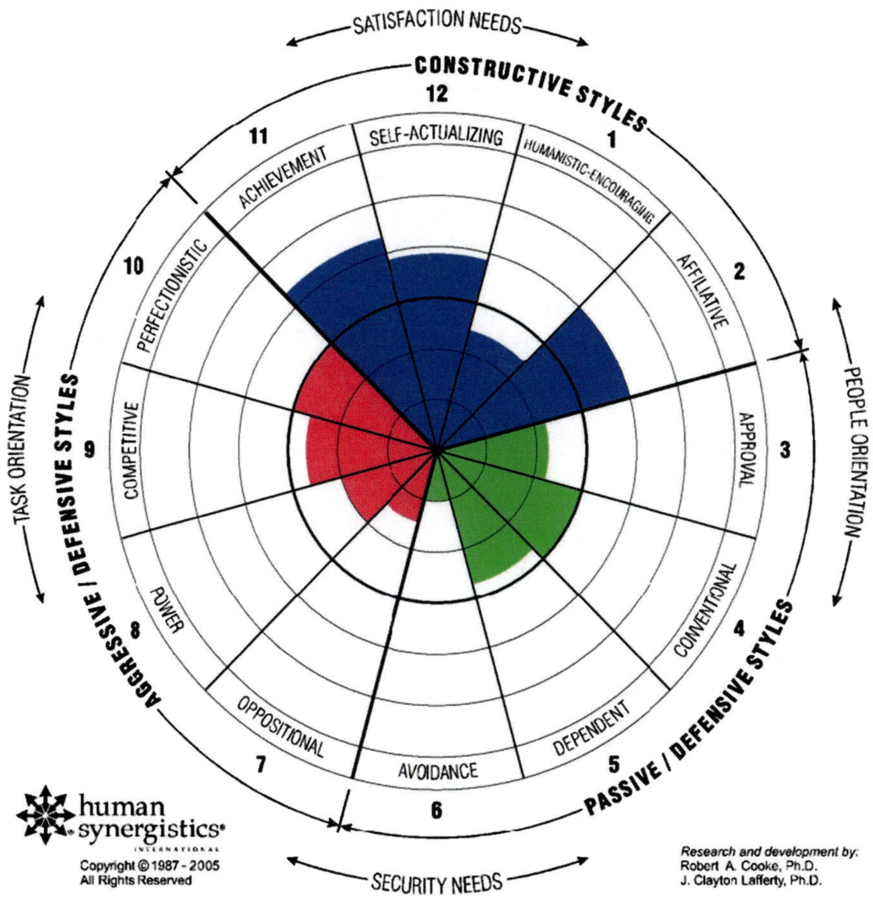

Fig. 19.3 Lifestyle inventory: different styles in personal need and orientation – constructive and (passive and aggressive) defensive styles (). [With permission of Doedijns Consulting BV, The Hague, The Netherlands]

The comprehensive set of 360° assessments provides the individual physician with tools to improve his/her level of self-regulation and development. The assessment indicators reflect on several areas relevant to medical leadership. The first two areas reflect on personal characteristics and include being knowledgeable of own emotions, being in control of one's personal emotions, and taking note of emotions of others. These attributes, also known as "emotional intelligence" support a climate of reasonableness and calmness influencing fellow team members and colleagues (Cooke 1987; Wong 2007; Goleman 2002; Harolds 2004). Physicians able to recognize and deal with their own emotions and those of others and to use this knowledge to change things for the better are "emotionally awake" (Harolds 2011). Thirdly, a novel scale on leadership capabilities that empower collaborations between teams and people is used (Chesluk 2012). Additionally, a scale on reflective skills is included to assess "the habitual and judicious use of communication, knowledge, technical skills, clinical reasoning, emotions, values, and reflection in daily practice for the benefit of the individuals and communities being served" by participating physicians (Aukes 2008).

All individual physicians participating in the program are debriefed on each of their 360° assessment. During one-on-one coaching sessions, they receive their personal leadership framework 360° feedback, followed by one of more additional coaching sessions. In a mono-disciplinary peer-to-peer coaching setting, initially facilitated by the external physician (medical leadership coach), physicians learn with and from each other, typically in sync with experiences physicians have during the parallel multidisciplinary team interventions. Physicians can undertake additional training in specific development areas identified. Over time the effects of individual and team-based activities are monitored with a follow-up measurement, typically after 1–1.5 year.

Active engagement of physicians is based not only on merely motivation. Physicians need to be facilitated as the professionals they are: trained in and disposed to performing on a level of excellence. Since medical leadership development is a relative novelty in medical education, future research will deliver deeper insight in its finesses, in particular in the constitution and development of medical *team* leadership competencies.

19.5 Conclusions and Future Considerations

Quality and service orientation and continuously striving for excellence are central in the current trends and influences healthcare is facing globally. Like any other division in healthcare, medical (nuclear) imaging services are increasingly challenged to perform based on excellent teamwork and leadership. To reach and remain performing on an acceptable and compatible level, medical (nuclear) imaging teams require training to learn how to work together, understand each other's role and build on mutual trust. New comprehensive teamwork systems like TeamSTEPPS offer innovative teams evidence based and ready to use tools and instruments.

Additionally, teams also require an effective administrative structure and leadership. Based on a concise organizational philosophy, management should

Table 19.3 Key physician leadership qualities and characteristics (Harolds 2004)

1. Integrity
2. Trustworthiness
3. Temperament
4. Competence and personal mastery
5. Professionalism
6. Inspiring and motivational
7. Win-win approach
8. Good communication
9. Focus on excellence
10. Networking and socializing
11. Love for people

specifically promote the continuous development of teamwork and leadership skills and behavior. The roles of the clinical imaging services leadership are well defined (The Royal College 2012). This also goes for physician leadership qualities and characteristics in this medical discipline (Harolds 2004) (Table 19.3).

Actively engaging physicians is founded in (re)inviting them in becoming "shareholders" in teamwork initiatives of the team(s) they lead. Based on their intrinsic leadership as team member with the medical end-responsibility, nuclear medicine physicians should be further equipped in their role as "coaching team leaders."

With the fast pace with which innovations in nuclear medicine emerge, we can only guess what this will ask for future teams working in such complex healthcare domain. Innovations in this field of expertise will not only bring about new therapies and interventions. Novel technologies and the empowerment of patients and their families soon might make them the most important team members on our teams. This too will ask for excellent teamwork based on reflectiveness and mindfulness, in close relation with them and all other disciplines that are shareholders in excellent medical nuclear imaging.[3]

References

Aukes LC, Geertsma J, Cohen-Schotanus J, Zwierstra RP, Slaets JP. The development of a scale to measure personal reflection in medical practice and education. Med Teach. 2007;29(2–3):177–82.

Baker DP, Gustafson S, Beaubien JM, Salas E, Barach P. Medical teamwork and patient safety: the evidence-based relation. Washington, DC: American Institutes for Research; 2003.

Baker D, Day R, Salas E. Teamwork as an essential component of high-reliability organizations. Health Serv Res. 2006;41(4 Pt 2):1576–98.

Baker DP, Krokos KJ, Amodeo AM. TeamSTEPPS teamwork attitudes questionnaire (T-TAQ) manual. Washington, DC: American Institutes for Research; 2008.

Beach TA, Karen G, Dam HQ, Manzone TA. Ensuring safe and quality medication use in nuclear medicine: a collaborative team achieves compliance with medication management standards. J Nucl Med Technol. 2012;40:1–10.

Blumenthal DM, Bernard K, Bohnen J, Bohmer R. Addressing the leadership gap in medicine: Residents' need for systematic leadership development training. Acad Med. 2012;87(4):513–22.

Borrill CS, Carletta J, Carter AJ, et al. The effectiveness of health care teams in the National Health Service. Aston Centre for Health Service Organisational Research, University of Aston, Human Communications Research Centre, Universities of Glasgow and Edinburgh, Psychological Therapies Research Centre, University of Leeds. 2001.

Bridges DR, Davidson RA, Odegard PG, Maki IV, Tomkowiak J. Interprofessional collaboration: three best practice models of interprofessional education. Med Educ Online. 2011;16:10.

Chesluk BJ, Bernabeo E, Hess B, Lynn LA, Reddy S, Holmboe ES. A new tool to give hospitalists feedback to improve interprofessional teamwork and advance patient care. Health Aff. 2012;31(11):2485–92.

Clancy CM, Tornberg DN. TeamSTEPPS: assuring optimal teamwork in clinical settings. Am Med Qual. 2007;22(3):214–7.

[3] TeamSTEPPS is a registered trademark of the US Department of Defense, Falls Church, VA, and the Agency for Healthcare Research and Quality (an agency of the US Department of Health and Human Services), Rockville, MD.

Clark J. Medical leadership and engagement: no longer an optional extra. J Health Organ Manag. 2012;26(4–5):437–43.

Cooke RA, Lafferty JC, Rousseau DM. Thinking and behavioral styles: consistency between self-descriptions and descriptions by others. Educ Psychol Meas. 1987;47:815–23.

Degeling P, Maxwell S, Iedema R, Hunter D. Making clinical governance work. British Medical Journal. 2004;329:679–82.

Denis JL, et al. Exploring the dynamics of physician engagement and leadership for health system improvement. Canadian foundation for healthcare improvement. 2013. (See: http://www.cfhi-fcass.ca). Site view: 30 Oct 2014.

Dickson G, Tholl B, editors. Bringing leadership to life in health: LEADS in a caring environment. Berlin: Springer; 2014.

EANM. European association of nuclear medicine. Technologist Committee and Technologist Education Subcommittee. Vienna, Austria. 2006. www.eanm.org.

EFQM (European Foundation for Quality Management). 2014. http://www.efqm.org/. Site view: 30 Oct 2014.

Godfrey M, Nelson E, Batalden P, et al. Clinical microsystems action guide. Hanover, NH: Trustees of Dartmouth College; 2004. Available at Clinical Microsystems Action Guide. Site view: 30 Oct 2014.

Goleman B, McKee A. Primal leadership: realizing the power of emotional intelligence. Boston: Harvard Business Press; 2002.

Greaves C, Gilmore J, Bernhardt L, Ross L. Reducing imaging waiting times: enhanced roles and service-redesign. Int J Health Care Qual Assur. 2013;26(3):195–202.

Harolds J. Selected important characteristics for enlightened medical leaders. J Am Coll Radiol. 2004;1:338–42.

Harolds JA. Tips for leaders, Part I. Basic principles of leadership. Clin Nucl Med. 2011;36:694–5.

IAEA. Nuclear security culture: implementing guide. Vienna: International Atomic Energy Agency; 2008. p. 2008.

JCI (Joint Commission International). 2014. http://www.jointcommissioninternational.org. Site view: 30 Oct 2014.

Keijser WA. Teamwork, leadership & TeamSTEPPS™: A Dutch Culture of Continuous Improvement. Presentation. 2014. National TeamSTEPPS Conference, Minn/StPaul, Minn, USA – June 11–12 2014. http://www.teamsteppsportal.org. Site view: 30 Oct 2014.

Keijser WA, van der Schrieck-de Loos EM. 2013. TeamSHOPP: een cultuur continu gericht op verbeteren. IGO Proceedings 2013. (1003–10). [in Dutch].

Khatri N, Brown GD, Hicks LL. From a blame culture to a just culture in health care. Health Care Manage Rev. 2009;34(4):312–22.

Kirkpatrick DL, Kirkpatrick JD. Evaluating training programs. San Francisco: Berrett Koehler Publishers; 1994.

Kitajima M, Kitagawa Y, Fujii H, Mukai M, Kubo A. Credentialing of nuclear medicine physicians, surgeons, and pathologists as a multidisciplinary team for selective sentinel lymphadenectomy. Cancer Treat Res. 2005;127:253–67.

Klein Ikkink AJ, Keijser WA, Krooneman-Smits IAM, Mariani M, Scheeren TWL, Struys MMRF, Beens EJ. Multidisciplinary teamwork, leadership and TeamSTEPPS. Towards a Culture of Continuous Improvement. First experiences in cardio-thoracic surgical teams in UMC Groningen. Poster Presentation. International Forum on Quality and Safety in Healthcare. London, United Kingdom, April 2013.

Klugman R, Gitkind MJ, Walsh KE. The physician quality officer model: 5 year follow up. Am J Med Qual. 2015;30(5):454–8.

Kohn LT, Corrigan JM, Donaldson MS. To err is human. Building a safer health system. Washington, DC: National Academy Press; 2000. (Report).

Kotter JP, Rathgeber H. Our iceberg is melting: changing and succeeding under any conditions. New York: St Martin's Press; 2006.

Reinertsen JL, Gosfield AG, Rupp W, Whittington JW. Engaging physicians in a shared quality agenda. IHI innovation series white paper. Cambridge, MA: Institute for Healthcare Improvement; 2007.

Rohren E. Physician – technologist interactions: the importance of team. Collimator Newsletter. 2012;1(2):1.

Salas E, Sims DE, Burke CS. Is there a big 5 in teamwork? Small Group Research. 2005;36(5):555–99.

TeamSTEPPS 2.0 Core Curriculum. Agency for healthcare research and quality, Rockville. http://www.ahrq.gov/professionals/education/curriculum-tools/teamstepps/instructor/index.html. Site view: 30 Oct 2014.

The Royal College of Radiologists and the Society and College of Radiographers. Team working in clinical imaging. London: The Royal College of Radiologists and the Society and College of Radiographers; 2012.

Tuttle M, Robbins R, Larson SM, Strauss HW. Challenging cases in thyroid cancer: a multidisciplinary approach. Eur J Nucl Mol Imaging. 2004;31(4):605–12.

UK Government. 2014. https://www.gov.uk/government/uploads/system/uploads/attachment_data/file/308513/shortageoccupationlistapril14.pdf. Site view: 30 Oct 2014.

VWS Veiligheid Management System. 2014. http://www.vmszorg.nl. Site view: 30 Oct 2014.

Wong CS, Foo M, Want C, Wong P. The feasibility of training and development of EI: an exploratory study in Singapore, Hong Kong and Taiwan. Intelligence. 2007;35(2):141–50.

The Safety Management System: Implementation for Nuclear Medicine

20

Jitze Medema and Walter Noordzij

Abstract

In the Netherlands, 5.7% of the 1.3 million people in hospitals suffer from unintended damage to health, which – in the majority of cases – can be explained by human factors such as knowledge, behaviors, or skills. Reduction of this unintentional and avoidable damage is highly necessary. A safety management system (SMS) embeds patient safety in healthcare practice. Using this system, hospitals continuously identify risks, implement improvements, and establish, evaluate, and modify policy. The healthcare inspectorate has the supervising role to control the (progress of) implementation of the SMS themes in all Dutch hospitals.

Demonstrable patient safety in each healthcare processes is a task for every employee. Compliance to the system and if necessary adjustment of agreements make the full circle of plan-do-check-act round.

This chapter focuses on the development of the SMS in general, the implementation of ten safety themes in our university medical center, and application of the three most important safety themes on the department of Nuclear Medicine and Molecular Imaging.

20.1 Introduction: Brief History of the Development of the Dutch Safety Management System for Hospitals

In the Netherlands, 5.7% of the 1.3 million people in hospitals suffer from unintended damage to health, which – in the majority of cases – can be explained by human factors such as knowledge, behaviors, or skills. Reduction of this unintentional and

J. Medema (✉) • W. Noordzij, MD, PhD
Department of Nuclear Medicine and Molecular Imaging, University of Groningen, University Medical Center Groningen, PO Box 30.001, Groningen 9700 RB, The Netherlands
e-mail: j.medema@umcg.nl

A.W.J.M. Glaudemans et al. (eds.), *Quality in Nuclear Medicine*,
DOI 10.1007/978-3-319-33531-5_20

avoidable damage is highly necessary. A safety management system (SMS) embeds patient safety in healthcare practice. Using this system, hospitals continuously identify risks, implement improvements, and establish, evaluate, and modify policy. The basic requirements for an SMS are set out in the Netherlands Technical Agreement (NTA) 8009, "Safety management system for hospitals and organizations which administer hospital care" (NTA 8009). This NTA provides an overview of the essential aspects which should be addressed in the development of an SMS. In addition, the NTA 8009 forms the basis for external review of hospitals' patient safety policies.

The starting point for developing a SMS for hospitals was the report "Here you'll work safely, or you won't work here" (Willems 2004), by the president-director of Shell, the Netherlands. In this report, Shell provides recommendations for the improvement of patient (and employee) safety in a healthcare setting, based on experiences with their own SMS. Based on this report, a healthcare SMS should consist of a risk assessment, a system for incident reporting (in a safe way), a method for incident analysis, and a system to manage the resulting recommendations and improvement measures. In fact, these requirements reflect the cycle of improvement: plan-do-check-act. The report further states that the message of working safely should be carried out actively by the board of directors of the healthcare institution and that all employees should fully comply to the system.

Based on this report, a SMS pilot was introduced in 2007. This project was implemented with the joint collaboration of the Dutch Association of Hospitals, the Dutch Federation of University Medical Centers, Society of Medical Specialists, and the Dutch Association of Nurses and Caregivers. Knowledge and experience of the basic requirements for leadership, employees, patient participation, risk assessments, and changes and improvements were gained during this project. The experiences from this pilot project were combined with requirements for communication, third party management, and control measures, to eventually form the basics of the NTA 8009:2007 (NEN 2011).

20.2 From Technical Agreement to Ten Safety Themes

In 2008, the national SMS safety program was launched to secure patient safety in daily practice and to reduce hospital accidents by 50 %. According to this safety program, hospitals were required to have implemented a certified and accredited safety management system which conforms with the requirements of NTA 8009:2007 by the end of 2012. Research into patient safety led to the identification of eleven themes, which can support the reduction of unintended, preventable harm in hospitals. Each theme was translated into a target objective and a practical guide. These practical guides are based on available literature, existing guidelines and (inter)national "good practices." The eleven themes are: (1) preventing hospital infections after surgery, (2) preventing line sepsis and severe sepsis treatment, (3) early recognition and treatment of the vital endangered patient, (4) medication verification at admission and discharge, (5) identification of vulnerable older people, (6) optimal care in acute coronary syndromes, (7) early recognition and treatment of pain, (8) high-risk medication: preparing and administering parenteralia, (9) exchange of and in patients, (10) prevention of renal insufficiency in intravenous use of iodine contrast agents, and (11) safe care for sick children. In fact, the last theme contains a more condensed application of 6 of the 10 themes for adults (Veiligheidsprogramma – Thema's 2013).

20.3 Integration of Safety Themes in Quality Management System

The board of directors of the University Medical Center Groningen (UMCG) has decided to integrate the safety themes into the hospital quality management system, which is based on the ISO 9001 criteria. Furthermore, the board of directors of the UMCG has set up a program team to coordinate the implementation within the UMCG. This program team is subdivided into theme-specific teams, which are responsible for the identification and informing of per theme relevant departments, initiation and coordination of the recommendations per theme, and reporting the progress back to the program team. The program team eventually coordinates the coherence between the themes and reports the status to the board of directors. To be certain of continuous awareness of the SMS themes, the UMCG has organized the awareness program "Demonstrable safe care: I'm doing it," has developed e-learning applications of each SMS theme, and organizes an annual "week of patient safety," with special interest for a symposium and presentations of new innovations and applications rewarded as "best practices."

The healthcare inspectorate (Inspectie voor de Gezondheidszorg, IGZ) has the supervising role to control the (progress of) implementation of the SMS themes in all hospitals (Van der Wal 2009). Using a specially designed inspection instrument ("safety management system in hospitals"), the progress of the themes was examined. The developments in the UMCG were audited by IGZ. Moreover, the UMCG was rewarded with a Hospital Certificate Patient Safety System in 2012 as well as certification according to NTA8009:2007.

20.4 Implementation of Safety Themes at the Department of Nuclear Medicine and Molecular Imaging

Since 2009, the department of Nuclear Medicine and Molecular Imaging (NIMMI) of the UMCG has successfully implemented the basic elements of the UMCG SMS. As part of the implementation, the basic elements are taken up into the quality policy and quality operation manual. Patient safety is also part of the annual management review of the department. In addition, risk analyses, using Hierarchical Task Analyses, are performed on each primary process (production of radionuclides, production of radiopharmaceuticals, performing diagnostics, therapy, bioanalysis, and reporting diagnostics). Moreover, the department has implemented a local emergency plan in case of calamities, installed a commission for decentralized (anonymous) incident reporting (DIM), developed a purchase process of medical devices with a focus on training of skills, and created a safety culture according to an awareness policy for employees with attention to patient safety in consultation and work consultation. "Based on incidents or calamities discussed in the DIM meetings, we can decide to use a system approached tool to identify basic causes of the specific incident(s): "Prevention and Recovery Information System for Monitoring and Analysis (PRISMA)"

Furthermore, the department of NMMI has identified three of the eleven SMS themes for implementation in daily practice: exchange of and in patients, high-risk medication: preparing and administering parenteralia, and prevention of renal insufficiency in patients who underwent a diagnostic CT with intravenous use of iodine contrast agents.

To reduce patient exchange, an identification and verification procedure at critical patient transfer moments was introduced in the UMCG. For the department of NMMI, these transfer moments occur at presentation on the outpatient clinic, preparation for the investigation (or treatment), and at the moment of the investigation (or treatment). On all these critical moments, the employee has to be certain that he or she is dealing with the correct patient, and both register and act if not. Mandatory questions are answered on the case-record form (CRF, Fig. 20.1), which consists of 16 items.

Investigation		**Check date of birth**	Signature
		Does the patient agree with the investigation? Y / N	
Acquisition	Signature	**Pregnancy?**	N / Y / not applicable
Processing	Signature	**Breast feeding?**	N / Y / not applicable.

Suspicion of (child) abuse / neglect / unsafety? **N / Y**
If yes, what are the arguments?
....
....
....
....

Sticker radiopharmaceutical	**Radiofarmaceutical**		Siganture **check**	Signature **administration**
	Date			
	Dose (MBq)			
	Place of injection			
	Time			
Evt. tweede sticker radiopharmaceutical	**Other medication**			
		Time	Siganture **check**	Signature **administration**
	Stannous chloride			
	Furosemide			
	Chloral hydrate			

Fig. 20.1 Part of the case-record form with parameters that are checked in each patient

Definition high risk patient UMCG criteria	**Definition high risk patient SMS criteria**
eGFR < 30 mL/min/1,73 m^2	eGFR < 45 mL/min/1,73 m^2
eGFR < 45 mL/min/1,73 m^2 and diabetes mellitus	eGFR < 60 mL/min/1,73 m^2 and diabetes mellitus
eGFR < 45 mL/min/1,73 m^2 and two or more risk factors	eGFR < 60 mL/min/1,73 m^2 and two or more risk factors
Kahler's or Waldenström's disease with light chains in urine	Kahler's or Waldenström's disease with light chains in urine

Normal risk: all situations others than high risk. Risk factors: peripheral vascular disease, heart failure, age > 75, anemia (Hb<8.3 for males en <7.5 mmol/l for females), symptomatic hypotension, contrastvolume > 150 mL, dehydration, use of diuretics en nefrotoxic medication (for example NSAIDs).

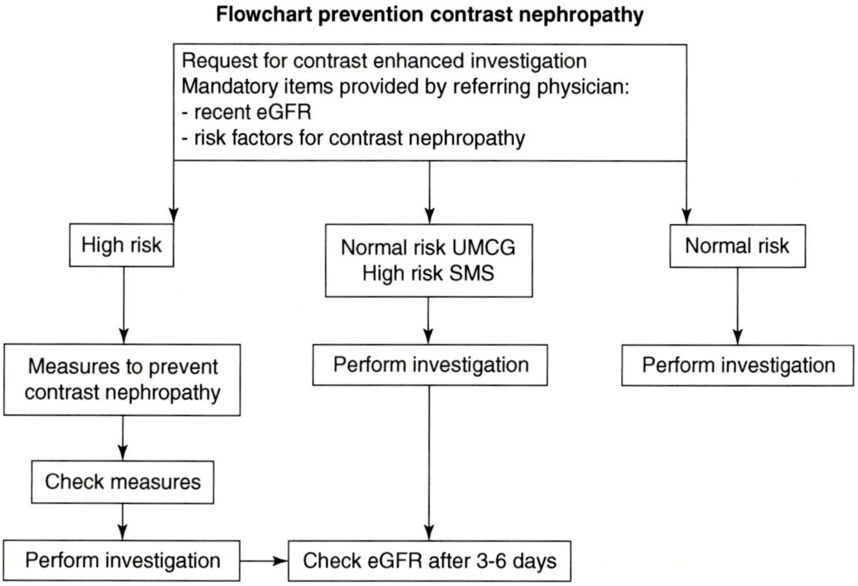

Fig. 20.2 Risk assessment contrast nephropathy

Radiopharmaceuticals are considered high-risk medication. Production and preparation of radiopharmaceuticals occur according to Good Manufacturing Practice (GMP) guidelines, in which SMS is incorporated that contains independent double check of the product and the syringe label. When administering a radiopharmaceutical to a patient on the department of NMMI, the employee should perform and register a double check to be certain he or she is dealing with the correct patient and the correct dose of the correct radiopharmaceutical for this investigation or therapy.

Prevention of renal insufficiency in intravenous use of iodine contrast agents during CT imaging procedures is the last SMS theme that was identified for implementation on our department. Contrast nephropathy can be prevented by early identification of all patients with elevated risk of contrast nephropathy and introduction of adequate measures to prevent its occurrence in high-risk patients. Therefore, for each patient that is referred for a CT using intravenous contrast agents, the estimated glomerular filtration rate (eGFR) should be known and should not be older than 12 months at the time of the planned CT. Three distant ranges of eGFR values are defined, and the combination of this eGFR value and other predefined risk factors determines the risk of contrast nephropathy and the measures to prevent (Fig. 20.2). The risk of contrast nephropathy is established at three different time points: when the patient is referred, the day before the investigation, and the moment of administration of the contrast agent. If eventually the eGFR does not allow contrast agent administration at the time of investigation, the patient will not undergo a contrast-enhanced CT.

20.5 Compliance

It is important to comply to the agreements from the SMS themes. Different tools to test the compliance are used on the department of NMMI. One of these tools is the monthly CRF sample survey. Despite that performing a sample survey is not part of regulations, it has been taken up in the quality management system of the department. During a sample survey, all CRF's (up to 50) of one randomly chosen day are retrospectively analyzed on completeness. The results of the analysis are discussed in the weekly management board meetings of the department and in the different section-specific meetings. Figure 20.3) shows the co-workers' compliance of answering all CRF items, during a time span of more than 2 years. It appears that a quick-win in compliance is easily established after the introduction of the sample survey. However 100% compliance remains a challange.

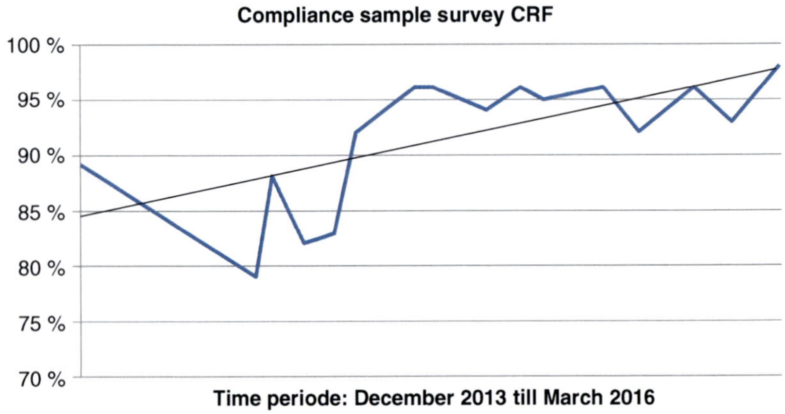

Fig. 20.3

Table 20.1 Parameters of the decentralized incident reporting system of the department of nuclear medicine and molecular medicine

DIM reports	2014	2013	2012	2011	2010	2009
Number of reports	29	65	47	26	15	9
Cases closed	28	65	47	25	15	9
Incidents > 6 months open	0	0	0	2	0	0
PRISMA	0	2	1	0	0	1
Risks of the incidents	**2014**	**2013**	**2012**	**2011**	**2010**	**2009**
Small	10	22	21	8	2	4
Moderate	17	36	22	12	6	4
Severe	2	7	3	6	7	1
Very severe			1			
Calamity						

Table 20.2 Decentralized incidents and the relation to safety management system themes

DIM reports vs. SMS themes	2014	2013	2012
Preventing hospital infections after surgery			
Preventing line sepsis and severe sepsis treatment			
Early recognition and treatment of the vital endangered patient			
Medication verification at admission and discharge			
Identification of vulnerable older people			
Optimal care in acute coronary syndromes			
Early recognition and treatment of pain			
High-risk medication: preparing and administering parenteralia	4	2	5
Exchange of and in patients	3	7	4
Prevention of renal insufficiency in intravenous use of iodine contrast agent	2	2	6
Safe care for sick children			1
Other (planning and daily patient care)	20	54	31

Another tool is the DIM system. Reports are first discussed in the department's own DIM meeting (Tables 20.1 and 20.2). Necessary improvements in patient safety are discussed and suggested towards the responsible employee of the concerning primary process. Furthermore, the reports, results, and actions are discussed in both the weekly management board meetings and in the different section-specific meetings.

The hospital uses clinical performance indicators (CPIs) for the compliance to the SMS themes (Table 20.3). These CPIs are conducted by the healthcare inspectorate.

Table 20.3 Clinical performance indicators (CPI) for the compliance to the safety management system (SMS) themes: nationwide, healthcare inspectorate indicators, hospital (UMCG)-wide indicators, and department (NMMI)-specific implementation

SMS theme	Nationwide SMS CPI	Inspectorate indicator	UMCG	NMMI
Prevention renal insufficiency	1. % of patients in which eGFR is known before contrast agent administration 2. % of high-risk patients hydrated before contrast agent administration	Centralized registration of eGFR within the hospital	1. % of patients in which eGFR is known before contrast agent administration 2. % of high-risk patients hydrated before contrast agent administration	Sample survey once every month both items
High-risk medication	1. Annual report of all hospital incidents 2. % correctly performed procedures concerning preparation and administration of parenteralia	Registration system for (near) accidents concerning preparation and administration of parenteralia	Report and analysis of medication accidents followed by actions Two systems: Incident reporting system Central registration of medication errors	Number of incident reports
Exchange of and in patients	Demonstrable patient identification and verification in centralized system Reporting (near) exchange in centralized system Number of exchanges of patient, place, side, and intervention per 1000 elective procedures	Demonstrable patient identification and verification at "critical" moments	Insight into number of exchanges of patient, place, side, and intervention per 1000 elective procedures and diagnostic procedures	Number of incident reports Monthly sample survey case-record form

Last, once every 3 years, the department is audited internally and every year externally for each primary process. All abovementioned tools for compliance are discussed and actions are evaluated.

Conclusions

The implementation of the SMS in the UMCG and consequences for the department of NMMI help to identify risks and implement improvements and should help to reduce unintended damage to patients. Demonstrable patient safety in each primary process is a task for every employee. Compliance to the agreements and if necessary adjustment of the agreements make the full circle of plan-do-check-act round.

References

NEN. NTA 8009 (English) Safety management system for hospitals and organizations which administer hospital care. Delft: Netherlands Standardization Institute; 2011.

Van der Wal G. Invoering veiligheidsmanagementsysteem in ziekenhuizen komt op gang. 2009. http://www.google.nl/url?sa=t&rct=j&q=&esrc=s&source=web&cd=1&cad=rja&uact=8&ved=0CCYQFjAAahUKEwjnh9Xp8Z3HAhWjZ9sKHcm5C-s&url=http%3A%2F%2Fwww.medischetechnologie.nl%2Fdownload.php%3Frefid%3D737&ei=5ETIVeeFFaPP7QbJ867YDg&usg=AFQjCNE0STkXUGaEs4Jk5UmG5YhDFJpBPA&bvm=bv.99804247,d.ZGU. Accessed 08 Aug 2015

Willems R. Hier werk je veilig, of je werkt hier niet. Sneller beter – De veiligheid in de zorg. Eindrapportage Shell Nederland. 2004. http://www.vmszorg.nl/_library/14216/rapport_rein_willems_2004.pdf. Accessed 08 Aug 2015.

VMS Veiligheidprogramma. 2013. Thema's http://www.vmszorg.nl/themas Accessed 08 Aug 2015.

Risk Management Systems

21

Alexander van der Star

Abstract

In general, most European countries have quality and safety provisions for health services addressed within their own national legislation. However, how are patients and professionals informed to, i.e. ensure them that the care in their hospital is of high quality? The number of reported incidents is at most a global indicator for 'how safe the hospital is for the patient'. Only a fully implemented reliable system for quality and safety management will ensure that goals set are achieved. Risk assessment can be an effective approach to encourage awareness and cultural change.

This chapter deals with methods for systematic estimation and reduction of risks. Within the context of this book, the focus will be on processes and patient safety. After an introduction on the systematic approach of risk management, in general, two complementary models for risk assessment applicable in healthcare organisations will be explained.

21.1 Quality or Risk Management?

Quality and safety of care is a complex concept with numerous dimensions. It can involve structures, processes and outcomes and deals with effectiveness, safety and patient centeredness. Hospitals are faced with major challenges due to increasing complexity and technological developments.

An effective quality management system is risk based. To improve quality, it is necessary to identify and control risks, e.g. the workers, the patient and the

A. van der Star, ME, MSc, MSHE
Department for Quality and Patientsafety, University Medical Center Groningen, University of Groningen, Groningen, The Netherlands
e-mail: vanderstar50@hotmail.com

A.W.J.M. Glaudemans et al. (eds.), *Quality in Nuclear Medicine*,
DOI 10.1007/978-3-319-33531-5_21

organisation. Failures and incidents can be held accountable for the fact that output does not fulfil the expectations or requirements. Output may affect continuity, finance, quality, safety standards, etc. Risk management therefore requires to have a greater impact on the policy and operations of organisations, much more than it has till now. In particular, on the operational level, hospitals are quite vulnerable for disturbances and (near) incidents with a negative effect on the efficiency and efficacy of an organisation. It is obvious that this generates a lot of waste in terms of money and capacity.

21.2 Risk Management Retrospective

For a long time, risks and safety have been correlated with the chemical industry, nuclear power plants, aviation and heavy industries like shipyards, construction and metal works. Common sense about safety was the human factor – reckless behaviour – which was the most important explanation for the occurrence of incidents. In a study by Greenwood and Woods, it was found that accidents were unevenly distributed among workers, with a relatively small proportion of workers accounting for most of the accidents (Greenwood et al. 1919). Their theory is known as the accident-proneness theory. Nowadays, in safety science, this theory is obsolete. However, the underlying idea that certain people attract accidents is still alive. In 1931, Heinrich reported that 88% of the accidents are caused by 'unsafe acts of persons'. Based on his research, he developed what often is referred to as Heinrich's accident triangle or pyramid. In a group of 330 accidents, 300 will result in no injuries, 29 will result in minor injuries and one will result in a major injury. Although there maybe reservations about Heinrich's data and conclusions, his theories espoused 80 years ago are still considered applicable today (Heinrich 1931).

Another widely used theory for accident causation also developed by Heinrich (1931) is the 'Domino Theory'. According to this theory, an 'accident' is one factor in a sequence that may lead to an injury. The factors can be visualised as a series of dominoes standing on edge; when one falls, the linkage required for a chain reaction is completed. Each of the factors is dependent on the preceding factor. Bird and Loftus developed this theory further and included the influence of management in accident causation (Jr et al. 1976).

In the early eighties, disasters in Mexico City (LPG-disaster, >500 fatalities) and Bhopal (Union Carbide India, 3787 fatalities) have given a boost to consider the performance of safety and risk management. In the same time, no serious large-scale incidents in hospitals were reported. Severe adverse events in health care in the 1980s and the 1990s concerned the pharmaceutical industries (Josefson 2003; Meers et al. 1973).

Concerning medical errors, this has been significantly addressed at individual level during the past few decades. This suits well with the obsolete thinking about safety, developed at the beginning of the last century. Patient safety however is a broader ambition that requires thinking beyond the individual patient to consider the

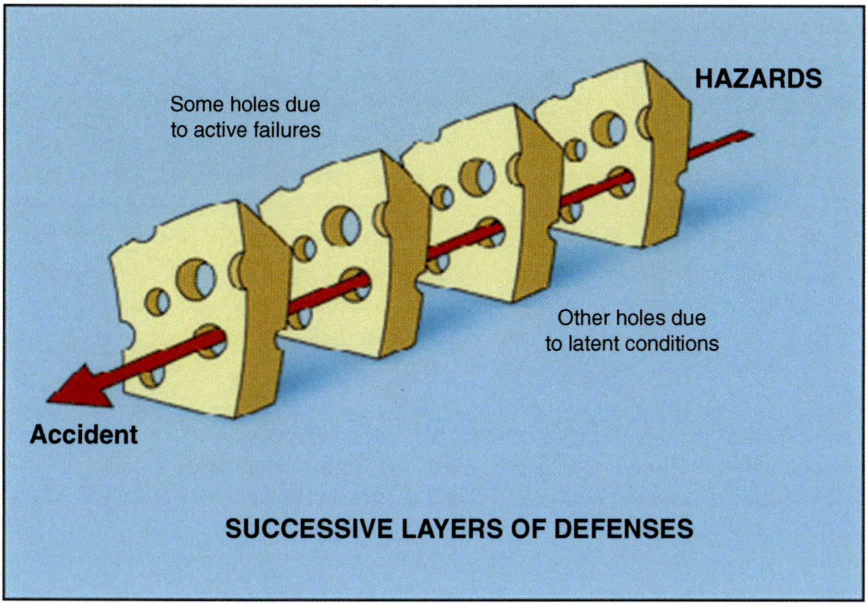

Fig. 21.1 "Swiss cheese" model (Reason 1991)

characteristics of the whole system of health care (Vincent C. Patient safety. John Wiley and Sons 2011).

Evaluation of and research on severe industrial incidents and incidents in the transport sector reveal that organisational and managerial aspects are of imminent importance. Reason (1997) developed the Swiss cheese model (Reason 2000). This model has become one of the standards in health care. Defences, barriers, organisational procedures and administrative controls have the function to protect organisations from accidents. The model shows (Fig. 21.1) that in reality defence layers are not intact and more like Swiss cheese. Nearly always a combination of latent conditions and active failures is involved in bringing a hazard into an accident (The original source for the Swiss Cheese illustration is: "Swiss Cheese" Model – James Reason 1991).

In modern safety management, the system approach is leading. Tripod Delta Safety management system is an example of such an approach. Developed in the late 1990s, the approach focuses on the formal design of processes and their operational weakness. Things can be perfectly organised on paper but cannot work in 'real life'. It seems then necessary to analyse how things are done in addition to how things are formalised. According to Cambon (and others), this aspect refers to the 'operational' facet of safety management systems (SMS). Building up the operational performance of a SMS actually strengthens the overall resilience of the organisation (Hollnagel and Rigaud Eric 2006).

The two methods discussed later in this chapter deal with both processes as operational weakness.

21.3 Risk Management in Health Care

21.3.1 Awareness

The publication of *To Err is Human* (Kohn et al. 1999) can be seen as a turning point in discussing publicly avoidable medical errors. All over the world, especially in developed counties, national initiatives and programmes have already been started, the aim being focused on the reduction of avoidable death in hospitals.

Certified bodies and accreditation institutes make requirements for patient safety as part of their schedules. Inspectorates review health-care organisations and take measures like closing down in case of severe nonconformities. Last but not least, health-care insurance companies require accountability based on quality and safety indicators. Governmental and public pressure have given a strong boost to the health-care sector to take their responsibility. Disadvantage is that a lot of organisations are more focused on 'damage' instead of 'Demming' control.

Elements of a safety policy for health care involves proactive risk analysis (what can go wrong, how severe is that and what can be done to prevent), a blame fair reporting, analysing incidents and a system to manage improvements and recommendations (quality management system).

21.3.2 Cultural Change

Why does it require great effort for the health-care sector to set up a risk management system? This has multiple reasons. First, the sector is confronted with complexity. Besides complex tasks and medical procedures, one can distinguish technical and organisational complexity. Technically, the health-care sector has to deal with system dependency and interactions, requirements concerning safety, reliability and continuity and technology-driven changes of medical equipment. The organisational complexity concerns aspects like increasing of multidisciplinary work, communication and training and implementation of new systems and medical technology. For example, in technical complex surgery, surgeons use more often robots. When robots were introduced, the FDA came to the conclusion that applying robots in health care is unsafe and incidents are under reported (Cooper et al. 2013). Or, an increasing high-tech E-world and the disappearance of a "Paper world" give challenges to the health-care sector but imply also risk to the patient.

Secondly, until recently, safety in the perspective of health care was the territory of the professional and has a strong operational focus. Clinical and nursing staff did not acknowledge or were not aware of the risks for patents, professionals and the health-care sector in general. In their opinion, the great majority of clinical staff have always been safety conscious in their personal practice. It is organised by professional groups, based on professional standards and not discussed publicly by health-care professionals. Medical errors were almost never addressed in medical journals (Patient 2011).

Thirdly, according to Mintzbergs structure of organisations (Mintzberg 1993), health-care organisations are defined as a professional bureaucracy. In a professional bureaucracy, the dominant factor is the operational core: the professional. The primarily mechanism of coordination is standardisation of skills. This structure is adequate in case of complex, nonroutine tasks. In contrary, in a machine bureaucracy, the dominant factor is the technostructure: experts on quality, safety, process control, etc. The primarily mechanism of coordination is standardisation of processes. Characteristic for this type of organisations are the formal rules and procedures. For the majority, a health-care organisation can be considered as a machine bureaucracy. For the (medical) professional, this is hard to accept.

Finally, for too long, the health-care sector has denied the importance of applying human factors engineering and organisational design in a way that human failure has been captured or does not result in any harm to the patient.

Finally, pitfalls and prejudices are still an obstacle in achieving an effective cultural change. Quotes like 'we do our work well', 'tasks are laid down in procedures and instructions' and 'everybody makes a mistake sometimes' do not change the mind-set to patient safety.

21.4 Risk Assessment

In the development of its business processes, health-care organisations have always considered patient safety as a dedicated part of the process. As stated earlier, the sector did believe that professional standards, a professional approach and defences were adequate. The paradigm shift to be made is that people may make mistakes and processes should be designed in a way that human failure is captured or does not result in any harm to the patient. Risk assessment techniques help professionals to get insights in the weakness of the health-care process. There are two techniques considered applicable in the health-care sector: Failure Modes and Effects Analysis and Hierarchical Task Analysis.

Failure Modes and Effects Analysis (FMEA) is an assessment approach to apply in existing situations or to analyse new chains of care on its performance and potential failure modes. Hierarchical Task Analysis (HTA) (Stanton Neville 2006) HTA is a methodology based upon the theory of human performance. HTA describes systematically how work is organised in order to meet the overall objective of the task. It is a goal-based analysis of a system. Top-down subtasks and their conditions are revealed. The result is a hierarchy of operations, including subtasks, human performance of the worker within the system and the plans and conditions which are necessary to undertake these operations.

21.4.1 Failure Modes and Effects Analysis (FMEA)

Risk management on the process level means identifying identification, reduction and control of predictable risks with a view to increase the chance the results wanted will be reached. Failure Modes and Effects Analysis (FMEA) is an adequate approach for risk management on the process level. It was developed in the late 1940s by the US Army and improved and extended over the decades. There are different types of FMEA Analysis. Health care is specially concerned with the process FMEA (Yue 2012).

Fig. 21.2 Process FMEA

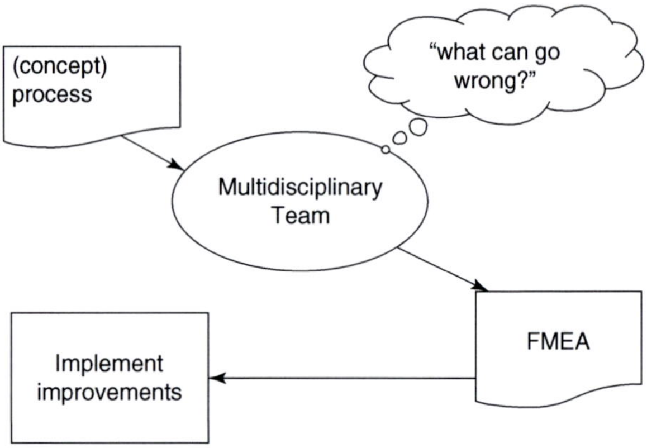

FMEA is a systematic prospective risk analysis technique, in which processes are mapped by a team (Fig. 21.2).

Starting point is often the existing situation. Analysing risks to the patient in the care process is an important part of the approach and brings into focus the dependency chain. Systematically, the process and subprocesses are reviewed to identify failure modes and their causes and to assess their potential impact. The results are listed in an FMEA worksheet. Near incidents, caused by technical, organisational and human factors are detected and can be controlled by taking appropriate actions. The approach is pretty intensive and therefore specially used to assess critical processes.

A failure mode defines the ways (modes) in which an (sub)process might fail. Failures are errors or inadequate actions, especially ones that affect the patient and worker. Examples of failure modes in the sub process 'preparing a patient for intravenous infusion with nuclide 131I' are:

- Wrong patient
- Select incorrect nuclide
- Incorrect infusion parameters
- Connection site not sterilised
- Inadequate protection against radiation for the worker

The failures will have a direct impact for the patient and the worker.

Based on the Swiss cheese model, adverse events are mostly the result of unexpected events or impropriate defences. Figure 21.3 gives an oversight of the different factors that contribute to the rise of an event (Henriksen et al. 2008).

Barriers and defences are of special interest in relation to safety. Only few people understand that only physical barriers and defences are safe proof. All others are only functional or symbolic (procedure, instruction) and are vulnerable.

The FMEA team also assesses severity (S), occurrence/frequency (O) and detection (D). For conducting FMEA, there are different worksheets available. An example, based on the Dutch safety programme VMSZorg, is given in Table 21.1.

The multiplication of S, O and D gives the Risk Priority Number (RPN). This is a measure that helps to identify the critical failure modes related to the process. A

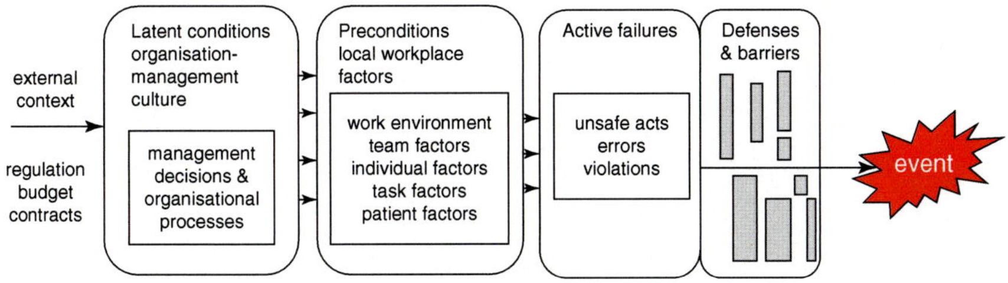

Fig. 21.3 Levels of defence (Based on Reason 1990)

RPN >10 implicates that action has to be taken. Although RPN is used to assess risks, it has no meaning in itself. In case of a high severity rate, action is always required. Interventions undertaken reduce the occurrence of these failure modes or limit its effect. Potts and others (Potts Henry et al. 2014) assessed the validity of prospective hazard analysis methods. Potts came to the conclusion that FMEA raised important hazards. The scope of the process included had a considerable influence on the outputs.

The HFMEA team should consist of all disciplines involved. Discussions in a multidisciplinary team about the performance of their daily tasks from a risk perspective are a valuable side effect. Data from sources, e.g. incident reports, quality and safety audits, performance indicators etc., should be used to complete the view of risk in a system.

21.4.2 Hierarchic Task Analysis (HTA)

Safety is dynamic and often on short-time scales in hospitals. When services and conditions in one link of the chain have limited effect on other parts of the chain of care, the system is called loosely coupled.

Tamuz and others (Tamuz and Harrison 2006) stated that loose coupling of routine activities enables providers to identify problems and intervene before they can cause harm. Similarly, changes in one unit do not necessarily affect others. A tight coupling system however is much more vulnerable for deviations and disturbances. In combination with interactive complexity, tight coupling can give rise to major system failure. Examples in health care of this type of process are the diagnostic processes using short-lived nuclides in nuclear medicine and complex medical interventions.

HTA is of added value to improve safety of the diagnostic process or intervention; firstly, because the HTA is specifically focussing on risks surrounding the patient and, secondly, because the HTA is focused to perform the task correctly. The HTA carried out provides insight into the processes and is an investment to improve processes, where possible, supported by (custom) procedures and automation. An important aspect of an HTA is to generate awareness among employees about the critical activities in their work process.

The HTA approach, developed in the 1950s, was first published by Annett et al. (1967). HTA is still frequently used for training and human reliability assessment as well as for process (re)design.

Table 21.1 FMEA Worksheet

Process step	Potential failure mode	Potential effect	Severity	Potential cause	Occurrence (frequently)	Detectable	RPN	Eliminate, control, accept	Description action	Result	Responsibility	Approval of management

There are different ways described to conduct a HTA. The process for carrying out the HTA is the following:

1. What is the overall goal of the task?
2. Give a general description of the task which, when carried out, will achieve this goal. This will be the first level of the HTA.
3. What are the subtasks which, when carried out, will achieve the operation at the top level. This will form the second level of the HTA.
4. How are the subtasks to be carried out? (e.g. in what order). This will be the plan for the second level of the HTA.
5. Taking each of the subtasks in turn, what actions have to be carried out in order to complete the suboperations?
6. How are the actions to be carried out?

When step 6 is reached, the stop rule needs to be considered, i.e. "does the bottom level of the HTA show the activities that need to be performed to carry out the supervision". If this criteria is reached, then further levels of the HTA are not required and a line can be drawn underneath this action to show this.

The HTA results in a schedule that can be transformed into a graphic scheme.

When a HTA is finished, observation in 'reality' is necessary to check the outcome. Not every observation gives rise to a recommendation. Recommendations are used to improve the HTA.

As an example, the scheme below (Fig. 21.4) shows a HTA of the insertion of a chest drain (tube thoracostomy). Modern types of chest tube are placed using the Seldinger technique, which implies that a blunt guidewire is passed over a trocar, over which the chest tube is then inserted (BTS guidelines for the insertion of a chest drain). The procedure is carried out by a medical doctor (intensivist) and an intensive care nurse. During the execution of the HTA, the medical staff became aware that they were not adequately informed about the exact working mechanism of the medical device and the necessity to apply risk assessment before starting the insertion. Also they were not aware of critical manipulations during the entire procedure. Based on the results of the HTA, it can be understood how fatalities previously occurred.

Another representation of (a part of) the HTA is shown in Table 21.2.

Conclusion

In order to achieve an adequate risk management system and to become a highly reliable organisation, a safety system approach is required. Transparency of all the included processes is a necessity to avoid operational dangers.

Nuclear medicine should be leading the way in health care. Nuclear medicine shares important characteristics with high-reliability organisations by their complexity, exact task performance, low incident rates and compliance to strict regulations. Also, they can learn a lot from the nuclear industries.

The challenge facing nuclear medicine is managing complex, demanding technologies and to avoid major failures that could paralyse the organisation and harm the patient and the workers irreversibly.

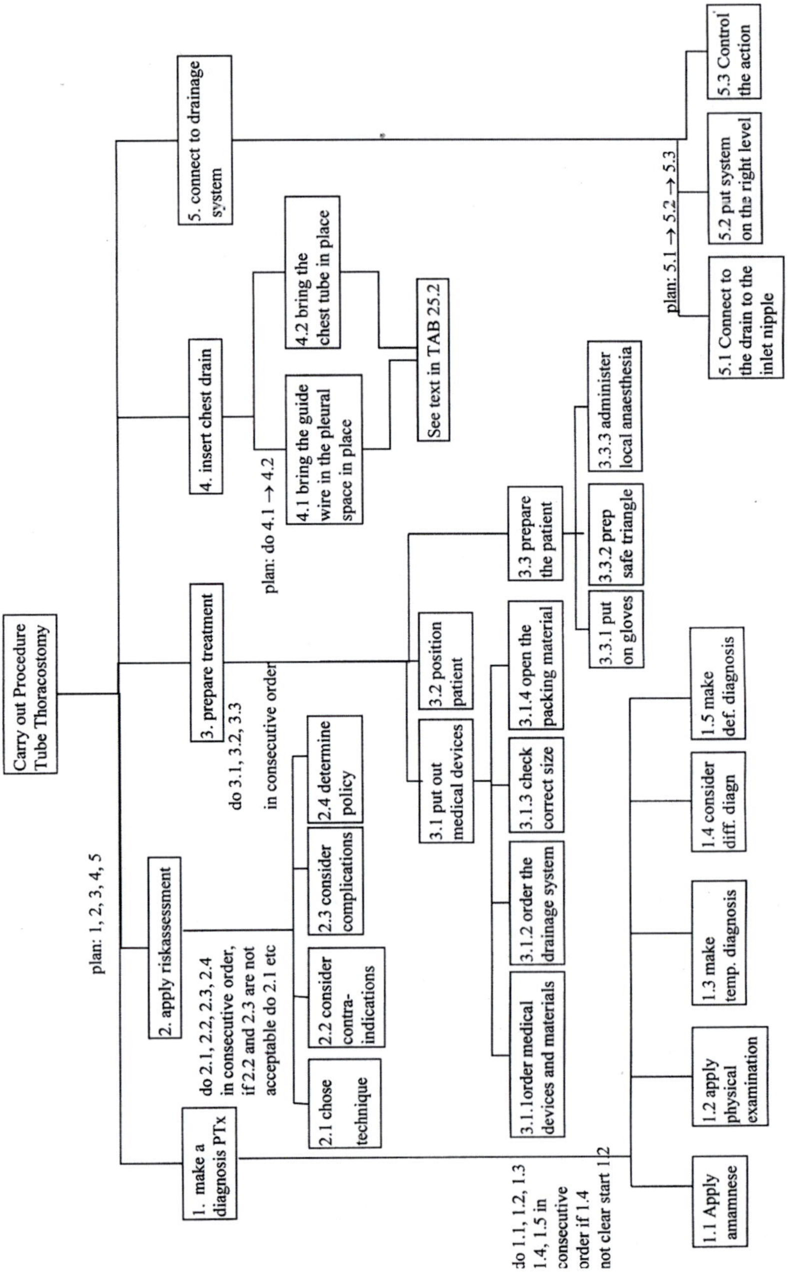

Fig. 21.4 Results of a HTA Procedure Tube Thoracostomy

Table 21.2 Tabular presentation of (a part of) a HTA (task 4)

No.	Task	Plan	No.	Subtask	Plan	No.	Suboperation
4	Insert chest drain	Plan: do 4.1 → 4.2	4.1	Bring the guide wire in the pleural space in place	4.1.1 → 4.1.2 → 4.1.3 →4.1.4 → 4.1.5 → 4.1.6 → 4.1.7 → 4.1.8	4.1.1	Make incision
						4.1.2	Administer additional anaesthesia
						4.1.3	Advance the introducer needle in the pleural space
						4.1.4	Check the angle of insertion
						4.1.5	Check the aspiration of air to confirm the needle's position in the pleural space
						4.1.6	Advance the 'J' end in the pleural space
						4.1.7	Remove the needle, leaving the wire
						4.1.8	Administer additional anaesthesia
			4.2	Bring the chest tube in place	do 4.2.1, 4.2.2 in consecutive order and repeat twice: with a medium and a large dilatator; then do 4.2.3, 4.2.4, 4.2.5	4.2.1	Insert the small dilatator through the costal muscle
						4.2.2	Continue insertion for 5 cm by rotating the dilatator
						4.2.3	Advance the chest inserter/chest tube assembly into the pleural space
						4.2.4	Remove the wire guide and chest tube inserter
						4.2.5	Secure the chest tube to the skin

Subsequently, risk management as described above can play an important role and contribute to successfully managing the business.

References

Annett J, Duncan KD. Task analysis and training design occup. Psychol. 1967;41:211–21.

Bird Jr F, et al. Loss control management. Loganville: Institute Press; 1976. p. 33–5.

BTS guidelines for the insertion of a chest drain. Laws D, Neville E, Duffy J, on behalf of the British Thoracic Society Pleural Disease Group, a subgroup of the British Thoracic Society Standards of Care Committee Thorax. 2003;58(Suppl II):ii53–ii59

Cooper Michol A, et al. Underreporting of Robotic Surgery Complications. Journal for Healthcare Quality. 2013. Article first published online. http://qap2.onlinelibrary.wiley.com/doi/10.1111/jhq.12036/references.

Greenwood M, Woods HM. The incidence of industrial accidents upon individuals with special reference to multiple accidents. Industrial Fatigue Research Board, Medical Research Committee. 1919. Report No. 4. Her Majesty's Stationery Office, London.

Heinrich HW. Industrial accident prevention: a scientific approach. New York: McGraw-Hill; 1931. In: Hollnagel E. Safer complex industrial environments: a human factors approach. CRC Press. 2009.

Henriksen K, et al. Editors understanding adverse events: a human factors framework. In: Patient safety and quality: an evidence-based handbook for nurses. Rockville: Agency for Healthcare Research and Quality (US); 2008. Chapter 5. Advances in Patient Safety.

Hollnagel E, Rigaud E. Proceedings of the second Resilience engineering symposium. 2006. Antibes-Juan-les-Pins, Mines Paris, les presses. 8–10 Nov 2006.

Josefson D. Haemophilia patients launch action against Bayer over contaminated blood products. Br Med J. 2003;14:326.

Kohn LT, et al. To err is human: building a safer health system. Washington DC: National Academy Press Institute of Medicine; 1999.

Meers PD, et al. Intravenous infusion of contaminated dextrose solution: the devonport incident. Lancet. 1973;2:1189–92.

Mintzberg Henry. Structure in fives: designing effective organizations. Englewood Cliffs: Prentice-Hall, Inc. vii 312. p. 1993.

Patient VC. Safety. New York: Wiley; 2011.

Potts Henry WW, et al. Assessing the validity of prospective hazard analysis methods: a comparison of two techniques. BMC Health Serv Res. 2014;14:41.

Reason, J. Managing the Risks of Organizational Accidents, Aldershot: Ashgate; 1997. ISBN 1840141042.

Reason J. Human error: models and management. Br Med J. 2000;320:768–70.

Stanton Neville A. Hierarchical task analysis: developments, applications, and extensions. Appl Ergon. 2006;37(1):55–79.

Tamuz MI, Harrison MI. Improving patient safety in hospitals: contributions of high-reliability theory and normal accident theory. Health Serv Res. 2006;41(4 Pt 2):1654–76.

The original source for the Swiss Cheese illustration is: "Swiss Cheese" Model – James Reason, 1991. The book reference is: Reason J. Human Error. New York: Cambridge University Press; 1990.

Vincent C. Patient safety. New York: John Wiley & Sons; 2011.

Yue Ying Kwan. A healthcare failure mode and effect analysis on the safety of secondary infusions. Institute of biomaterials and biomedical engineering, University of Toronto. 2012.

Quality Aspects in Daily Management in Nuclear Medicine

22

Annegrit Wijker, Jitze Medema, and Robert Siepelinga

Abstract

This chapter describes examples of how quality aspects are involved in routine daily management at a department of nuclear medicine, in this case the department of nuclear medicine and molecular imaging of the University Medical Center Groningen, the Netherlands.

Before writing about this relationship between management and quality, there is a need to explain both topics separately.

22.1 Management

Many different definitions of the word "management" exist. Management can be defined as "the management of the organization and coordination of the organization activities according to the guidelines to achieve bright described targets" (Verkooijen and Moeke 2013). Another definition is based on Daft (2000): "The attainment of organizational goals in an effective and efficient manner through planning, organizing, leading and controlling."

There are two important concepts in this definition of Daft (2000): (1) the four functions of planning, organizing, leading, and controlling and (2) the attainment of organizational goals in an effective and efficient manner. Managers use a wide variety of skills to perform these functions, such as conceptual, human, and technical skills.

Four management functions can be distinguished (Daft 2000):

A. Wijker (✉) • J. Medema • R. Siepelinga
Department of Nuclear Medicine and Molecular Imaging, University of Groningen, University Medical Center Groningen, Hanzeplein 1, Groningen, RB 9700, The Netherlands
e-mail: a.wijker@umcg.nl

A.W.J.M. Glaudemans et al. (eds.), *Quality in Nuclear Medicine*,
DOI 10.1007/978-3-319-33531-5_22

1. *Planning*: the management function concerned with defining goals for future organizational performance and deciding on the tasks and resource use needed to attain them
2. *Organizing*: the management function concerned with assigning tasks, grouping tasks into departments, and allocating resources to departments
3. *Leading*: the management function that involves the use of influence to motivate employees to achieve the organization's goals
4. *Controlling*: the management function concerned with monitoring employees' activities, keeping the organization on track toward its goals, and making corrections as needed

It's the manager's responsibility to achieve high performances and accomplish the organization's goals in an efficient and effective manner.

Organizational effectiveness is the degree to which the organization achieves the stated goals. Organizational efficiency is the use of minimal resources like raw materials, money, and people, to produce the desired volume of output manner (Daft 2000).

22.2 Quality

Quality is a term that also can be defined in different ways (van Dam and Marcus 1999). The traditional business economic definition of quality correlates with the technical specifications of a product. This can be called the *technological* quality. According to Garvin (1984), quality can be translated to five modalities, namely, transcendence approach, product approach, customer approach, protocol approach, and value approach. This can be managed by quality control, quality assurance, and learning organization.

One of the ideas to improve product quality is derived from the PDCA cycle, conducted by Deming (Gupta 2006a and 2006b). The PDCA cycle of Deming (1985, 1994) consists of four steps to improve processes in an organization. The abbreviation stands for Plan, Do, Check, Act. Recently, the cycle is also being introduced in healthcare (Carter 1996; Mori and Takebayashi 2002); Platje et al. (1994) and even developed an additional component, namely, management (Fig. 22.1), which indicates that the management is in the middle of the processes. The action component will be the function of management.

Combining quality and the four management functions of Daft (2000), we see that the four phases of the cycle matches the management functions. We can conclude that:

- The planning function matches the Plan phase of the cycle.
- The organization function matches the Do phase.
- The leading function matches the Act phase.
- The controlling function matches the Check phase.

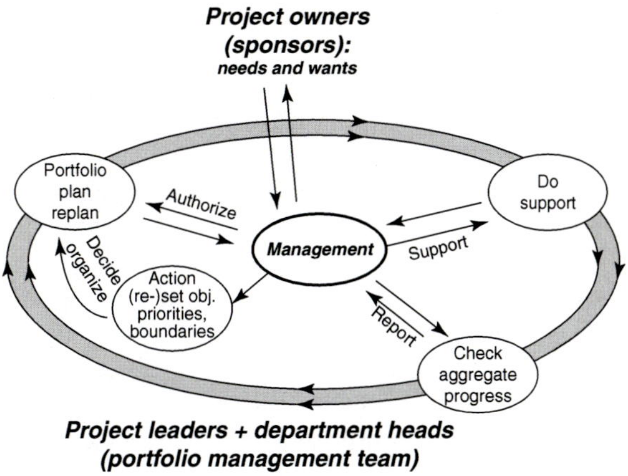

Fig. 22.1 Planning cycle for portfolio of projects

Based on these conclusions, we think that to our opinion, management is the key performance for guiding the quality of a company or department. We will now show an example of this as part of daily management in the department of nuclear medicine and molecular imaging of the University Medical Center Groningen, the Netherlands.

22.3 The Use of (Key) Performance Indicators

The department of nuclear medicine and molecular imaging is part of the University Medical Center Groningen. Therefore the department distracted her mission, vision, and strategy from the mission, vision, and strategy of the hospital, written by the board of directors in the document "building the future of health 2020 Raad van Bestuur UMCG (2014). Bouwen aan de toekomst van gezondheid 2020. Groningen." The department aspires to attain three key goals:

- Excellent healthcare
- Excellent research
- Excellent educational programs

The department defined (key) performance indicators ((K)PIs) that help to correct if the defined strategy and the implementation of matching plans did not lead to the intended results (Verkooijen and Moeke 2013). In total, the department formulated 42 performance indicators of which the most important nine indicators are being monitored monthly and being presented in a digital dashboard. All 42 indicators are derived from the translation of the strategy by using the Balanced Scorecard (Kaplan and Norton 2007) and the A3-method (Doeleman et al. 2010).

The performance indicators help to monitor the implementation of the strategy. An often used method for performing research on strategy is the value disciplines model of Treacy and Wiersema (Verkooijen and Moeke 2013) which describes three generic value disciplines:

- Operational excellence: focus on efficiency and streamlining operations
- Product leadership: focus on development and innovation,
- Customer intimacy: focus on delivering products and services above customer expectations

Any company must choose one of the value disciplines and act upon it consequently and vigorously.

The department decided to choose product leadership as value discipline, since her main focus is the development and translation of new radiopharmaceuticals. In other words, the department needs to stimulate innovation and development of state-of-the-art products and services.

In this light, all performance indicators were classified to the three value disciplines for checking if the (K)PIs were monitoring our strategy. The results are presented below (Table 22.1).

We noticed that our strategy of product leadership was not monitored adequately because of the lack of good performance indicators. As a consequence, we performed research on better indicators and choose new ones to improve our monitoring and our possibilities to correct.

22.4 Correcting Based on Performance Indicators

As mentioned before, performance indicators help the management to correct when the intended results were not achieved and to implement a switch in strategy to finally achieve the intended goal.

This is illustrated by the following examples.

Example 1: Changing Administration into Patient Care Logistics
The traditional administration section of the department of nuclear medicine and molecular imaging did not achieve the intended goals. Based on the key performance indicators of the administration (KPI 1–5), the management of the department found that the number of incidents was rising, that the amount of people in the waiting list was increasing, and that the occupancy rate of the cameras was decreasing. With these arguments, the management tried to convince the management of the hospital to change the traditional administration into patient care logistics with higher qualified personnel for the planning. With these people, it should be possible to achieve an integrated planning of the department with all kind of benefits as a consequence. After the approval, the new people reached a great result. The waiting list decreased to almost zero, the occupancy rates rose to the reached target, and fewer patients were sent home because of a bad planning. Figure 22.2 shows the percentage of scan requests that were planned within 48 h after the placement of the order by the referring clinician.

Table 22.1 Classification of performance indicators of the department divided into the value disciplines of Treacy en Wiersema

Product leadership	Customer intimacy	Operational excellence
Number of professors	KPI 1 – time between order and making an appointment	Number of quality certificates
Number of PhDs/postdocs	KPI 2 – time between getting an order and scanning the patient	KPI 3 – no shows and cancellations within 24 h
Number of principal investigators	KPI 7 – waiting time <15 min	KPI 4 – occupancy camera's PET and SPECT
Percentage of staff that followed the BROK course (GCP course)	KPI 8 – time between scan and report	KPI 5 – occupancy per camera
Number and quality of publications (impact factor, Q1 publications)	External complaints	KPI 6 – production number of scans
Different research cash flows	Accessibility by telephone	KPI 9 – finances
Research production (scans)	Satisfaction of staff	KPI 10 – reliability of the production of radiopharmaceuticals
	Satisfaction of internal customers	Absence due to sickness
	Satisfaction of patients	Yearly performance evaluations with the staff
	Satisfaction of PhDs	Company accidents
	Patient participation projects	Medical incidents
		Medical complications
		Internal complaints
		Healthcare failure mode and effects analysis (HFMEA) – "covenant"
		Risk inventarization
		Staff indicators
		Staff manning
		Investments
		Administration of documents
		Down time cyclotron
		Down time cameras
		Number of apprenticeships
		Number of teaching hours
		Percentage of teachers with BKO (education quality)

Example 2: Changing the Planning of Nuclear Medicine Specialists on Making Reports

Implementing the PDCA at the department provided feedback by discussing the outcomes of the weekly, daily, and yearly key performance indications in management meetings and provides information about results. Questionnaires for referring

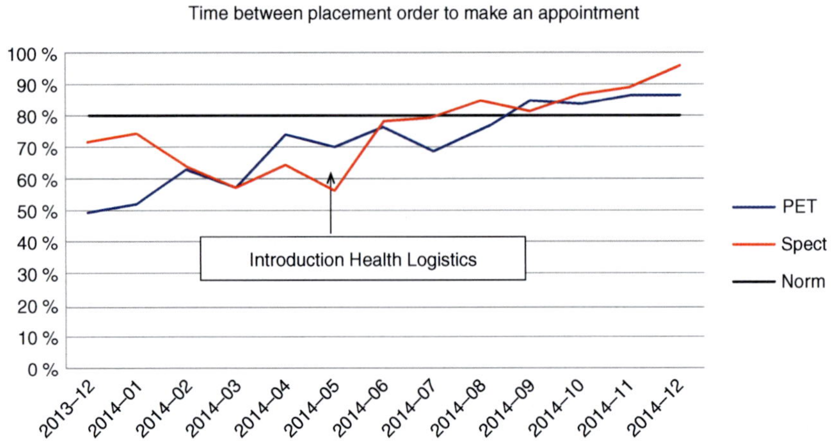

Fig. 22.2 Time between placing an order and making an appointment. The goal is to plan more than 80 % of the orders within 2 working days

clinicians taught us that they were not completely satisfied with the timelines before they received the scan reports. So, KPI 8 was implemented which measured the timelines between the acquisition of the scan and the report into the patient systems. It was showed that fewer reports were finalized within 24 h that what the nuclear medicine specialists thought based on their feelings. Together, they changed their way of working and planning of clinical duties, which resulted in a fast decrease of time between acquisition and report (now > 90 % of the reports is finalized within 24 h, Fig. 22.3). Analyzing the facts presented by the KPI provided solutions to improve the results and helped stimulating the doctors to improve their work speed.

Example 3: Filling in the CRF Correctly

Random survey of case record forms (CRFs) needed to be performed because of the legislation on Good Clinical Practices. The standard is 100 %, so everything has to be documented on the CRF. In Fig. 22.4, the percentage of complete documentation of the CRFs is showed. What you see is a fast increase from 80 to approximately 95 %; however, it was found very difficult to reach the goal of 100 %. This is an example of the 80/20 rule; improving the last percentages is really hard. Analyzing this KPI shows that it is important to also consequently monitor the results, even if the intended results were not reached. Right now, we are discussing in the department if we are going to accept this level or if we need to search for another method of filling in the forms.

Within the department, the key performance indicators are such an important tool to measure the performance of the department that the management of the department collects these figures now for already more than 10 years.

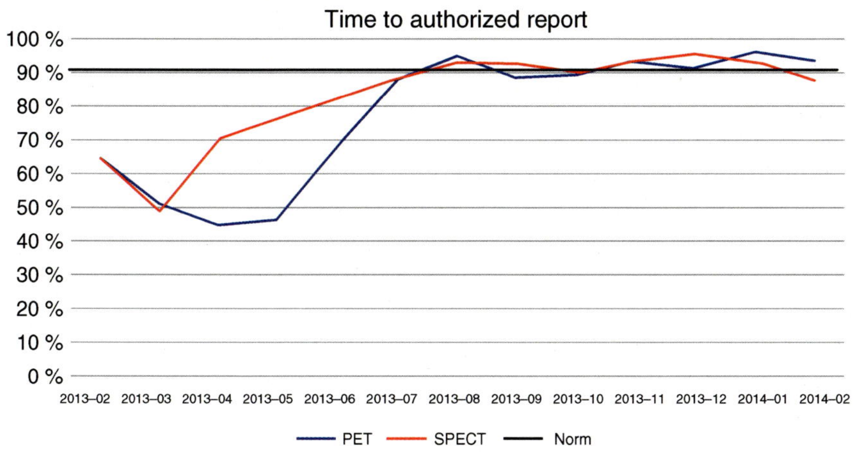

Fig. 22.3 Time to authorize report. The goal is to authorize 90 % of the reports within 24 h

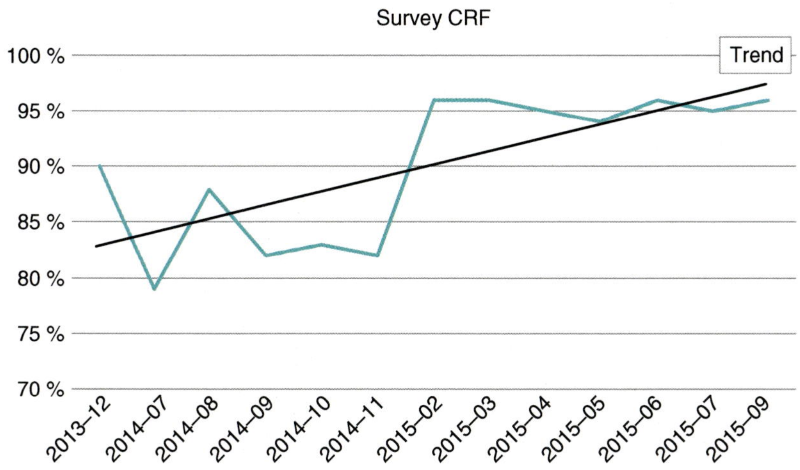

Fig. 22.4 The amount of correct filling in CRFs. No goal is set up to now

22.5 Monitoring Is More than Monitoring with Key Performance Indicators

However, monitoring is more than just following the (K)PIs. In the daily routine, all kinds of quality instruments are imbedded to continuously improve the department.

The following quality instruments are routinely being used by the department:

Management function *plan*:

- Brainstorm sessions on scenario planning and strategy
- Multiannual planning (5 years) including contemplated activities
- "A3" – annual plan including monitoring

- Accreditation by the European Board of Nuclear Medicine (UEMS/EBNM)
- EARL-EANM accreditation

Management function *do*:

- Hierarchic task analysis (HTA)
- Risk inventarizations and evaluations (RI&E)
- Portfolio personnel
- Team SHOPP (see Chap. 21)
- Lean Six Sigma (projects and game)
- Update and standardization of medical protocols

Management function *check*:

- Benchmarks on, for instance, research quality
- Multiannual planning (5 years) including contemplated activities
- "Mirror" meeting for confronting staff with experiences of patients
- Internal and external audits ISO 9001
- (Periodically) Inspections (by the Dutch Society of Nuclear Medicine, Health Government, GMP)
- Walkarounds
- Quick scan dress code
- Monitoring GCP
- Self inspections (GMP, information safety)
- Position monitoring INK/EFQM
- Scores audit systematics INK
- Self evaluation reports INK/EFQM
- Exit interview

Management function *act*:

- Deviation measurements (good manufacturing practice)
- Prevention and Recovery Information System for Monitoring and Analysis (PRISMA)
- Management review ISO 9001

Many of these instruments produce possibilities for improvements. The activities needed to be done to improve are written on a list with the name "improve and correct" list. This list will be regularly evaluated so we will finally succeed in our strategy.

Below are three instruments explained in depth.

22.5.1 Brainstorm Sessions on Scenario Planning and Strategy (*Plan*)

As an organization to maintain in ever-changing circumstances and to be able to seize new opportunities, an organization will have to learn, and the knowledge must be constantly updated with new knowledge and new skills.

A way of learning is "learning from the future" by means of scenario planning. Scenarios are descriptions of alternative hypothetical futures that display different perspectives on developments from the past, in the present and for the future that can serve as a basis for taking action.

Scenario planning is of multiple images or events occurring in the future might do. By means of group sessions, in which collective is speculation about future, the borders can be shifted and the implicit knowledge from different perspectives. It is noted that for a successful application of scenario planning, the corporate culture plays a crucial role.

22.5.2 Hierarchic Task Analysis (*Do*)

The backbone of our risk management is the risk assessment and evaluation (RAE). It serves as a master checklist and inventory that takes the primary processes, as already defined for the ISO 9001, as input and tracks whether the presence of, e.g., risk analysis and work instructions is covered. This approach is highly compatible with the IAEA "Quality Management audits in Nuclear Medicine Practices." The risk analysis of processes is performed through a hierarchic task analysis (HTA). Processes are analyzed by subdividing into sub-tasks. A risk assessment, such as SAFER/HFMEA or, when quantitative risk analysis is possible, the Fine-Kinney model is subsequently applied in order to evaluate the sub-task and formulate corrective action when required.

22.5.3 Walkaround NMMI (*Check*)

A walkaround is a short visit on the work floor by colleagues. The workplace is seen as the place where the added value is. It is very important that colleagues have the experience that takes place at the other sections especially in multidisciplinary organizations such as the NMMI. You get understanding for each other and it improves internal communication.

The target is multiple:

- Identify and register problems and waste.
- Contribution for the collegiality.

Background:

It is known that the best proposals arise from interaction with the workplace. Here, the people who have daily contact with the customers, the material, and the protocols. Their practical experience makes a valuable contribution to solving problems and initiates improvement projects.

Motto is: look and ask your colleagues with respect.

The conditions for a walkaround:

- Focus on one location.
- It is not announced.
- Up to 1 h.
- By two persons, e.g., manager and employee, another location.
- Frequency: location every year one visit.
- Report: three best practices and three points for improvement.

22.5.4 Quick Scan Dress Code (*Check*)

The dress code is based on the personal hygiene. The visit is unannounced, and sitting in the waiting room of the NMMI, the inspector will watch the first ten employees in corporate clothing and will be included for the quick scan. The zero measurement was in 2013. The standard is 100 % compliance.

The frequency is every 3 months.

The following six items are observed:

- Nails are free from nail polish (also no transparent nail polish).
- Hair is correct; short hair or long hair is pinned up or tied up.
- Hands and wrists are free of jewelry (watches, rings, and bracelets).
- White jacket (long and short) be worn closed.
- When jacket has short sleeves, the forearms are free of own clothing.
- The employee carries correct hospital clothing.

22.5.5 Exit Interview (*Check*)

Procedure NMMI:

1. When it is known that an employee, who worked for the department for more than a year, will leave, this will be reported to the management.
2. The staff member quality will make an appointment with the employee for the exit interview. Participation to the exit interview is voluntary.
3. The exit interview takes place after finalization of the dismissal procedure and before the actual leave of the employee.
4. The exit interview will be a personal interview (maximal 1 h), taken by the staff member quality.
5. Together with the employee, the questions on the question form exit interview NGMB will be answered. The direct supervisor does not participate in the interview.
6. The management will receive the information filled in on the question form.
7. The question form will be stored until 2 years after the employee has left, in a separate folder (not in the personnel file), and destroyed hereafter.

Reporting:

- Signals deriving from the exit interview will be discussed with the management and direct supervisor and converted to action points as soon as possible.
- The staff member quality will evaluate the exit interview yearly and the outcome will be reported in the management review (anonymously).

22.5.6 Prevention and Recovery Information System for Monitoring and Analysis (*Act*)

The PRISMA method provides a systematic analysis that provides insight into the emergence of (near) incidents. Incidents are analyzed by the underlying causes in a logical way to organize into a cause tree and then classification rather than the causes of the incident. This means that further defined is what technical-, organization-, human-, and patient-related root causes played a role at the time that the incident occurred. Understanding these basic causes makes it possible to determine the most effective improvement. The retrospective analysis of the PRISMA method has eventually become a proactive operation.

The PRISMA method is ideally suited to identify trends and patterns to find the causes of multiple incidents. The method also helps you improve measures to prevent incidents in the future.

The PRISMA consists of the following components:

- Incident description in chronological order
- Causes tree
- Classification of causes
- Preventive actions

Conclusion

Quality management is embedded in our routine daily practice. Implementing and controlling of KPIs helped us to achieve intended goals by constantly adapting to reach these goals. Quality management is now part of our thinking. Attitude and behavior of employees can be supported by instruments and creating a culture of continuous improvement.

References

Carter J. Small-scale study using the PDCA cycle. In: Gift R, Kinney C, Shortell S, editors. Today's management methods: a guide for the health care executive. New York: Wiley, John & Sons, Inc; 1996. p. 209–22.

Daft RL. Management. 5th ed. Orlando Harcourt College Publishers; 2000. p. 7–11.

Dam, van N.H.M. & Marcus, J.A. Een praktijkgerichte benadering van management en organisatie. Derde druk, Houten, Educatieve Partners Nederland bv. 1999. p. 534.

Deming WE. The new economics: for industry, government, education. Cambridge: MIT, Center for Advanced Educational Services; 1994. p. 132.
Deming E. Transformation of western style of management. Interfaces; 1985. 15:p. 6.
Doeleman H, Heumen van L, Diepenmaat M. A3 methodiek: naar jaarplannen met meer focus en bezieling – en minder papier. TNO Management Consultants/Dienst Justitiële Inrichtingen, 2010.
Gupta P. PDCA's beginnings. Qual Prog. 2006a;39:47.
Gupta P. Beyond PDCA–A new process management model. Qual Prog. 2006b;39:45.
Kaplan RS, Norton DP. Using the balanced scorecard as a strategic management system, Harvard Business Review, July–August, 2007, p. 150–161.
Mori K, Takebayashi T. The introduction of an occupational health management system for solving issues in occupational health activities in Japan. Ind Health. 2002;40:167.
Platje A, Wadman S. From Plan-Do-Check-Action to PIDCAM: The further evolution of the Deming-wheel. Int J Proj Manage. 1998;16(4):201–8.
Platje A, Seidel H, Wadman S. Project and portfolio planning cycle: project-based management for the multiproject challenge. Int J Proj Manage. 1994;12(2):100–6.
Verkooijen L, Moeke D. Bedrijfsvoering voor zorg en welzijn: juiste zorg op het juiste moment (eerste druk), Groningen/Houten: Noordhoff Uitgevers; 2013.

23 Measuring Performance and Service Quality in Health Care

Paul Gemmel

23.1 Performance Measurement

The goal of performance measurement is to inform managers on the performance of their organization. As measuring all performance aspects within an organization is both unfeasible and irrelevant, most organizations select a number of performance indicators based on the organization's objectives. According to Bauer (2004), "quantifiable metrics which reflect the performance of an organization in achieving its goals and objectives" (p. 63) can be considered as "key performance indicators" (KPIs). These performance indicators are not a goal in itself but provide a basis for the organization's "management control system," id est the data gathering system in function of helping and coordinating the planning process and the control of decisions throughout the organization (Jorissen 1994). In general, performance measurement enables the organization's management to follow up, coordinate, control, and improve certain aspects of organizational activities (Kollberg et al. 2005).

In the profit sector, short-term financial indicators were dominant in the past, but today the importance of nonfinancial indicators (such as quality and operational indicators) has increased. This resulted in an extended range of performance indicators (Jorissen 1994). In the health-care sector, ensuring quality has been an important issue for years (Rooney and van Ostenberg 1999), but financial measurement was the dominant mechanism of control until the 1990s (Aidemark 2001). The focus on financial performance, however, failed to provide a "big picture" assessment of the overall performance (Tarantino 2003).

P. Gemmel
Professor in Service Management and Management of Health Organizations,
Faculty of Economics and Business Management, Ghent University,
Tweekerkenstraat 2, Ghent 9000, Belgium
e-mail: Paul.Gemmel@UGent.be

A.W.J.M. Glaudemans et al. (eds.), *Quality in Nuclear Medicine*,
DOI 10.1007/978-3-319-33531-5_23

In recent years, performance measurement in function of quality improvement became more important in the health-care sector, as a result of lapses in quality of care, safety issues, and low consumer satisfaction (Ten Asbroek et al. 2004; Becker Formisano and Roger 2006) and as a result of medical progresses (Bothner et al. 2003; Ten Asbroek et al. 2004; OECD 2005) and changing delivery and environment in medicine (Becker et al. 2006). Wollersheim et al. (2006) even argue that the ultimate goal of performance measurement is to make the quality of health care more transparent and to improve health-care quality.

23.2 Performance Measurement in Function of Quality Improvement

Quality has been studied for years, and this has led to a plethora of publications in books, academic journals, and trade journals. The result of these publications is many different definitions of quality which are not always consistent nor coherent. In a review article on the definitions of quality, Reeves and Bednar (1994) recognize four categories of quality definitions based on what concept is behind them:

- Quality is excellence.
- Quality is value.
- Quality is conformance to specification.
- Quality is meeting and exceeding customer's expectations.

23.2.1 Quality Is Excellence

The real root of this category of quality definitions lies in the ancient Greek time. Philosophers Socrates, Plato, and Aristotle mentioned "excellence" as an absolute ideal to achieve (Reeves and Bednar 1994). The idea of excellence is still very popular because this idea is reflected into the framework for business excellence of the European Foundation for Quality Management (EFQM). The EFQM Excellence Model is a nonprescriptive framework, covering many approaches to achieve sustainable organizational excellence (de Cleyn et al. 2004; Rusjan 2005; Gemmel et al. 2013). Excellence can be defined as the outstanding practice in managing the organization and achieving results based on fundamental concepts, which include results orientation, customer focus, leadership and constancy of purpose, processes and facts, involvement of people, continuous improvement and innovation, mutually beneficial partnerships, and public responsibility. Behaviors, activities, or initiatives based on these concepts are often referred to as quality management (Rusjan 2005). The EFQM model has been widely diffused in health care. For instance, it has been used as the basic framework for the accreditation of hospitals by The Netherlands Institute for Accreditation in Healthcare (NIAZ).

23.2.2 Quality Is Value

From an economic point of view, value can be seen as an equation incorporating the features and benefits of the products or services for the customer, as compared with the price (or cost) of obtaining this product or service. Feigenbaum (1951) (as mentioned in Reeves and Bednar 1994, p. 420) introduced the idea that the notion of value must be included in any quality definition: "Quality does not have the popular meaning of 'best' in any absolute sense. It means 'best for certain customers' conditions. These conditions are (a) the actual use and (b) the selling price of the product. Product quality cannot be thought of apart from the product cost." Value is a very popular managerial concept, also in health care. According to Porter and Lee (2013), the overarching goal for all stakeholders in health care must be improving value for patients "where value is defined as the health outcomes achieved that matter to patients relative to the cost of achieving those outcomes" (Porter and Lee 2013). This means that outcomes and costs must be considered together to create value in a health-care context.

23.2.3 Quality Is Conformance to Specifications

While the previous categories of quality definition are subjective, Shewhart and later Juran have introduced a more objective or engineering way of looking at quality. This more engineering point of view includes two important steps. The first one is to translate the "wants" of the customer into "physical" characteristics of the product manufactured to satisfy these wants (Shewhart 1931). Quality function deployment (QFD) has been proposed as a technique for translating customer requirements into the product design as well as in the design and operation of production systems (Evans and Dean 2000). QFD is successfully used by manufacturers of electronics, clothing, appliances, and construction equipment (Evans and Dean 2000, p. 98) and is increasingly used in the service sector (Gemmel 2013). The second step is then to "set up ways and means of obtaining a product which will differ from the arbitrarily set standards for these quality characteristics by no more than may be left to chance" (Shewhart 1931, p. 44). This gave birth to more statistical oriented techniques such as statistical process control (SPC). The purpose of statistical process control is trying to keep the variation of processes under control by detecting assignable causes (as opposed to common or unassignable causes). This kind of thinking has led to the still very popular Six Sigma programs, originally developed by Motorola. The basic idea behind Six Sigma is to limit the number of defects as much as possible. Since then, Six Sigma programs have combined statistical and nonstatistical methods in order to improve businesses, also in health care. For instance, Mount Carmel Health in Columbus, Ohio, was one of the first health-care organizations to implement Six Sigma through its entire organization (Revere and Black 2003). One of its first Six Sigma projects sought to achieve timely and accurate reimbursement. For Mount Carmel Health, "process improvements attained through

Six Sigma resulted in an $857,000 gain in net income" (Revere and Black 2003, p. 380). Consequently Mount Carmel Health, through Six Sigma, improved its financial stability (Woodard 2005).

23.2.4 Quality Is Meeting and Exceeding Customer's Expectations

Although Shewhart and Juran also recognize the importance of customer wants in defining quality, they gave no advice on how to assess these wants. As to Berry et al., customers assess quality "by comparing what they want or expect and what they actually get or perceive they are getting" (Berry et al. 1988). So quality has something to do with expectations and performance as actually perceived by the customer. This definition of quality is based on the so-called paradigm of disconfirmation (Carvalho and Leite 1999). A customer is only satisfied when the actual performance is equal or better than expected. The actual judgment of the discrepancy between expectations and actual performance is described as perceived service quality (Dagger et al. 2007). Of course an important question is to identify the components (called service quality dimensions) for which customers have expectations and perceive performance. In the next paragraphs, we will focus on this definition of quality.

23.3 Service Quality in Health Care

CIHI (2006) confirms that monitoring patient perceptions of the hospital care they received is an essential component when measuring the quality of services provided in hospitals. Four indicators are made up of a varying number of individual questionnaire items: communication, consideration, responsiveness, and the overall impressions. These four indicators integrate several indicators of other authors and will be used as a framework.

Communication refers to "patients' view about the amount and quality of information and communications they received about their condition, treatment, and preparation for discharge and care at home, and whether they felt family and friends were given sufficient information" (CIHI 2006, p. 34). Information is a success factor of customer satisfaction (Aidemark, 2001). *Consideration* refers to "patients' view about whether they were treated with respect, dignity, and courtesy" (CIHI 2006, p. 34). This corresponds with one of the indicators of Ten Asbroek et al. (2004), namely, "patient centeredness." *Responsiveness* refers to "patients' assessments of the extent to which they got the care they needed in hospital and how coordinated and integrated that care was when it was delivered" (CIHI 2006, p. 34). Ten Asbroek et al. (2004) also situate effectiveness within this perspective. Readmission and waiting time, quality, service, and price are interesting indicators within this perspective (Muntinga and Lagerveld 2003). Aidemark (2001) adds availability as success factor. Important is that responsiveness assesses thus the perception of the efficiency and effectiveness of health care and not the efficiency itself. *The overall impression* refers to "patients' view of their overall hospital experience, including the overall quality of care and services they received at the hospital, and their confidence in the doctors and nurses who cared for them" (CIHI 2006, p. 34). Patient safety (Ten Asbroek et al. 2004) is an aspect that may be integrated within the overall impression, as well as security and covering (Aidemark 2001).

However, identifying what customers value (personal attention, on time delivery, innovative products) is also part of the consumer perspective. In the profit sector, customers' values need to be measured, because customer satisfaction contributes to the financial performance (Kershaw and Kershaw 2001). According to Aidemark (2001), links between the perspective of consumer and finance are missing. Instead, emphasis on the perspective of consumers leads to increased activity and expenses, especially in connection with a buying and selling system where professionals are paid to expand health treatment. DuMoulin (2007) argues that performance measures should address dimensions of health performance that the consumer values. Patients may thus not be overvalued, neither neglected, since patient centeredness is considered as important. It will be necessary to give patients the opportunity to bring some elements forward.

23.4 Tools for Measuring Service Quality

Performance measures should reflect dimensions of health performance that the consumer values. A very well-known tool to capture and measure these dimensions is Servqual. Servqual identifies the service quality dimensions having an impact on the attitude of the customer toward the organization. This attitude represents a long-run, overall evaluation of the service provided. Parasuraman et al. (1985) originally listed ten determinants or dimensions of service quality (see Exhibit 23.1).

Exhibit 23.1: Ten Components of Service Quality

1. Reliability involves consistency of performance and dependability. It also means that the firm performs the service right the first time and keeps its promises. Some specific examples it may involve are:
   - Accuracy in billing
   - Performing the service at the designated time
2. Responsiveness concerns the willingness or readiness of employees to provide service. It may involve:
   - Mailing a transaction slip immediately
   - Calling the customer back quickly
   - Giving prompt service (e.g., setting up appointments quickly)
3. Competence means possession of the skills and knowledge required to perform the service. It involves:
   - Knowledge and skill of the contact personnel
   - Knowledge and skill of operational support personnel
   - Research capability of the organization

4. Access involves approachability and ease of contact. It may mean:
   - The service is easily accessible by telephone
   - Waiting time to receive service is not excessive
   - Convenient hours of operation and convenient location of the service facility
5. Courtesy involves politeness, respect, consideration, and friendliness of contact personnel (including receptionists, telephone operators, etc.) It includes:
   - Consideration for the customer's property
   - Clean and neat appearance of public contact personnel
6. Communication means keeping customers informed in language they can understand and listening to them. It may mean that the company has to adjust its language for different customers. It may involve:
   - Explaining the service itself and how much the service will cost
   - Explaining the trade-offs between service and cost
   - Assuring the consumer that a problem will be handled
7. Credibility involves trustworthiness, believability, and honesty. It involves having the customer's best interests at heart. Contributing to credibility are:
   - Company name and reputation
   - Personal characteristics of the contact personnel
   - The degree of hard-sell involved in interactions with the customer
8. Security is the freedom from danger, risk, or doubt. It may involve:
   - Physical safety
   - Financial security and confidentiality
9. Understanding/knowing the customer involves making the effort to understand the customer's needs. It involves:
   - Learning the customer's specific requirements
   - Providing individual attention
10. Tangibles include the physical evidence of the service:
    - Physical facilities and appearance of personnel
    - Tools or equipment used to provide the service
    - Physical representations of the service, such as a plastic credit card

Source: Buttle (1996)

This list was made up as a result of focus group studies with service providers and customers and is sufficiently generic to cover a variety of services in different sectors. Based on further study, Parasuraman et al. (1988) were able to reduce the ten quality dimensions to five (Parasuraman et al. 1988):

- Reliability: the ability to perform the promised service reliably and accurately
- Assurance: the knowledge and courtesy of employees and their ability to inspire trust and confidence in consumers
- Tangibles: the physical facilities, the equipment, and the appearance of personnel

- Empathy: the extent to which caring, individualized attention was provided to consumers
- Responsiveness: willingness to help consumers and provide prompt service

Using this tool, service quality was measured as the difference between the consumers' perceptions and expectations of the service, quoted on 22 statements that represented the Servqual dimensions (Parasuraman et al. 1985). However, Patterson and Johnson (1993) state that service quality is neither directly nor indirectly influenced by expectations. Perception alone appears to be a strong predictor of service quality (Cronin and Taylor 1992; Parasuraman 1995). Later, Parasuraman (1995) argues that the perception-only approach to measuring quality is even more acceptable from a predictive validity point of view, as it explains considerable variance in overall service quality ratings. Moreover, it is regarded as impractical to ask participants to complete two surveys. Since its development, Servqual has been used in several healthcare settings (Parasuraman et al. 1994a, b). In Exhibit 23.2, Servqual was used to measure the service quality at an outpatient nuclear medicine clinic.

Exhibit 23.2: Measuring Service Quality at an Outpatient Nuclear Medicine Clinic
A survey comprising 22 questions was taken to measure patients' perception of service quality on a 7-point scale. The survey was based on the original Servqual items. Altogether, 416 patients received the questionnaire, of which 259 were completed and returned (response rate: 62 per cent). Using factor analysis, it became clear that the items could be grouped into five dimensions. Table 23.1 shows these dimensions, the different items, and the average and the standard deviation of their scores on the dimensions (De Man et al. 2002). Four items were not retained in the analysis due to a large number of missing values.

When looking at the results, a first observation is that the dimensions in this study are not the same as in the basic Servqual framework. It is generally accepted that different service environments can generate different service dimensions. A second observation is that only the perception part of the Servqual was measured. Expectations were deliberately not measured because of considerable disagreement about the added value of measuring expectations when perceptions are already measured.

As to the results (see Table 23.1), we can conclude that patients give the highest score to the tangibles-assurance and convenience dimension. They have the perception that the opening hours are convenient and that employees care about their patients. The lowest scoring items are all situated within the responsiveness dimension. Patients perceive that they do not get prompt service and that they do not know when the service will be performed. One of the problems patients are confronted with in a hospital outpatient clinic is the waiting time. To better serve customers, management needs to pay more attention to the responsiveness dimension.

Table 23.1 The results of a Servqual perception measurement in a nuclear medicine clinic

Item analysis of patients' service quality perception	
Item in each dimension	Mean and standard deviation (SD) of patients' perceptions
Tangibles-Assurance	
Has up-to-date equipment	5.99 (SD 5 1.04)
Physical facilities are visually appealing	4.88 (SD 5 1.60)
Employees are neat in appearance	6.13 (SD 5 0.91)
Physical facilities in accordance with service	5.17 (SD 5 1.49)
Shows sincere interest in solving your problems	5.99 (SD 5 1.07)
Employees can be trusted	5.95 (SD 5 0.99)
Feels safe in your interaction with employees	6.08 (SD 5 0.93)
Reliability	
When promises to do something, it does so	5.50 (SD 5 1.38)
Provides services at the time it promises	5.35 (SD 5 1.56)
Responsiveness	
Tells you when the services will be performed	4.68 (SD 5 1.88)
Gives prompt services	4.65 (SD 5 1.83)
Personnel is always willing to help	5.77 (SD 5 1.44)
Never too busy to respond to your requests	4.61 (SD 5 1.83)
Empathy	
Gives individual attention	5.01 (SD 5 1.68)
Employees give personal attention	5.35 (SD 5 1.52)
Employees understand your specific needs	5.03 (SD 5 1.57)
Convenience	
Has operating hours convenient to you	5.65 (SD 5 1.41)
Has your best interests at heart	5.90 (SD 5 1.40)
Not included in the analysis	
The personnel perform the service right the first time	
The department keeps its records accurately	
The personnel are consistently courteous	
The personnel get adequate support from the University Hospital	

Source: De Man et al. (2002)

Although Servqual seems to be a useful tool for measuring service quality in health care, the application of this tool to the context of an outpatient nuclear medicine learns that it is difficult to replicate the five original dimensions, namely, reliability, empathy, tangibles, responsiveness, and assurance across different service contexts. From a practice point of view, this means that studies measuring service quality using the Servqual tool cannot rely on its five-dimensional structure without further investigation. Based on an extensive research of service quality in the health care and in the marketing literature, Dagger et al. (2007) find that the Servqual dimensions should be considered as descriptors of four more overarching dimensions: interpersonal quality, technical quality, environmental quality, and administrative quality. Exhibit 23.3 describes these different dimensions and their subdimensions. Dagger et al. (2007) have further developed a scale which can be used to monitor and improve the quality of service delivered to patients.

The performance indicators as identified in the earlier mentioned CIHI study (2006, p. 34) can be linked to these four overarching dimensions. Communication and consideration are part of the interpersonal quality, responsiveness as defined by the CIHI study (2006) can be linked to administrative quality, and the overall impression can be related to technical quality and environmental quality. Although tested in a the context of oncology clinics, the scale of Dagger et al. (2007) seems to describe a comprehensive set of dimensions and subdimensions in health care.

Exhibit 23.3: The Overarching Dimensions of Service Quality in Healthcare and Their Sub-dimensions

Interpersonal quality reflects the relationship developed and the dyadic interplay between a service provider and a user:

- *Interaction*: the attitude and behavior of a service provider in a service setting.
- *Relationship*: the closeness and strength of the relationship developed between a provider and a customer.

Technical quality involves the outcomes achieved and the technical competence of a service provider:

- *Expertise*: the ability of a service provider to adhere to high standards of service provision.
- *Outcome*: what a consumer receives as a result of his or her interactions with a service firm.

Environment quality defines the complex mix of environmental features that shape consumer service perceptions:

- *Atmosphere* refers to the intangible, background characteristics of the service environment. These elements generally exist below consumers' level of awareness, thus affecting the pleasantness of the surroundings.
- *Tangibles* refer to the physical elements of the service environment that exist at the forefront of awareness. This comprises the design, function, lay-out of the environment and the signs, symbols, and artifacts found in the environment.

Administrative quality refers to elements that facilitate the production of a core service while adding value to a customer's use of the service. Facilitating services are essential to the delivery and consumption of a core service. Supporting elements augment the service but are not necessary to core service delivery.

- *Timeliness*: waiting lists, waiting time, hours of operations.
- *Operation*: general administration and the co-ordination, integration and organizaiton of medical care.
- *Support*: an augmented service element that adds value to the core service.

Source: Dagger et al. (2007)

Conclusion

In this chapter, we emphasized the importance of measuring performance in an organization. It is quite clear that in health care, the ultimate goal of performance measurement is to make the quality of health care more transparent and to improve health care quality. To make the quality of health care transparent, one should be aware of the many definitions of quality. In this paper, we further expand on quality defined as "meeting and exceeding customer expectations" or service quality. Service quality itself is again a multidimensional construct which can be measured with several tools such as Servqual. Although these tools seem to be useful in healthcare contexts such as an outpatient nuclear medicine clinic, there is still some work to adapt the tools to this specific environment.

References

Aidemark L-G. The meaning of balanced scorecards in the health care organisation. Financ Account Manage. 2001;17(1):23–40.

Bauer K. KPIs – the metrics that drive performance management. DM Rev. 2004;14(9):63–4.

Becker B, Formisano A, Roger MD. Strategic planning for departmental divisions in an academic health care centre. Am J Med. 2006;199(4):357–65.

Berry LL, Parasuraman A, Zeithaml V. The service-quality puzzle. Bus Horiz. 1988;31:35–44.

Bothner U, Brinkman A, Gebhard F, Isenmann R, Mohl U, Schwilk B. Balanced scorecard: tool or toy im Krankenhaus? Anaesthesist. 2003;52:947–56.

Buttle F. Servqual: review, critique, research agenda. Eur J Mark. 1996;30(1):8–32.

Canadian Institute for Health Information [CIHI] (2006). Hospital Report 2006: Acute Care. http://www.hospitalreport.ca/downloads/2006/AC/acute_report_2006.pdf. Accessed 20 Apr 2007.

Carvalho De FA, Leite VF. Attribute importance in service quality: an empirical test of the PBZ conjecture in Brazil. Int J Serv Ind Manage. 1999;10(5):487–504.

Cronin JJ, Taylor SA. Measuring service quality: a reexamination and extension. J Mar Sci. 1992;56:55–68.

Dagger TS, Sweeney JC, Johnson LW. A hierarchical model of health service quality: scale development and investigation of an integrated model. J Serv Res. 2007;10(2):123–42.

de Cleyn W, Linnanen L, Panapanaan V, Timmers J, van Marrewijk M, Wuisman I. A phase-wise development approach to business excellence: towards an innovative, stakeholder-oriented assessment tool for organizational excellence and CSR. J Bus Ethics. 2004;55(2):83–98.

De Man S, Gemmel P, Vlerick P, Van Rijk P, Dierckx R. Patients' and personnel's perceptions of service quality and patient satisfaction in nuclear medicine. Eur J Nucl Med Mol Imaging. 2002;29(9):1109–17.

DuMoulin J. URAC introduces performance-based measures applicable to health plans and care management vendors. Manag Care Outlook. 2007;20(6):11–2.

Evans JR, Dean JW. Total quality: management, organization and strategy. Canada: South-Western College Publishing, Thomson Learning; 2000.

Feigenbaum AV. Quality control: principles, practice and administration. New York: McGraw-Hill; 1951.

Gemmel P. Service process design. In: Gemmel P, Van Looy B, Van Dierdonck R, editors. Service management: an integrated approach. 3rd ed. London: Pearson; 2013.

Jorissen A. Prestatiemeting. Naar een betere beheersing van bedrijfsactiviteiten. Antwerpen – Appeldoorn: MAKLU Uitgevers; 1994.

Kershaw R, Kershaw S. Developing a balanced scorecard to implement strategy at St. Winter: Elsewhere Hospital. Management accounting quarterly; 2001: p. 28–35.

Kollberg B, Elg M, Lindmark J. Design and implementation of a performance measurement system in Swedish health care services: a multiple case study of 6 development teams. Qual Manag Health Care. 2005;14(2):95–111.

Muntinga MA, Lagerveld NJ. Managementmodellen voor kwaliteit. Deventer: Kluwer; 2003.

OECD Health at a Glance: OECD Indicators – 2005 Edition. 2005. http://www.oecd.org/dataoecd/49/13/35618688.pdf. Accessed 23 Apr 2007.

Parasuraman A. Measuring and monitoring service quality. In: Glynn WJ, Barnes JG, editors. Understanding services management: integrating marketing, organizational behavior and human resource management. Chichester: John Wiley & sons; 1995. p. 143–77.

Parasuraman A, Zeithaml VA, Berry LL. A conceptual model of service quality and implications for further research. J Mar Sci. 1985;49:45–50.

Parasuraman A, Zeithaml VA, Berry LL. SERVQUAL: a multi-item scale for measuring consumer perceptions of service quality. J Retail. 1988;64:12–37.

Parasuraman A, Zeithaml VA, Berry LL. Alternative scales for measuring service quality comparative: assessment based on psychometric and diagnostic criteria. J Retail. 1994a;70(3):201–30.

Parasuraman A, Zeithaml VA, Berry LL. Reassessment of expectations as a comparison standard in measuring service quality: implications for further research. J Mar Sci. 1994b;58(1): 111–24.

Patterson PG, Johnson LW. Disconfirmation of expectations and the gap model of service quality: an integrated paradigm. J Retail. 1993;64:12–40.

Porter ME, Lee TH. The strategy that will fix health care. Harv Bus Rev. 2013;91(10):50–70.

Revere L, Black K. Integrating Six Sigma with total quality management: a case example for measuring medication errors. J Healthc Manag. 2003;48(6):377–91.

Reeves CA, Bednar DA. Defining quality: alternatives and applications. Acad Manage Rev. 1994;19(3):419–45.

Rooney AN, van Ostenberg PR. Licensure, accreditation, and certification: approaches to health services quality. Center for Human Services. 1999. http://www.qaproject.org/pubs/PDFs/accredmon.pdf. Accessed 11 May 2007.

Rusjan B. Usefulness of the EFQM Excellence Model: theoretical explanation of some conceptual and methodological issues. Total Qual Manage. 2005;16(3):363–80.

Shewhart WA. Economic control of quality of manufactured product. New York: D. Van Nostrand C; 1931.

Tarantino DP. Using the balanced scorecard as a performance management tool. Physician Exec. 2003;29:69–72.

Ten Asbroek AHA, Arah OA, Geelhoed J, Custer T, Delnoij DM, Klazinga NS. Developing a national performance indicator framework for the Dutch health system. Int J Qual Health Care. 2004;16(1):165–71.

Wollersheim H, Faber MJ, Grol RPTM, Dondorp WJ, Struijs AJ. Vertrouwen in verantwoorde zorg?: effecten van en morele vragen bij het gebruik van prestatie-indicatoren. Den Haag: Centrum voor Ethiek en Gezondheid; 2006.

Woodard TD. Addressing variation in hospital quality: is Six Sigma the answer? J Healthc Manag. 2005;50(4):226–36.

No-Show with Particular Emphasis on Nuclear Medicine

24

Katinka Lauwerens-Daniëls and Johann Freese

Abstract

No-show causes disruption of normal clinic flow, resulting in longer waiting times for diagnostic appointments for other patients, wasted resources and reduced efficiency. In nuclear medicine the consequences are far-reaching due to the additional high costs of radiopharmaceuticals, time of the high educated staff and the reservation of expensive camera time. Investigating no-show asks for a clear definition suitable a for nuclear medicine ward. There are different ways to address the problem like using a reminder system (letters/telephone call/text messages) or introducing a fine for no-show.

24.1 Definition

Missed appointments are referred to as "no-shows". No-show patients are patients who fail to appear without cancelling (or rescheduling) their scheduled appointment (Lauwerens 2003). To concrete the definition to a practical definition we could add the time into the definition: cancelling, for example, 24 h in advance. No-show influences the capacity, the finances and the management of a department, especially a department of nuclear medicine. On a daily basis, caretakers are confronted with patients who fail to appear. On a yearly base, costs are being made and there is no revenue for it.

K. Lauwerens-Daniëls (✉)
Department of Nuclear Medicine, Erasmus Medical Center,
s-Gravendijkwal 230, Rotterdam, CE 3015, The Netherlands
e-mail: k.lauwerens@erasmusmc.nl

J. Freese, MBA
Director Work Force Holland BV, Groningen, RM 9700, The Netherlands

A.W.J.M. Glaudemans et al. (eds.), *Quality in Nuclear Medicine*,
DOI 10.1007/978-3-319-33531-5_24

24.2 Severeness

The severeness of no-show can be explained through international research. A national American survey shows that most outpatient clinics have a no-show percentage of more than 20 %. Especially investigations in the United States show that missed outpatient appointments have significant implications on continuity of health care, residency education and productivity (Hixon et al. 1999). Since medical manpower is scarce, it should be used to the maximum. Efficiency, quality and continuity of care are the main objects. Optimal use of scarce medical manpower is thwarted because of patients not showing up for their appointments (Hixon et al. 1999). In various investigations there is a big variety in no-show numbers. Investigators suspect that the variation should partially be described to the use of different definitions of no-show and the different ways of registration of no-show (Geest et al. 1998).

Some patients cancel their appointment so tardy, that it becomes impossible to plan another patient. In addition the treatment of a no-show patient is delayed. Fewer resources are available for a ward. Investigation in literature shows that only 34 % of the patients arrive on time, the rest come late or not at all (Xakellis and Benett 2001). This raises the question: who are those patients? General characteristics of chronic non-attenders include male gender, age <40 years, low socioeconomic status and referral by a high-volume general practitioner. Longer intervals between scheduling and appointments also predict nonattendance (Stubbs et al. 2012).

24.3 Scheduling

The increased demand and the complexity in the procedure protocols make the scheduling of patients and resources in nuclear medicine a challenging problem. Nuclear medicine procedures require the administration of a radiopharmaceutical to the patient and involve multiple sequential steps. Each procedure step requires several resources such as technologists, nurses, equipment (gamma cameras and Positron Emission Tomography (PET) cameras) and sometimes a treadmill. Radiopharmaceuticals have to be managed carefully and their delivery requires a well-planned lead time (Perez et al. 2013). For scheduling problems mathematic models have been introduced in healthcare. The main goal of these models is introducing an optimal outpatient appointment scheduling. In these models no-show is allowed to happen (Kaandorp and Koole 2007).

In nuclear medicine a considerable amount of effort goes into planning an appointment. As a consequence no-shows at a nuclear medicine department can't be taken for granted. Patients who fail to come to their nuclear diagnostic appointments cause disruption of normal clinic flow, resulting in longer waiting times for diagnostic appointments for other patients, wasted resources and reduced efficiency. The second reason is the high costs of radiopharmaceuticals; they are ordered or produced on site specially for a patient. These radiopharmaceuticals are ordered in advance; they are expensive, very specific, not durable and have very a specific time window. Also the duration of the examination (camera-time) lies between 10 and 240 min; this makes it difficult to overbook patients as is done scheduling using the mathematic models which are discussed above.

An example of wasted resources is the cost for a PET-CT scan including staff time and use of imaging machinery; the costs vary between 650 and 1100 pounds per scan. With contrast enhancement CT, the cost is estimated to be 20 % higher. The duration lies between 20 and 40 min per scan (Brush et al. 2011).

Therefore preventing no-show is an important issue in nuclear medicine. Preferably cancellations are communicated more than 48 h in advance, so that the radiopharmaceutical order can be cancelled. There are different ways to address the problem like using a reminder system or introducing a fine for no-show.

24.4 Fine

Economic incentives, such as imposing a fine, should ideally stimulate patients to either appear at their scheduled appointments or to cancel them. Patients should be informed in advance about the fine system if they don't show up for their appointment. Legal systems must allow to introduce a system of compensation. Wards shouldn't be forced to charge a fine. Depending on the situation, they should be able not to.

Complete compensation for hospitals is not preferable, because then hospitals would not be stimulated to develop an efficient system for scheduling appointments. A system of compensation entails costs for implementation and execution. Besides, a patient is entitled to the possibility of appeal which has to be developed as well. The realisation of this system of compensation has various drawbacks. By introducing a system of compensation, hospitals may face patient claims for lack of service in return, since hospital communication towards the patient especially concerning scheduled appointments still leaves a lot to be desired (Lauwerens 2003). A study describing process improvement shows that no-show can be eliminated by improving written and verbal information (Upshaw et al. 2013).

24.5 Reminders

The costs of developing and introducing a reminder system are expected to be considerably lower than developing a system of compensation concerning no-show (Quattlebaum et al. 1994). Different kinds of reminders are in use. There are written reminders such as letters and text messages for mobile phones. Hospitals also use verbal reminders such as an automated telephone call or a personal one by a staff member.

Using a system by which patients receive a reminder may reduce the number of no-show patients at least to 50 %. Sending a reminder letter 2 weeks in advance has proven to be the most effective method in the past (Hixon et al. 1999). It is also very much appreciated by patients (Moser 1994). A meta-analysis with combined evidence from randomised controlled trials shows that the use of SMS reminders increases the likelihood of attendance at clinical appointments by 50 %, compared to no appointment reminders. In this analysis 18 papers were included, and the interventions represented a wide variety of countries, mostly Europe, but also including Malaysia, China, Brazil, the United States and Australia (Guy et al. 2012). The delay between sending and receiving an SMS message is minimal compared with traditional methods such as letters (Da Costa et al. 2010).

Cancellation rates in groups that receive a reminder are significantly higher. The clinical staff reminder by telephone significantly reduced the no-show rate. Although an automated reminder system is less effective in some studies, it likely has a cost advantage making it more attractive (Parikh et al. 2010). In other studies text messaging or telephone reminders are equivalent in reducing the proportion of missed appointments. The rates of attendance are slightly higher following telephone reminders, indicating that direct personal contact with the patient may therefore be more effective to increase attendance rates. Automated text message reminders however are cost-effective (0.07 Euro/text message), mostly because of the additional administrative resources that were needed for the telephone reminders. Still, the efficacy of text messaging depends on the penetration rate of mobile phones and may therefore vary from one context to another (Junod Perron et al. 2013). In a systematic review of the English literature (1999–2009), it was showed that all interventions seem to improve attendance, but at varying costs. Aggregate analysis of the various reminder systems showed the greatest reduction in no-show with telephone reminders, followed by text messaging/SMS and mail reminders. Cost analyses suggest text messaging to be most cost-effective, but its applicability may be limited by technology penetration (Stubbs et al. 2012).

In nuclear medicine the costs of wasted resources are higher than those made in a clinical department for primary outpatient care on which the studies above recall. The reason is that the consequences are far-reaching due to the additional costs of radiopharmaceuticals, the booked time of the highly educated staff and the reservation of expensive camera time. By reducing no-show, besides using the appointment time to provide care to the patient, the facility avoids wasting resources (Da Costa et al. 2010). One of the negative effects of reminders, whether a phone or text message, is that they shift the responsibility of attendance away from the patient to the organisation (Fairhurst and Sheikh 2008).

24.6 Conclusion

Reminders can reduce no-show by 50 %, but it induces a higher rate of cancelled appointments.Sending a text-message as a reminder more than 48 h in advance is a useful strategy to reduce no-show and limit additional costs for a nuclear medicine ward. Increasing the reminder delay may help to reallocate these cancelled appointments more efficiently.

24.7 How to Address No-Show: A Case Study

No-show, is it a problem anyway? And if it is, how do you qualify and quantify this problem? Isn't it nice to have a spare hour to do some unfinished business from yesterday? For an occasion it may give the workforce some relief on stress. The following practical example gives an illustration on how no-show can be handled.

24.7.1 Introduction

This practical example addresses a company that conducts individual psychodiagnostic research for people with occupational disabilities. The purpose is to determine whether people should work in a "protected environment" and is commissioned by the government (UWV). This service can be well compared with the kind of service delivered by healthcare, for instance, nuclear medicine. Certain conditions must be met in order to have insight in your operational process. These conditions are:

- A description of the work process; this work process can be used to produce several products.
- A separate protocol for each product.
- The work process is made up of successive operations. Of each activity the time and the cost per unit of time is known.
- The influence of "no-show" is known for each activity.

24.7.2 A Case Study

In this case study no-show is an existing problem. Within the old procedure, a no-show was actively managed by the company staff. Clients were called to confirm their appointment, after they received a written invitation, in order to conduct their psychodiagnostic research. This call was made 3 days before the research took place. Due to this effort, the no-show was 11 %, during the entire contract (between 2009 and 2012). The no-show was thus slightly above the norm of 10 %. This norm was set as a goal by the management.

In 2013 a new procedure was introduced/contract was signed. Due to modified laws and regulations, the contract volume is expected to decrease from 10,000 to 5,000 individual psychodiagnostic researches. The company therefore needs to be supplied from fewer locations. This means that the travel time increases for clients.

In practice, the no-show appears to increase to 90–9 % for the first 3 months of 2013. The management wants to take measures to reduce no-show. Not only research is necessary, the company should also have an understanding of the consequences of no-show. This case shows in a few steps the financial consequences of no-show and the possibilities to manage no-show.

24.7.3 Activity-Based Costing

It is often wrongly thought that only an economist/specialist is involved in being able to make a service. Supporting tasks are often disregarded in business matters. Activity-based costing considers a service as consecutive activities (Atkinson et al. 1997). Without planning activity, sending an invitation or an invoice, etc., there will be no service delivered. Naturally, it is of critical importance to check if each step is actually necessary and adds value to a service.

24.7.4 Processes and Protocols

This company works with a generic core process; all services are going through the same process steps and are identical. Within this workflow, each product has its own protocol. A psychodiagnostic research for this particular contract partner consists of the following activities:

- Registering orders
- Planning activity
- Performing service
- Finishing orders
- Invoice
- Archive

The psychodiagnostic research works according to the following protocol:

Activity (generic process)	Standard time in hours (protocol)	Hourly	Value added activity	Influence no-show	Value no-show
Registering orders	0.125	€22.67[a]	€2.83	100 %	€2.83
Planning activity	0.5	€22.67[a]	€11.33	100 %	€11.33
Performing service	2.5	€46.40[b]	€116,-	40 %	€46.40
Finishing orders	0.2	€22.67[a]	€4.53	50 %	€2.27
Invoice	0.13	€22.67[a]	€3.02	0 %	
Archive	0.07	€22.67[a]	€1.51	0 %	
Total			€139.23		€62.83
Impact no-show (29 %)					€18.22

[a]Based on 1.500 h per year and an annual income of €34.000,-
[b]Based on 1.250 h per year and an annual income of €58.000,-

The psychodiagnostic research has one standard modality and was sold for € 325,-, with a project volume of 4,800 per year.

The influence of no-show varies per activity (process step). Some activities should be carried out again (registering orders and planning activity); other activities provide part time loss (perform service and finishing orders). Part of the added value is not explained by this core process. These are housing (11 %), office expenses (5 %), transport (4 %), personnel staff and general management (6 %), other costs

(4 %) and profit (16 %), all of which are not explained by this core process. The budget available to provide this service is €175.50 (54 % of €325,-).

24.7.5 Size and Costs of No-Show

The size of no-show will be continuously measured and recorded in a management information system. As a result, the size is a percentage and is also known as a total. The size of the no-show in the project is 9–90 %. Because the costs per step are known, it is now possible to calculate the costs of no-show for the organisation. The costs of no-show (29 %) with unchanged policies amount to € 87.464, – (4.800 × €18.22) at a project volume of € 1,560,000, – (4.800 x €325,-).

24.7.6 Analysis of No-Show

Calling clients is executed from a list of agreements/appointments. The percentage of the coefficients that will be called is stored. Management's decision to assess whether there is a link between achieving a client by phone and no-show initiated research. This research took a week and was performed under 156 people who were planned in April and May for their psychodiagnostic research. Of the people that have been achieved (89 persons) 83 persons appeared on their appointment. The no-show was 7 %. Of persons who were not reached (67), 35 people appeared on their appointment. The no-show in this group was forty-eight percent (48 %) This study shows a clear link between accessibility and show. Management has a tool at hand to come within their maximum standard of 10 % no-show.

24.7.7 Measures Taken by This Company

- If no phone number is known to the notification, the notification will be returned to the client (contract partner).
- Planning and invitation activity will be reversed. Only when it appears that a client can be reached by telephone, it is also planned.

By reversing activity, as a measure, there are no additional costs involved. However, consultation with the contract partner is necessary because of a change in the time of acceptance of clients.

24.7.8 Expected Yield of Measures

In this example it is expected that the cost of no-show will diminish to €21.112,- at a no-show level of 7 %. The yield of measures therefore is about €66.000,- (€87.464,- - €21.112,-).

References

Atkinson AA, Banker RD, Kaplan RS, Young SM. Management accounting. Prentice Hall. 1997. p. 269–6.

Brush J, Boyd K, Chappell F, Crawford F, Dozier M, Fenwick E, et al. The value of FDG positron emission tomography/computerised tomography (PET/CT) in pre-operative staging of colorectal cancer: a systematic review and economic evaluation. Health Technol Assess 2011;15(35). From: Department of Health. A framework for the development of positron emission tomography (PET) services in England 2005. and National Cancer Research Institute. A framework for PET research in the UK. 2007.

Da Costa TM, Salomão PL, Martha AS, Pisa IT, Sigulem D. The impact of short message service text messages sent as appointment reminders to patients' cell phones at outpatient clinics in São Paulo, Brazil. Int J of Med Inform. 2010;79:65–70.

Fairhurst A, Sheikh K. Texting appointment reminders to repeated non-attenders in primary car: randomised controlled study. Qual Saf Health Care. 2008;17(5):373–6.

Geest van der L, Colenberg S, Scholten C, Rapport No Show in ziekenhuizen in de Amsterdamse regio, Research voor Beleid/SIGRA, Leiden/Amsterdam, maart 1998.

Guy R, Hocking J, Wand H, Stott S, Ali H, Kaldor J. How effective are short message service reminders at increasing clinic attendance? A meta-analysis and systematic review. Health Serv Res. 2012;47(2):614–32.

Hixon AL, Chapman RW, Nuovo J. Failure to keep clinic appointments: implications for residency education and productivity. Fam Med. 1999;9:627–30.

Junod Perron JN, Dao MD, Righini NC, Humair JP, Broers B, Narring F, Haller DM, Gaspoz JM. Text-messaging versus telephone reminders to reduce missed appointments in an academic primary care clinic: a randomized controlled trial. BMC Health Serv Res. 2013;13:125.

Quattlebaum TG, Darden PM, Sperry JB. Effectiveness of Computer-Generated Appointment Reminders. Pediatrics. 1991;4:80–5.

Kaandorp GC, Koole G. Optimal outpatient appointment scheduling, Health Care Manage Sci, Springer science + Business Media. 2007;10:217–29.

Lauwerens K. No-show: inkomstenderving in de ziekenhuissector door verzuim van poliklinische patienten, Rotterdam: Erasmus Universiteit; 2003.

Moser SE. Effectiveness of post card appointment reminders. Family Practice Res Journal. 1994;3:281–8.

Parikh A, Gupta K, Wilson AC, Fields K, Cosgrove NM, Kostis JB. The effectiveness of outpatient appointment reminder systems in reducing No-show rates. Am J Med. 2010;123(6):542–8.

Pérez E, Ntaimo L, Malavé CO, Bailey C, McCormack P. Stochastic online appointment scheduling of multi-step sequential procedures in nuclear medicine. Health Care Manag Sci. 2013;16:281–99.

Stubbs ND, Geraci SA, Stephenson PL, Jones DB, Sanders S. Methods to reduce outpatient Non-attendance. Am J Med Sci. 2012;344(3):211–9.

Upshaw C, Lee RB, Rivard AL. Process improvement decreases no show rates for pediatric cardiac MR imaging with anesthesia. J Cardiovasc Magn Reson. 2013;15 suppl 1:283.

Xakellis GC, Benett A. Improving clinic efficiency of a family medicine teaching clinic. Fam Med. 2001;7:533–8.

Part VI

Organisations

The Role of the Medical Ethics Review Board in the Netherlands: Focus on Clinical Studies Utilizing Radiopharmaceuticals and Imaging

25

Hendrikus H. Boersma and Anne M.J. Paans

Abstract

In this chapter the role and function of ethical review boards (ERBs) are discussed, combined with an overview on the organization of clinical trial ethics review in the Netherlands. The roles of the different members of the ERB and their functions are described, and the role of ERB study protocol review is compared to the situation abroad.

25.1 Introduction

According to the declaration of Helsinki (Declaration of Helsinki 2013) and many other regulations (e.g., EU and US legislation), prospective ethical review of clinical trial protocols and related documents is a requirement before any patient related proceedings considering this kind of research can take place. Under the Dutch Law, the judgment of a governmentally accredited ethical review board (ERB) is mandatory to start with clinical investigations according to the Dutch Law on research

H.H. Boersma, PharmD, PhD (✉)
Department of Nuclear Medicine and Molecular Imaging EB 70, University of Groningen, University Medical Center Groningen, Groningen, The Netherlands

Department of Clinical Pharmacy and Pharmacology, University of Groningen, University Medical Center Groningen, Groningen, RB, P.O. Box 30.001, NL-9700, The Netherlands
e-mail: h.h.boersma@umcg.nl

A.M.J. Paans
Department of Nuclear Medicine and Molecular Imaging EB 70, University of Groningen, University Medical Center Groningen, Groningen, The Netherlands

A.W.J.M. Glaudemans et al. (eds.), *Quality in Nuclear Medicine*,
DOI 10.1007/978-3-319-33531-5_25

with human subjects. In this concise chapter we will give special attention toward the medical ethics review process in the Netherlands with a special focus on radiopharmaceuticals and imaging.

25.2 ERB Organization in the Netherlands

In the Netherlands, the government is involved in the CCMO, the Dutch Central Committee on Research Involving Human Subjects. The CCMO should be regarded as a certifying body for all recognized ERBs. Furthermore, the CCMO (CCMO, www.ccmo.nl) functions as an ERB itself by performing ethics review study protocols requiring specialized knowledge, such as those concerning gene therapy, drug abuse, and research involving minors and mentally disabled subjects. Also, they serve as the appeal ERB for unapproved study protocols which were rejected by the regular ERB. Although ERBs are independent, currently most ERBs are affiliated to university hospitals as well as to larger community hospitals. One of the big differences of the Dutch approach of medical ethics review is the absence of health inspectorate medication quality review for the approval of study medication. By the involvement of a hospital pharmacist and a clinical pharmacologist, this part of the study review is done by the ERB. Depending on the speed of inspectorates, this generally means that the investigator has a less high hurdle to take as compared to the quality review of the diverse national health inspectorates. This does not mean that Dutch health inspectors are neglecting the GMP/GCP domain. In the Netherlands, the health inspectorate plays a crucial role in the EU GMP approval of production sites for study medication. Furthermore, they perform GCP inspection visits, thereby auditing the real life performance status of ongoing as well as closed clinical studies. The latter is not a task of the Dutch ERBs.

25.2.1 When Is the Judgment of an ERB Obligatory?

In the Netherlands, law defines clinical research with human subjects in a way, which requires not in all cases an ERB judgment. It actually depends on two questions whether the clinical study needs an ERB approval. Firstly, the ERB should evaluate whether the proposed protocol is scientific. There are many protocols containing objectives like "what is the added value of a novel medical procedure/technique which was introduced several years ago?" These protocols are regarded as evaluation of the care process and do not need an approval from the ERB, as the objectives are not per se scientific. Furthermore, many of these protocols do not require additional information from the subjects involved; it will be mainly based on gathered data during clinical practice. Of course, here the investigator has a responsibility toward privacy of the involved subjects and all other features involving patient integrity, but these are general hospital requirements which do need the involvement of an ERB.

Secondly, the reviewing ERB will evaluate to what extent human subjects are involved in a study. If the scientific research protocol is, for instance, only consisting of data research without any additional burden for the involved subjects, the approval of an ERB is not required. The same is the case for "simple" questionnaires which have no impact to the subjects involved. However, when a subject is asked to participate in a study protocol and should fill out a questionnaire on items with a highly emotional burden (such as "suicidal thoughts" or "how to cope up with the loss of a loved one"), an ERB approval is required. The same yields for any study in which the patient will participate and should follow any additional rules, give blood, take medication, and undergo biopsies, solely with the purpose of conducting a clinical study. It is evident that this way of regulating clinical studies contains quite some gray zones, which makes the ERB also serving as an advisory board to figure out whether ERB approval is needed or not.

25.2.2 ERB Review Process

Most ERBs meet several times per month to discuss the scheduled, individually reviewed protocols together with the other members. During each meeting new study protocols are discussed as well as amendments to existing studies. All requirements which are to be met by the ERB are laid down in the Dutch law on research with humans as well as the ERB's statutes.

Generally, the ERB looks at scientific and medical ethics aspects of a particular clinical study protocol. The committee poses questions toward each protocol, such as:

- Are the aims of the proposed or its study novel and scientifically sound?
- Does the study methodology answer the questions posed in the aims of the study?
- What is the statistical design of the study and does it fit to the needs of the study aims?
- Is the burden of the study justified/balanced by the severity of the studied disease?
- Is there an advantage for participants in the study, and, if yes, what is the exact gain?
- Does the study meet all ethical as well as juridical requirements?
- Are the investigators competent and sufficiently equipped to perform the study?
- What is the defined quality of the medication or radiopharmaceutical to be used?
- Are there any issues concerning quality assurance of the used medical devices (pacemakers, novel tested equipment)?
- Is the written patient information as well as the informed consent letter comprehensible for the average reader?
- Does the patient information contain all required information?
- Are all patient rights, such as well well-being and safety measures, taken into account in the study?

- Is an independent expert (mostly a physician) available to be consulted by subjects which desire additional information of the study?
- Is the accrual of patients performed correctly? Here, touting should be avoided.

After each meeting, the ERB writes for each single protocol a letter of explanation to the principal investigator, mostly with suggestions for further improvement. Sometimes, the study is judged as "being unsuitable" to be performed in the proposed way. For the latter, the ERB may even suggest that they will reject the study because of these reasons. In these cases, a meeting of a delegation from the ERB with the investigators is likely for further clarification of the objections of the ERB as well as to get feedback from the investigators. In many cases, the investigators rewrite their study protocol to meet the ERB criteria. In case the investigators do not agree with the ERB, they may submit the protocol to the CCMO for appeal.

25.2.3 ERB Additional Review of Studies Involving I onizing Radiation

In case of the use of radiopharmaceuticals or the use of radiation in general, the ERB has to pay special attention to the risks involved in the use of ionizing radiation also with respect to the legal aspects of this use. Within the Dutch law, the Dutch government has given the "Besluit Stralingsbescherming" (Regulations on Radiation Protection). These regulations are based on European regulations and will be similar to the regulations in other European countries of European Union. The general rule of the Dutch government is a limitation of the radiation dose to the general public of 1 mSv/y at maximum on the average. This means that next to the radiation dose due to the natural background and the dose due to medical diagnostic and therapeutical applications should be limited to 1 mSv/y on average for a normal member of the population. This limit is also valid for the (unborn) fetus if applicable. In the Netherlands the total natural background is about 1.6 mSv/y National Institute of Public Health and the Environment (RIVM) and due to medical diagnostic applications about 0.8 mSv/y has to be added (RIVM). The "Rijksinstituut voor Volksgezondheid en Milieu" keeps track of doses in the Netherlands (www.rivm.nl). For the evaluation of the extra risks in studies involving human volunteers, the Dutch government refers to the guidelines of the International Commission on Radiological Protection (ICRP). The ICRP has numerous publications in the field of radiation safety (www.icrp.org) including the radiation dose of radiopharmaceuticals used in the field of nuclear medicine (ICRP 53, 62, 80). The medical ERB has to evaluate the request for approval on the basis of the radiation dose given in the request which often is based on literature or an explicit calculation by a radiation safety expert. In order to have an estimate of the risk, the ICRP has published the "Radiation dose to patients from radiopharmaceuticals" in publication ICRP 62 in 1992. In Table 25.1 of ICRP 62, the different categories of risk are given; see also below. In practice it turns out that the radiation dose due to radiopharmaceuticals at the necessary dose in nearly all studies falls within the ICRP 62 Category IIb of risk

Table 25.1 Categories of risk according to ICRP 62

Risk category	Effective dose (mSv)	Level of risk	Social benefit
I	<0.1	Trivial	Minor
II:			
IIa	0.1–1	Minor to intermediate	Intermediate to moderate
IIb	1–10		
III	>10 (not deterministic)	Moderate	Substantial

(1–10 mSv). When longer lived (t1/2 in the order of days) radiopharmaceuticals are used, this category of risk is easily overstepped meaning a radiation dose of 10 mSv or more. In the case of patients involved in radiotherapeutic procedures, this general rule is of course not applicable and also the total body dose for this category of patients has to be taken into account in the evaluation. The ERB has to establish its own interpretation and evaluation in which a comparison has to be made between the level of social benefit to be achieved with the proposed study and the radiation dose involved. The simple conclusion that studies with radiopharmaceuticals cannot be performed is not correct because the radiation dose is not in contradiction with the general rule of the government where in the limitation of the extra dose to 1 mSv/y the term "on the average" is used. In practice this means that the bookkeeping on the radiation dose for patients has to be extended to studies with volunteers. In the case of a study with a volunteer, this bookkeeping has to be checked in order to inspect if the general rule of 1 mSv/y on the average is not overstepped.

25.2.4 Competences of the ERB

To get input of various disciplines, Dutch law requires individuals with different backgrounds to be a member of each ERB. The board consists of at least two physicians, a clinical pharmacologist, a clinical pharmacist, a lawyer, a representative for the participating subjects, a methodologist/statistician, an ethicist, a member with a nonscientific background, and a member with no direct affiliation with the connected institution. Each member of an ERB is approved based on their Curriculum Vitae (CV) by the CCMO.

25.3 Regulations

Each ERB in the Netherlands reviews each study protocol based on the applicable laws in the Netherlands, all available regulations in place for protection and proper participation of the subject (GCP, see Chap. 2), and proper quality of the study drugs (see Chap. 3 on GMP).

These regulations, for instance, require that the ERB be involved in the safety assessments of each reviewed and approved study. Every serious adverse event in a study is reported to the ERB. Also, the ERB judges whether the investigators of a are required to install a data safety monitoring board to monitor the study for all data-related inconsistencies and eventual upcoming risks for subjects who will participate in this study on a later moment. Furthermore, any study with additional risk will be asked to have an insurance of the study to be able to cover costs for any unexpected risk emerging from the study. Although it is good to have a certified insurance, proceeding to get access to reimbursement of these costs is very difficult. There are better solutions for this problem. For example, in Denmark, a clinical trial fund exists, which covers all costs from most harm, caused by participating in a clinical trial. The costs of participating in this fund are comparable to the payments for having the risk insured, and it is far more participant-friendly.

Conclusion

In the Netherlands, the ERB plays a major role in the review and approval of any scientifically based clinical study which involves participation of human subjects in a direct way. The way in which the ERBs are organized in the Dutch society makes those in principle more accessible compared to the situation in which larger governmental bodies are taking care of the review process. Furthermore, their competences are ensured in a strict way by the Dutch government, assuring a solid review process and good consultancy options for conduction of a clinical trial in the Netherlands.

References

Besluit Stralingsbescherming, National (Dutch) legislation based on the EU Directive 2013/59/Euratom:https://osha.europa.eu/nl/legislation/directives/directive-2013-59-euratom-protection--against-ionising-radiation. Assessed Dec 2015.

CCMO, CCMO-website: www.ccmo.nl. Assessed Dec 2015.

Declaration of Helsinki (2013) website: http://www.wma.net/en/30publications/10policies/b3/. Assessed Dec 2015.

Dutch State Institute for Public Health and environment. (Rijks Instituut voor Volksgezondheid en Milieu (RIVM)), http://www.rivm.nl/Onderwerpen/M/Medische_Stralingstoepassingen. Assessed Dec 2015.

EU-GCP http://ec.europa.eu/health/files/eudralex/vol-1/dir_2005_28/dir_2005_28_en.pdf. Assessed Dec 2015.

GMP http://ec.europa.eu/health/documents/eudralex/vol-4/index_en.htm. Assessed Dec 2015.

ICRP: International Committee on Radiological Protection. www.icrp.org. Assessed Dec 2015.

Quality Visits: Dutch Example (Dutch Society of Nuclear Medicine)

26

Joris van den Heuvel

Abbreviations

cGRPP	Current good radiopharmacy practice
EBCA	Evidence-based clinical audit
GMP	Good manufacturing practice
IFMS	Individual Performance Medical Specialist
NIV	Dutch Society of Internal Medicine
NVMBR	Dutch Society of Medical Imaging and Radiotherapy
NVNG	Dutch Society of Nuclear Medicine
NVVR	Dutch Society of Radiology
SMART	Specific measurable, achievable, results-focused, and time-bound
SMS/VMS	Safety management system
TCI	Team Climate Inventory

26.1 Definitions

CanMEDS: a framework for improving patient care by enhancing physician training. Developed by the Royal College in the 1990s, its main purpose is to define the necessary competencies for all areas of medical practice and provide a comprehensive foundation for medical education and practice in Canada.

Small-scale radiopharmacy: a facility where the small-scale preparation of radiopharmaceuticals is carried out under a license that is in accordance with national

J. van den Heuvel
Department of Clinical Pharmacy, OLVG Amsterdam, Amsterdam, The Netherlands
e-mail: j.vandenheuvel@slaz.nl

A.W.J.M. Glaudemans et al. (eds.), *Quality in Nuclear Medicine*,
DOI 10.1007/978-3-319-33531-5_26

regulations. The term small-scale radiopharmacy is not related to the size of the facility, that may vary in a broad range, but only to the kind of radiopharmaceutical preparation performed.

26.2 Introduction

The Dutch Society of Nuclear Medicine (NVNG) is a professional and scientific organization founded in 1968. It is a relatively small organization with currently 401 members. The NVNG has a multidisciplinary character, with nuclear medicine physicians, clinical physicists, radiopharmacists, and radiochemists as members.

The NVNG promotes science, technology, and application of nuclear medicine and defends their professional interests. Another objective of the NVNG is education of its members.

Quality visits in nuclear medicine go back for more than 20 years. In 1994 a first pilot was done by the NVNG. Currently, quality visits have a prominent role in the quality policy of all scientific organizations of medical specialists in the Netherlands. Quality visits are of great importance: participation is obligatory for re-registration of medical specialists and in order to obtain recognition for nuclear medicine physician residency training.

It is important to stress that quality visits are meant to improve patient care, not to punish or detect "rotten apples."

Currently there is still a lot of attention for the performance of physicians and quality of healthcare, not only within the medical profession itself but also in politics and the media. It is a dynamic field. This chapter will describe how quality visits of nuclear medicine departments are done and how it is evolving.

26.3 Legal Framework

In the Netherlands, nuclear medicine physicians, as well as other medical specialists, are registered with the Royal Dutch Medical Association. After registration specialists can use their professional title. The initial registration is valid for 5 years. Following this period, you need to re-register. Requirements for re-registration are a sufficient number of working hours, proven advancement of expertise, and participation in a quality visit. Participation in a quality visit is a requirement for re-registration since 2005.

In the early 1990s, an agreement was reached with the government that the medical profession itself would be responsible for medical quality policy; the government creates the necessary enabling conditions and monitors quality via the Healthcare Inspectorate. The Dutch Society of Nuclear Medicine had several pilots in 1994 and officially started quality visits in 1995.

In May 2015, a draft decision has been published by the College of Medical Specialists (CGS) with a revision of reregistration requirements. New topics are development of personal performance and functioning of the professional group.

Scientific organizations and medical specialists have time until January 2019 to have a system in place for assessment of individual and team performance.

26.4 Practical Organization of Quality Visits

The "Quality Visiting Committee" of the Dutch Society of Nuclear Medicine visits all nuclear medicine departments in the Netherlands. Quality visits are done every 5 years.

An ad hoc committee is put together for every quality visit. This is a multidisciplinary team, composed of two nuclear medicine physicians, one clinical physicist, one radiopharmacist, and a secretary. One nuclear medicine physician is member of the Quality Visiting Committee and is chairman of the ad hoc committee. The radiopharmacist is not part of the team if there is no radiopharmacy department.

Before the audit, the department fills in a questionnaire based upon the quality guidelines of nuclear medicine. The ad hoc committee visits the department and interviews various stakeholders such as the board of directors and peer physicians. At the end of the day, the committee gives feedback of their findings. A final version of the report will be determined by the Quality Visiting Committee itself. The audited department then responds to the given recommendations.

The Dutch Health Ministry and the Federation of Medical Specialists agreed upon a fixed amount reserved for quality projects. Until 1st January 2016, all quality visits performed by the NVNG were fully financed by this "quality fund." From this date forward, the quality fund cannot be used anymore to pay quality visits but is used to finance other kinds of quality projects. Hospitals have to pay for the audit themselves.

26.5 Quality Framework

The NVNG published new quality guidelines in 2014. The former guideline needed an update. There was a demand for tools to evaluate medical care and professional performance. In the new concept of quality visits, there is a shift from a global assessment of structures and prerequisites to a more specific evaluation of care and outcome of care.

The Federation of Medical Specialists worked on a new model for quality visits (Fossen et al. 2005). In 2012, the federation published another guideline: *valuation system for quality visits* (Fossen et al. 2012). All scientific organizations of medical specialists adopted these guidelines.

The NVNG adopted these recommendations. New instruments are developed, for example, a Quick Scan for group performance. At the same time, the NVNG wanted a standardized method of judgment, and also this is introduced.

The "Quality Committee" of the NVNG drafted this guideline. The Quality Committee is also a multidisciplinary team. This guideline is approved by the Dutch Society of Nuclear Medicine (NVNG), the Dutch Society of Hospital Pharmacy (NVZA), and the Dutch Society of Clinical Physics (NVKF).

The quality framework of the Dutch Society of Nuclear Medicine (NVNG) sets out recommendations based on eight quality domains:

1. Evaluation of care
2. Team performance
3. Patient perspective
4. Professional development
5. Personal provisions
6. Facilities
7. Radiopharmacy
8. Clinical physics

Domain 1 Evaluation of Care
Evaluation of care consists of several questions regarding the quality system. Evaluation of patient files, audits, adherence to guidelines, recording complications, quality indicators, risk assessments, and validation of equipment are some of the themes questioned.

Domain 2 Team Performance
Questions regarding structure of organization and team performance are asked in this domain. Team performance can be evaluated by a Quick Scan, a tool developed by the NVNG to assess and evaluate team performance. Another tool to evaluate team performance can be used too.

Domain 3 Patient Perspective
Patient satisfaction is an important indicator for quality in healthcare. Patient risks, complaints, patient safety, and waiting lists are topics in this domain.
There is also a check on adherence to the safety management system (SMS, VMS in Dutch). SMS embeds patient safety in healthcare practice. SMS is a system through which hospitals continuously identify risks; implement improvements; and establish, evaluate, and modify policy. One theme of the SMS is the parenteral administration of medication.

Domain 4 Professional Development
Are expertise and skills up to date?
Is there a system in place to assess and evaluate personal performance?

Domain 5 Personal
Is there enough personnel to do all the work in the nuclear medicine department?

Domain 6 Facilities
Facilities have to be up to date and in accordance with the legislation in force.

Domain 7 Radiopharmacy

Preparations of radiopharmaceuticals are subject to several regulations and rules. It involves adherence to regulations on radiation protection as well as to appropriate rules of working under aseptic conditions. For small-scale preparations at hospital pharmacies, the Dutch Society of Hospital Pharmacy issued a guideline "good manufacturing practice in hospitals" (GMP-z in Dutch). GMP-z is in accordance with European GMP regulation but addresses specific issues with preparation of radiopharmaceuticals in a hospital setting. This guideline is accepted by the inspectorate. Other guidelines and regulations are monographs in the European Pharmacopoeia, the Nuclear Energy Act, and EANM guideline current good radiopharmaceutical practice (cGRPP).

Domain 8 Clinical Physics

Clinical physicists have responsibility regarding maintenance and validation of equipment and software and play an important role in radiation protection. Responsibilities regarding these aspects and procedures on technical failures of equipment are examples of items in the quality guideline.

In these guidelines there is more focus upon team and personal performance, patient perspective has a more prominent place, and new tools are introduced to evaluate care (e.g., the existence of prospective risk assessments). Nuclear medicine departments are supposed to do these evaluations themselves and follow the plan-do-check-act (PDCA) cycle.

26.6 Valuation Method

A recent recommendation is to have a standardized method of judgment. The goal of standardization of judgment is obvious, that is, decreasing subjectivity and making a judgment predictable. Valuation is done by a five-point scale. Quality visits are done every 5 years, and it is a peer review. With this valuation system, feedback can be asked between quality visits. This is an improvement (Table 26.1).

Table 26.1 Valuation method by a five-point scale

Scale	Corrective action
Target standard	Excellent, example for others
Basic standard	Good, this is the standard
Recommendation	Practice can be improved in one or more aspects. Correction within 5 years
Important advice	Practice had to be improved in one or more aspects. Correction within 2 years
Requirement	Critical flaws in essential aspects.
	Correction within the term stated by the committee, with a maximum of 6 months

Table 26.2 Example of standard "quality indicator"

Domain 1. Evaluation of care	
1.19 Quality indicators	
The department delivers data for quality indicators of the NVNG and the Dutch inspectorate. Moreover these quality indicators are analyzed by the department and actions for improvement can be demonstrated.	
1. Target standard	The department delivers data for quality indicators of the NVNG and the Dutch inspectorate. Moreover, these quality indicators are analyzed by the department and actions for improvement can be demonstrated. There is a procedure in a document management system. Actions for improvement are formulated in a SMART way. The department contributes to the development of nationwide quality indicators.
2. Basic standard	The department delivers data for quality indicators of the NVNG and the Dutch inspectorate. Moreover, these quality indicators are analyzed by the department and actions for improvement can be demonstrated. There is a procedure in a document management system.
3. Recommendation	The department delivers data for quality indicators of the NVNG and the Dutch inspectorate. Moreover, these quality indicators are analyzed by the department. However actions for improvement are not formulated.
4. Important advice	Department does not deliver data on a structural basis for quality indicators of the NVNG and Dutch inspectorate. Data are not analyzed.
5. Requirement	Department does not deliver data for quality indicators of the NVNG and Dutch inspectorate.

Target standards are best practices and will never lead to recommendations. Target standards can, for example, be derived from the best outcome of care. For example, the best score of 10–20 % of healthcare professionals.

An example of a standard with a five-point scale is shown below (Table 26.2).

26.7 New Instruments for Self-Evaluation

New instruments in the NVNG quality guidelines are self-evaluation tools. Evaluation needs to be done individually but also with the whole group. In 2016 the NVNG starts using these tools.

26.7.1 Individual Performance

More than 85 % of medical specialists in the Netherlands participate in a system of individual performance (IQ healthcare 2016).

There are various systems in place to evaluate individual performance of the medical specialist. Instruments used to support the medical specialist are, for example, Appraisal & Assessment (A&A) and Multi-Source Feedback (MSF). The Dutch Society of Nuclear Medicine does not impose a system but states that there should be a system in place to evaluate personal functioning. A&A is based upon the experiences of Mr. JW Rodney Peyton, a trauma surgeon who is responsible for the development of appraisal and assessment workshops on behalf of the Royal College of Surgeons in the United Kingdom. The medical specialist is responsible for evaluation and maintenance of his or her performance and functioning. Evaluative systems help the physicians to improve.

In 2014, the Dutch Federation of Medical Specialists published a guideline "Individual Performance Medical Specialists (IFMS)." This guideline explains how an effective system can be organized. It states that evaluation should be based upon CanMED competencies. Not only medical practice is assessed but also competencies such as communication skills, organizational skills, and ability to cooperate.

IFMS is an evaluative system to improve quality of professional performance of medical specialists. This is done by a periodic conversation where 360-degree feedback, self-reflection, and personal development plan (PDP) are discussed. A combination of these instruments is the most effective.

Multi-Source Feedback (MSF) is a questionnaire-based assessment method in which rates are evaluated by peers, patients, and coworkers on key performance behaviors. Reliable data can be generated with a reasonable number of respondents, and physicians will use the feedback to contemplate and initiate changes in practice.

Several prerequisites are necessary for an optimal working system:

- Safety
  - Safety of participants is guaranteed. Appraisee needs to have trust and respect for appraiser. To ensure this, best option is to have a medical specialist as an appraiser. Also, appraisees should be involved in their choice of appraiser.
- Organization
  - Appraisal systems should seek to minimize the time taken to prepare portfolios, complete documentation, and participate in the appraisal.
- Appraiser
  - A key for success is a competent and appropriately trained appraiser. Appraisers should be qualified and have enough experience. It is advised that each appraisee is not always assessed by the same appraiser.

A personal development plan (PDP) is the result of this system. The appraisee should formulate development goals.

26.7.2 Team Performance

A department of good nuclear medicine physicians, doesn't make a good department

In the old days, a healthcare professional did an individual consultation with a patient; nowadays multidisciplinary teams become the basis of work in the healthcare sector, mainly because of increasing complexity. The methods of performance evaluation shift as well, where team-based approaches gain interest.

Literature shows that there is a relation between team processes and team effectivity. Team processes refer to questions like *how team members interact with each other*? *Are you as a team member involved in decision-making*?

It is widely recognized that cooperation between professionals is essential for a good quality of care. A good cooperation between physicians has a positive influence on patient care, many believe. A team climate oriented towards innovation leads to better patient care (Shortell et al. 2005). Investigation also shows that cooperation between medical specialists can be better. Recommendations in quality visits often show recommendations upon this aspect.

In team-based approaches, the organization is not interested in the activities or effectiveness of individuals, but rather the outcome of the team. Emphasis is not on the individual but on the individual's relationship with the team.

The NVNG developed a so-called Quick Scan. It is a self-evaluation tool for teams. A standard of good team performance does not exist, but all scientific organizations agree that healthcare professionals should measure and improve team performance. The Quick Scan is developed at the end of the last century by other scientific organizations: the Dutch Society of Paediatrics, the Dutch Society of Surgery, and the Dutch Society of Obstetrics and Gynaecology. The Quick Scan is proven effective and actualized by other organizations such as the NVNG.

The Quick Scan consists of two types of questions; on the one hand, questions regarding structure of organization (hard side) and on the other hand, questions regarding communication and beliefs (soft side).

The questionnaire is divided in five sections:

- Shared objectives
- Structure of partnership
- Decision-making
- Communication and team climate
- Results and reputation

The Quick Scan gives a priority list on items of group performance which can be improved. These items are related to team effectiveness and job satisfaction.

Not every specialty uses the Quick Scan. The Dutch Society of Internal Medicine (NIV), for example, uses a tool called Team Climate Inventory (TCI). TCI is similar to the Quick Scan and is a validated instrument, not only used in healthcare organizations but also in the industry. The current standard of the NIV is that TCI should be used at least twice every 5 years. The NVNG states that evaluation of team performance has to be done periodically.

26.8 Future Perspectives

26.8.1 Radiology

In the year 2015, a joint residency training program in radiology and nuclear medicine started in the Netherlands. The advent of hybrid technologies, the growing interest of young residents in radiology and nuclear medicine training, and the interest of Dutch authorities in merging nuclear medicine and radiology all added importance to the goal of a single specialty.

Moreover, several departments of radiology and nuclear medicine already merged into a single Medical Imaging Department, and there are more to follow.

On the basis of these new developments, it would be logical to perform a quality visit together with the radiologists. At this very moment, the Dutch Society of Radiology and the Dutch Society of Nuclear Medicine are separate organizations, with separate quality visiting and quality committees.

26.8.2 Residency Programs

Residency programs are assessed separately from quality. With the new instruments developed for quality visits, these instruments might very well be suitable for assessment of residency programs. Pilot assessments have been done in hospitals with a residency program, and results are encouraging.

26.8.3 Audit Team

Quality visits are done by colleagues from another center, and this has to stay this way. But, as mentioned before, the focus of quality visits is not any more purely on medical topics. There is discussion whether one or more professional auditors should be added to the team. Assessment of other competences than merely medical requires differently trained auditors. This could be different between specialisms or even between departments, depending upon audit documentation received. Several scientific organizations are having this discussion; the NVNG did not take position yet.

26.8.4 Evidence-Based Clinical Audits (EBCA)

The most common definition of an evidence-based clinical audit is (Bullivant and Corbett-Nolan 2010):

> a quality improvement process that seeks to improve the patient care and outcomes through systematic review of care against explicit criteria and the implementation of change.[5]

The primary goal of an EBCA is to improve in a systematic way outcome of care by improving performance of caregivers and quality of care in general.

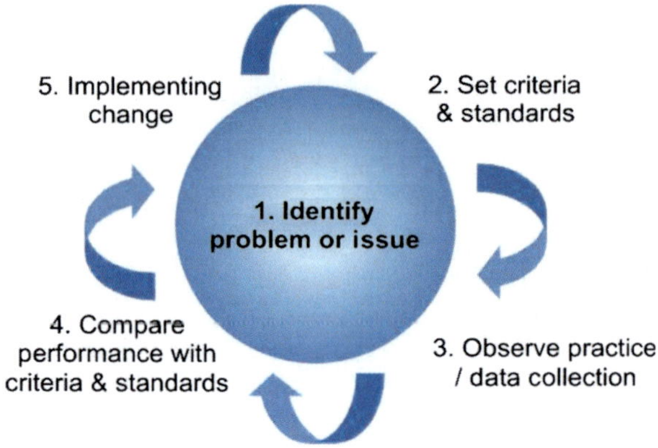

Fig. 26.1 Clinical audit cycle

EBCA uses (evidence-based) guidelines and promotes the use of it. Research shows that there is a discrepancy between existing guidelines and daily practice. An effective way to promote implementation of guidelines is giving active and structured feedback upon the care the patient actually received. This is what EBCA does.

There are two possible methods to perform an EBCA. The standard method is to select a group of patients and analyze the quality of care systematically. This is done retrospectively or prospectively by means of quality indicators. For example, select a group of patients with thyroid carcinoma and investigate if these patients are treated according to existing (evidence based) guidelines.

An alternative method is selecting patients with an unfavorable outcome of care, like a complication. By analyzing and evaluating these patients systematically, it is possible to improve care and prevent complications in the future.

EBCA is often done monodisciplinary but can also be used multidisciplinary (Fig. 26.1).

The NVNG did not set up a system for clinical audits yet. In the quality guideline, it is mentioned that you have to follow (evidence based) guidelines and that professionals have to argue and record why they deviate.

26.8.5 Imaging Technologists

To increase efficiency it is advisable to perform quality visits together with the Dutch Society of Radiology, but another option is to perform audits together with the Dutch Society of Medical Imaging and Radiotherapy (NVMBR). Imaging technologists are very well organized, and the Society has its own structure for quality visits.

This has been organized several times in the past, with success.

Conclusion

Concepts of quality and quality assessment have changed. Focus shifted from structures (*do we have a procedure*?) to processes (*how is this procedure being used*?) and outcome (*what is the result for the patient*?). The NVNG published new quality guidelines in 2014 in which new instruments are available to answer the right questions.

Key topics are evaluation of care processes, personal and group performance, and patient perspective. At the same time, a new, more objective, valuation system was introduced.

It is a dynamic field where new tools will be introduced in the near future, for example, clinical audits, and where organization of quality visits will change in an even more multidisciplinary way.

References

Bullivant J, Corbett-Nolan A. Clinical audit: a simple guide for NHS Boards & partners. Good Governance Institute, London. 2010.

Fossen JA, et al. Kwaliteitsvisitatie nieuwe stijl Handboek voor wetenschappelijke verenigingen. Van Zuiden Communications B.V. Postbus 2122, 2400 CC Alphen aan den Rijn. 2005.

Fossen JA, et al. Advisory Board quality visits. Valuation system for quality visits. Orde van Medisch Specialisten, Utrecht. 2012.

IQ Scientific Center for Quality of Healthcare. Sturen op verantwoord functioneren en omgaan met verminderd functioneren van zorgverleners. Published by Scientific Center for Quality of Healthcare (IQ healthcare), Radboudumc, Nijmegen. 2016

Shortell SM, Schmittdiel J, et al. An empirical assessment of high performing medical groups: results from a national study. Med Care Res Rev. 2005;62:407–34.

Quality Visits: The EANM/EARL FDG-PET/CT Accreditation Programme

27

Sabine Ettinger, Giorgio Testanera, Terez Sera, Ronald Boellaard, Fred Verzijlbergen, and Arturo Chiti

Abbreviations

AC-PET	Attenuation-corrected PET
CT	Computed tomography
FDG	[^{18}F]fluorodeoxyglucose
NAC-PET	Non-attenuation-corrected PET
PET	Positron emission tomography
QC	Quality control
SOP	Standard operating procedure
SUV	Standardised uptake value
VOI	Volume of interest

S. Ettinger
EANM Research Limited, European Association of Nuclear medicine, Vienna, Austria

G. Testanera • A. Chiti (✉)
Department of Nuclear Medicine, Humanitas Research Hospital, Milan, Italy
e-mail: arturo.chiti@cancercenter.humanitas.it

T. Sera
EANM Research Limited, European Association of Nuclear medicine, Vienna, Austria

Department of Nuclear Medicine, University of Szeged, Szeged, Hungary

R. Boellaard
Department of Radiology and Nuclear Medicine, VU University Medical Centre, Amsterdam, The Netherlands

F. Verzijlbergen
Department of Nuclear Medicine, University Medical Centre Rotterdam, Rotterdam, The Netherlands

A.W.J.M. Glaudemans et al. (eds.), *Quality in Nuclear Medicine*,
DOI 10.1007/978-3-319-33531-5_27

Personalised medicine will allow the stratification of patients into biological subgroups and thereby potentially improve the quality of care for every single patient. In this context, imaging biomarkers will play a significant role in identifying tumour characteristics which can influence clinical outcome.

Radiopharmaceutical distribution as evaluated with combined positron emission tomography/computed tomography (PET/CT) represents a powerful and useful imaging biomarker. A particular characteristic of PET/CT is its ability to provide quantitative information through image analysis. In order to be reproducible, quantitative measurements need to be standard. Accordingly, the nuclear medicine community is working to achieve standardisation of PET/CT imaging and to improve the quality of the images generated, both in clinical routine and in clinical trials.

In 2010, the European Association of Nuclear Medicine (EANM) initiated a programme for the accreditation of PET/CT scanners using [^{18}F]fluorodeoxyglucose (FDG) in order to support compliance with requirements regarding quality control and quality assurance of PET/CT systems. The programme, run within the scope of EANM Research Limited (EARL) activities, is based on the *FDG-PET and PET/CT: EANM procedure guidelines for tumour PET imaging: version 1.0*, published in the *European Journal of Nuclear Medicine and Molecular Imaging* (*EJNMMI*) in the same year (Boellaard et al. 2010). This widely accepted guideline aims to provide a minimum standard for the acquisition and interpretation of PET and PET/CT scans obtained with FDG.

The FDG-PET/CT accreditation ensures harmonised quantitative performance of PET/CT systems within a multicentre setting through the standardisation of acquisition and processing of PET/CT scans. This rigorous harmonisation of the imaging systems enables PET/CT sites to compare, exchange and combine FDG-PET/CT findings as data are collected and processed. Standardised uptake values (SUVs) can also be reliably used owing to the resultant reduction in inter-/intra-institute variability (Boellaard et al. 2013). The standardisation achieved by the accreditation programme relates to imaging procedures and methodology, including patient preparation, scan acquisition and image processing and analysis, which is of the utmost importance for quality assurance in daily clinical practice as well as in multicentre trials.

Starting at the end of 2010, EARL implemented a pilot accreditation programme in which 11 sites, with 12 PET/CT systems, participated. These sites needed to receive accreditation as a prerequisite for participation in EORTC 22071–24071: "Randomized, phase III trial of EGFR-antibody combined with adjuvant chemoradiation for patients with head and neck squamous cell carcinoma (HNSCC) at high risk of recurrence". Two of the 11 sites were asked to recalibrate their PET/CT systems and to adapt their image reconstruction settings before all of them received approval. After this pilot phase, EARL reviewed and revised all of its documents, administrative and technical procedures, online tools and analysis software. Furthermore, the specifications for SUV recovery coefficients, which are used as the basis for evaluation of quality controls (QCs) of image quality, were redefined. It was shown that comparable SUV recovery among sites and vendors is feasible (Boellaard et al. 2011).

In the meantime, the EANM has established a working group to review and update the EANM FDG-PET guidelines, ensuring that they reflect state of the art scientific knowledge. The new version is recently published (2015).

Both the EANM Board and the EARL Scientific Advisory Board have been providing advice regarding the FDG-PET/CT accreditation programme and are monitoring its development. As of March 2014, over 90 PET/CT centres located throughout Europe and beyond are participating in the programme, of which more than 80 have already been granted EARL accreditation.

In order to maintain and ensure this high-level service for the nuclear medicine and imaging community, EARL needs to charge a fee, which is due every year for each PET/CT system included in the programme. This fee covers quarterly analysis of QC documents by an EARL expert physicist, continuing support and scientific supervision of the sites throughout the year, the maintenance and updating of accreditation documents, and provision of software/hardware and server capabilities. A dedicated analysis and data server collects and stores the QC data from the sites and allows online access by the sites and by EARL. EARL is running the accreditation programme in such a way that costs are covered, taking into account the need for regular extensive QC checks that involve much time and effort. Sites can also rent a NEMA NU2-2007 phantom, which is required for the QC phantom measurements, from EARL at a specified cost.

27.1 Requirements and Procedures

Sites can join the accreditation programme at specified quarterly time points, which are consistent from year to year. After an expression of interest to EARL, sites receive the manual for EARL accreditation, in which all requirements and procedures are explained in detail. After receipt of payment, sites gain access to their "online box", which is a personal web area to be used for the submission of QC documents. This "online box" and the corresponding "admin area" have been programmed and designed in order to meet the needs of the sites and to allow professional and standardised handling of all steps within the programme. The QC documents must be submitted by a stipulated deadline within each quarter, in accordance with a timeline set out by EARL. An automated messaging system reminds sites of submission deadlines, and EARL is also automatically notified when sites submit QC documents, so that these can be checked immediately.

The "online box" contains the online questionnaire, which is designed to evaluate current QC procedures and identify the human resources and technology infrastructure within the imaging department in question. Submission of the online questionnaire, which needs to be updated in the first quarter of each year, is a prerequisite for submission of the QC documents.

EARL also offers a webinar, "Good clinical practice (GCP) in the imaging department: the clinical trials perspective", which is available in the "online box" and must be viewed by sites prior to further accreditation procedures. This webinar describes the importance of QC by showing practical examples of retrospective and prospective QC of PET/CT scans in multicentre clinical trials. The retrospective example is based on an EORTC imaging substudy, while the prospective example is taken from a 2011 publication from Binns et al. (2011). Additional webinars are being planned.

As a further step, the head of department needs to sign a statement confirming that all FDG-PET/CT oncology examinations, or at least all quantitative FDG-PET and PET/CT oncology examinations, will be performed strictly as described in the EANM imaging guideline. Additionally a signet policy, which defines the use of the accreditation signet, needs to be signed. These documents have to be submitted only once, at the start of the accreditation procedure.

After these initial steps, sites need to submit phantom images and corresponding data of two different QC phantom measurements, as explained in detail in the EANM imaging guideline and in the EARL Manual, which comprises the standardised operating procedures (SOPs). The QC phantom measurements must be submitted within 3 weeks after completion of the online questionnaire. EARL can provide assistance in performing these QC phantom measurements, via e-mail or telephone or through an onsite visit (at cost) by an EARL expert physicist, who will explain the required QC phantom measurements and guide sites through the procedures.

The "online box" contains two different scan report forms, one for the calibration QC and the other for the image quality QC phantom measurements. The calibration QC phantom measurements, which must be repeated every 3 months, provide information on the alignment between the PET/CT system and the dose calibrator. The image quality QC phantom measurements, which must be performed annually, check the level of the calibration, as well as the quantification, by measuring the activity concentrations and calculating the recovery coefficient as a function of sphere sizes of the NEMA phantom. Only the scan report form or forms due for submission in a particular quarter are made available online.

Sites need to submit three DICOM datasets for each set of calibration QC and image quality QC phantom measurements: non-attenuation-corrected PET (NAC-PET) data, attenuation-corrected PET (AC-PET) data and CT data. The phantom images of both QC phantom measurements need to be reconstructed using the same parameter settings, and after being approved by EARL, these parameters must be used every quarter. The accreditation manual provides instructions on saving and transporting DICOM datasets in order to ensure that images contain all the required information and that they can be analysed by EARL; for example, no type of DICOM compression should be used, and intermediate third-party systems, PACS or other locations should be avoided. Sites are asked to save all raw data for the QC phantom measurements on the PET/CT system at least until the QC results have been approved by EARL. The reason for this request is that sites may be asked to perform additional reconstructions using different settings if the results do not meet EARL's specifications.

27.2 Technical Aspects

Standardisation and harmonisation of quantitative measurements in nuclear medicine imaging require not only criteria for data (e.g. response) interpretation but also guidelines relating to user-/observer-related factors (uptake time, patient preparation, data analysis/interpretation), requirements for image data acquisition (activity, scan acquisition parameters, reconstruction settings) and rules for image/data analysis.

EARL accreditation establishes new standards for participating centres designed to promote the achievement of specific goals with respect to the quality of images generated in the department.

Owing to its widespread use in tumour response assessment studies, the standardised uptake value (SUV), defined as the activity concentration ratio in tissues, was selected as the measure for use in the EARL project to define the standards of scans.

Absolute SUV is used for definition of patient eligibility, patient stratification and lesion selection, while relative SUV (percentage changes from pretreatment values) can also be used to evaluate response to therapy.

As stated above, the main goal of the EANM guidelines and EARL accreditation is to standardise the quantification of PET examination procedures. Defining quantification as a combination of image resolution, image noise and data analysis methods, SUV_{max} can be considered as the standard in practice.

27.2.1 Multicentre QC and Calibration (EARL FDG-PET/CT Accreditation Version 2.1 2013)

EARL has suggested that QCs should be based on investigation to identify the highest common denominator in the performance of scanner calibration and SUV recovery.

The EARL project considers scanner performance harmonisation to be feasible on a large scale, but only with support and service from vendors. This means that their quality standards on PET scanners have to be met and that further external checks are necessary.

QCs need to comply with strict deadlines. While some QCs are to be performed and checked internally by department staff, others must be checked by the EARL team, as already stated. The different QCs include the following:

- Daily QC of PET or PET/CT camera performance conforming to the standard procedure specified by the manufacturer
- Calibration QC using a (cylindrical) phantom (15–30 cm diameter)
- "Adjusted" NEMA NU 2–2007 (Performance Measurements of Positron Emission Tomograph) Image Quality QC to measure recovery coefficients as a function of sphere size (= "effective image resolution")

- CT QC following recommendations of the European Society of Radiology and national law
- Miscellaneous QC (for activity metres, scales, alignment, etc.)

EANM Guidelines (Boellard et al. 2010) and EARL SOPs are tools designed for physicists and technologists that will enable them to perform QCs effectively.

27.2.2 Daily QC

The aim of daily QC is to confirm that the PET or PET/CT camera is operating correctly or, put another way, to identify detector failure and/or electronic drift. Most commercial systems are equipped with an automatic or semi-automatic procedure for performing daily QCs. For some PET and PET/CT systems, the daily QC includes tuning of hardware and/or settings. Both the procedure and its name may differ between PET and PET/CT systems. In all cases, all daily QC measures and/or daily set-up and tuning measurements should be performed according to the manufacturer's specifications. Users should check that the daily QC meets these specifications and that all tests are passed.

When available, a daily PET or PET/CT scan of a cylindrical phantom filled with a germanium-68 solution *may* be acquired. Inspection of uniformity and quantitative accuracy of the reconstructed image may help to identify technical failures not detected using the routine daily QC procedures. In addition, sinogram data may be visually inspected to check detector failures.

27.2.3 Calibration QC

The aim of calibration QC is to verify that the average activity concentration and/or SUV within the phantom is within 10 % of the expected value.

Calibration QC for EARL accreditation of PET and PET/CT requires a cylindrical calibration phantom of any dimension but with a precisely known volume (the phantom is preferably 20 cm in diameter and 20–30 cm long). All relevant information on the SOP needs to be recorded accurately, including the exact phantom volume, scanner hardware and software, exact doses and time of performance of every step.

It is necessary to prepare a 5- to 10-ml syringe with about 70 MBq FDG, providing the exact measured amount of FDG activity. The calibration phantom must be completely filled with water and then 10 ml is removed. The next step is to dispense the FDG into the phantom, ensuring that all activity is in the phantom by flushing the syringe a few times. It is compulsory to vigorously shake the phantom to homogenise activity throughout it. Once the phantom is ready, a PET or PET/CT scan consisting of at least two PET bed positions needs to be acquired. PET and PET/CT scan acquisition and reconstruction should be performed identically to patient studies as prescribed in the clinical protocol. However, somewhat longer acquisitions are recommended (e.g. 5–10 min per bed position), with inclusion of a standard transmission or (low-dose) CT for attenuation correction purposes.

Reconstructions should be performed with corrections for attenuation, scatter, normalisation, decay and dead time, i.e. all corrections required for quantification.

All procedures require great accuracy, and various pitfalls are possible:

- All clocks involved (dose calibrator, PET or PET/CT system) need to be synchronised with the official local time to within 1 min.
- Residual activity within the syringe will result in incorrect verification of PET or PET/CT system calibration.
- If count rates exceed the limits of the PET or PET/CT system to allow for accurate quantification due to high dead time or random fractions, QC with a lower FDG activity is suggested, perhaps with preparation of the phantom a couple of hours in advance to allow for radioactive decay.

27.2.4 Image Quality

The recovery coefficient is determined as a function of the sphere size using the maximum pixel value and A50 VOI.

As for calibration QC, all relevant information on the SOP must be recorded accurately, including the exact volume of the phantom, scanner hardware and software, exact doses and time of performance of every step. Use of the NEMA NU2-2007 phantom is compulsory for this QC.

Before starting, one needs two syringes each containing 20 MBq FDG at the expected phantom acquisition time. To prepare a solution for use in the spheres, a bottle must be filled with exactly 1,000 ml water, which is then mixed with the FDG contained in one of the syringes (20 MBq), flushing the syringe several times. It is important to homogenise the solution before proceeding to fill the spheres inside the phantom, and it is also important not to leave air inside the spheres. The next step is to remove 30 ml water from the background compartment of the phantom and to add 20 MBq FDG, flushing several times to ensure that all activity has been dispensed from the syringe into the phantom. At this point, the background compartment must be filled fully with water and the solution homogenised by shaking the phantom vigorously. It is now possible to acquire a routine quantitative whole-body FDG-PET scan of at least two PET bed positions (at least 5 min per bed position), covering the entire phantom, with use of standard acquisition parameters as specified in the guidelines. It is important to position the phantom so that the spheres are located at the centre of the axial field of view.

Reconstructions should be performed with corrections for attenuation, scatter, normalisation, decay and dead time, i.e. all corrections needed for quantification.

A calibrated well counter can be a useful tool for verifying the exact concentration of activity in the spheres and in the background of the phantom.

27.2.5 CT Quality Control

QC procedures for CT scanners (and of CT as part of PET/CT) are usually defined by the radiological societies and incorporated in the scanner (software). It is recommended that QC guidelines are followed as required by national law and/or as indicated by the (national) radiological societies.

27.2.6 CT Equipment

The following is a short list of additionally recommended QC measures, specifically applicable to PET or PET/CT systems:

- Alignment of PET and CT images on a PET/CT system should be checked in accordance with the procedure and frequency recommended by the manufacturer.
- Set-up and normalisation for both PET and CT should be performed in accordance with the procedure and frequency recommended by the manufacturer.
- All devices involved (PET and PET/CT cameras, dose calibrators, well counters, clocks, scales) should be maintained according to the manufacturer's recommendations. This includes preventive and corrective maintenance in order to ensure correct and accurate functioning of the devices.
- Calibration of the above-mentioned devices should always be performed or correct (cross)-calibration verified (by means of QC) after maintenance and software upgrades.
- Dose calibrators and well counters should be calibrated at least once per year.
- The accuracy of scales used to weigh patients should be checked.

27.2.7 Dataset Management

When sending images for external checking at the EARL office, after collection and reconstruction of the phantom images, it is important that the images are exported in DICOM format on a CD or DVD using the PET/CT console, thereby avoiding intermediate third-party systems such as PACS. This is essential to guarantee that the images meet the conformance statement of the PET or PET/CT scanner manufacturer.

For each QC measurement, three DICOM datasets (NAC-PET, AC-PET, CT) need to be generated and sent to EARL in one ZIP or RAR archive. EARL may request the performance of additional reconstructions using different settings. Raw data should be saved in either sinogram or list mode, including all other data files (normalisation, low-dose CT, etc.) required for quantitative image reconstruction.

These tasks, together with QC measurements performed for EARL accreditation or as part of daily routine in nuclear medicine departments, are among the competencies of physicists and technologists alike.

27.2.8 Note on Daily Practice and the Technologist's Role

In PET centres, technologists have the major role of acquiring images with PET and PET/CT scanners and ensuring that the acquired images meet the quality standards established by departmental criteria. This is also true for QC (in collaboration with physicists) and scans for clinical trials.

Working in an accredited site implies not only greater accuracy in standard daily practice but also a different mindset. Involvement in the accreditation procedure may help technologists to develop this new mindset and to raise operating standards.

SUV measurements present uncertainties that may result in resistance to their use in cancer therapy clinical trials. Possible causes of uncertainties are as follows (Boellard 2009):

Technical factors[1]
- Relative calibration between the PET scanner and dose calibrator (10 %)
- Residual activity in the syringe (5 %)
- Incorrect synchronisation of clocks (10 %)
- Injection vs. calibration time (10 %)
- Quality of administration (50 %)

Physics-related factors
- Scan acquisition parameters (15 %)
- Image reconstruction parameters (30 %)
- Use of contrast agents (15 %)
- ROI (50 %)

Biological factors
- Uptake period (15 %)
- Patient motion and breathing (30 %)
- Blood glucose levels (15 %)

It is evident that the above factors relate to every step of the workflow for PET scans, and it is the responsibility of technologists to minimise their impact for every single scan.

There is a great debate in Europe regarding the basic competencies and advanced practice of nuclear medicine technologists. A consensus document (Watersham-Rich et al. 2011) has distinguished two levels as follows:

1. Entry level:
   - A competence and skill set that is considered necessary to ensure that nuclear medicine procedures are conducted to an appropriate level.
   - The competence and skill set would be engendered during basic training/formative professional education.

[1] Percentages in parentheses indicate the typical maximum impact of the factor in question on SUV measurement.

2. Advanced practice:
   - A competence and skill set that is acquired after basic training.
   - The competence and skill set would be at a higher cognitive and clinical level than basic training/formative professional education.
   - The competence and skill set would seek to improve patient care and management.
   - The competence and skill set would seek to offer clinical career progression opportunities.

It is true that the technologist's role in EARL accreditation can be considered a basic competency, since it mainly relates to QCs, but meeting the high-quality standards required surely pushes technologists to improve their working skills. This improvement, often requiring a completely new skill set, can be considered at the higher cognitive level and fosters improvement of patient care and departmental efficiency. Therefore, the role of the technologist can be considered either basic or advanced depending on whether he or she is taking the lead in the process and can be a good starting point in further developing advanced practice in nuclear medicine departments.

27.3 Central Data Analysis and Accreditation Status

Dedicated software has been developed in order to ensure standardised analysis of QC documents at EARL headquarters. The software allows the automatic import of data from the scan report forms to the analysis tool, which minimises sources of error and further standardises and facilitates work procedures.

Analysis of the calibration QC phantom measurements reveals the cross-calibration factor between the PET/CT system and the dose calibrator. This factor needs to be within ±10% from 1. Furthermore, automatic volume of interest (VOI) placement and verification of inter- and intra-plane uniformity are performed. The image quality QC phantom measurements are analysed in order to determine the background calibration factor by using several VOIs placed in the uniform background compartment. The maximum allowable calibration deviation is again ±10% from 1. Additionally, the SUV recovery coefficients are calculated for each sphere. A cold spot recovery using a central insert to verify accuracy of scatter correction is also performed. The software automatically compares the results of both QC phantom analyses with the EARL specifications.

The results of the analysis of the QC phantom measurements, generated by the software, are saved and centrally stored within the online database. In this way, EARL can keep track of the performance of the sites and can issue additional notices to sites. This procedure also ensures transparency in the case of audits by organisations, pharmaceutical companies or contract research organisations (CROs) which have asked EARL to accredit sites participating in clinical trials. Moreover, the data can easily be used for reports and publications.

EARL provides quarterly feedback to sites concerning the results of QC phantom measurements. If the results meet the EARL standard requirements, EARL grants FDG-PET/CT accreditation to the sites. Approved sites are listed on the

EARL website as accredited PET/CT centres of excellence and are allowed to use the accreditation signet on their correspondence and website, which raises their visibility and status. Additionally, the sites annually receive an accreditation certificate and a signet sticker, which can be put on the PET/CT systems.

If the results are beyond the limits of the EARL standard requirements, sites receive a notice including proposals on how to comply with the requirements. The notice may, for example, recommend a change to the reconstruction algorithms or settings (filters, etc.), point out phantom-filling errors or provide further hints regarding the SOPs.

27.4 Multicentre Trials

Sites participating in a multicentre trial organised in collaboration with EARL must follow certain rules: First, they must ensure that all PET/CT systems used in the trial are accredited by EARL. Second, they are required to apply the EARL-approved parameter settings (used for processing of the QC phantom images) for the reconstruction of patient studies during the trial. The sites can, of course, apply additional reconstructions for other purposes, local use or diagnostic interpretations. The EANM provides recommendations for acquisition times per bed position in combination with dosage per kg patient weight for various types of PET/CT system in the EANM imaging guideline.

27.5 Collaboration with Other Societies, Organisations and Companies

EANM/EARL is collaborating with other professional societies, organisations and companies all over the world. The aim is to enhance the visibility and acceptance of the EARL FDG-PET/CT accreditation programme to the benefit of patients. Furthermore, EARL is keen to contribute to the global efforts being made to harmonise and standardise PET/CT procedures (Tatsch 2012). There is a high level of interest in collaboration and joint actions since EARL is highly valued for its professional set-up and experience, including the strong backing from the EANM.

The EARL FDG-PET/CT accreditation programme is strongly supported by the European Organisation for Research and Treatment of Cancer (EORTC) Imaging Group (IG), which was founded in 2009 to ensure standardisation of image acquisition and quality assurance for EORTC clinical trials with regard to computed tomography (CT), PET, MRI and other imaging modalities as they become available (DeSouza et al. 2012). The EORTC IG requires the EARL FDG-PET/CT accreditation for some of its imaging trials since the group recognises the importance and added value of PET/CT accreditation in the clinical trial setting. Moreover, the EORTC is advancing the development and inclusion of PET/CT imaging parts in their study design and trial protocols from the outset. The EORTC is promoting the EARL FDG-PET/CT accreditation within their scope of action.

EANM/EARL and the International Atomic Energy Agency (IAEA) are working together with regard to quality standards in nuclear medicine. Under the QUANUM

(Quality Management Audits in Nuclear Medicine Practices) programme, IAEA provides assistance in the field of nuclear medicine by evaluating the quality of all components related to the nuclear medicine practice of the institute undergoing an audit. A multidisciplinary team comprising a nuclear medicine physician, medical physicist, radiopharmacist, technologist and senior administrator carry out the audits. There are several checklists, such as the following: (1) strategies and policies; (2) administration and management; (3) human resources development; (4) radiation, regulation and safety compliance; (5) radiation protection of the patient; (6) evaluation and assurance of the quality system; (7) quality control for imaging equipment; (8) computer systems and data handling; (9) acceptance tests; (10) general aspects – clinical services; (11) summary of imaging diagnostic procedures; (12) summary of non-imaging diagnostic procedures; (13) general aspects – radionuclide therapy services; (14) summary of therapeutic procedures; (15) hospital radiopharmacy – operational level 1; (16) hospital radiopharmacy – operational level 2; and (17) tumour marker radioimmunoassay service against which the site is evaluated. The final report contains recommendations with corrective actions to be taken. If the site fulfils the criteria identified in the checklists, it receives proof from the IAEA that the audit was successful, with the recommendation that auditing should be performed on a regular basis – at least annually for internal audits and at least every 3 years for external audits (but IAEA does not provide a follow-up). As regards clinical research, the QUANUM programme is not meant to assess the eligibility of institutes for entry into cooperative clinical research studies. Therefore, under the collaboration between EARL and IAEA, IAEA recommends the EARL accreditation programme to the IAEA Member States on the occasion of QUANUM audits; this helps sites to join a network of excellence and to be prepared for involvement in clinical trials and helps EARL in establishing a worldwide harmonised quality standard. The IAEA already requires the EARL accreditation for some of its coordinated research projects (CRP), including PET/CT.

EANM/EARL is aware of the different harmonisation and standardisation efforts regarding PET/CT worldwide and is eager to contribute to a possible alignment of accreditation programmes. To this end, discussions are being held with the Society of Nuclear Medicine and Molecular Imaging (SNMMI) Clinical Trials Network (CTN). Furthermore, the Japanese Society of Nuclear Medicine (JSNM) has adopted the basis of the EARL accreditation programme. The Italian Lymphoma Foundation (FIL), Lymphoma Study Association (LYSA) and GELA (Groupe d'Etude des Lymphomes de l'Adulte, i.e. Adult Lymphoma Study Group) are further groups that have taken the EANM imaging guideline as the basis for PET/CT QC within their studies. The Society of Nuclear Medicine, India (SNMI) and the Brazilian Society of Nuclear Medicine (Sociedade Brasileira de Medicina Nuclear/SBMN) have also expressed great interest in the EARL FDG-PET/CT accreditation programme.

The EANM imaging guideline is widely accepted and is also well represented within the draft of the Uniform Protocols for Imaging in Clinical Trials (UPICT), established by the Quantitative Imaging Biomarkers Alliance (QIBA). EANM/EARL participated in these efforts in order to contribute to the development of widely accepted, consistent imaging and imaging quality protocols.

EARL is collaborating with the three main vendors of PET/CT systems, namely, GE Healthcare, Siemens and Philips, who are working on the implementation of EARL-compliant protocols. This should enable customers easily to select the EARL-required acquisition and reconstruction settings. This support is highly valued and further strengthens the practical implementation of the accreditation programme.

Furthermore, an increasing number of CROs and pharmaceutical companies are accepting and requiring EARL FDG-PET/CT accreditation for their clinical trials (e.g. ICON Medical Imaging, BetaCure EC Project, IAEA project on FDG-PET/CT in radiation treatment planning) since they are aware of the necessity of this accreditation programme for the successful conduct of clinical studies in terms of accurate, reproducible and quantitative assessment of data.

Conclusions

The EANM/EARL accreditation programme represents a successful model for the implementation of a system to improve quality in clinical trials and clinical practice. The cost of the process is negligible compared with the benefits that can be conferred by such a programme.

The programme is going to be extended, with application of quality accreditation not only to other fluorine-18-labelled radiopharmaceuticals but also to radiopharmaceuticals labelled with other radionuclides, such as zirconium-89 or gallium-68.

Other future activities for the EARL accreditation programme will be related to the standardisation of advanced imaging techniques, the use of PET/MR scanners and therapeutic applications of radiopharmaceuticals.

References

Boellaard R, O'Doherty MJ, Weber WA, et al. FDG PET and PET/CT: EANM procedure guidelines for tumour PET imaging: version 1.0. Eur J Nucl Med Mol Imaging. 2010;37(1):181–200.

Boellaard R, Hristova I, Ettinger S, et al. EARL FDG-PET/CT accreditation program: feasibility, overview and results of first 55 successfully accredited sites. J Nucl Med. 2013;54 Suppl 2:2052.

Boellaard R, Hristova I, Ettinger S, et al. Initial experience with the EANM accreditation procedure of FDG PET/CT devices. Eur J Cancer. 2011;47 Suppl 4:S8.

Binns DS, Pirzkall A, Yu W, et al. Compliance with PET acquisition protocols for therapeutic monitoring of erlotinib therapy in an international trial for patients with non-small cell lung cancer. Eur J Nucl Med Mol Imaging. 2011;38:642–50.

Following subchapters refers to Manual for EARL FDG-PET/CT Accreditation Version 2.1. 2013.

Boellard R et al. FDG PET and PET/CT: EANM procedure guidelines for tumour PET imaging: version 1.0. Eur J Nucl Med Mol Imag. 2010;37(1):181–200.

Boellard R. J Nucl Med Suppl Issue 2009;50(11S). J Nucl Med. 2009 May;50 Suppl 1:11S–20S.

Watersham-Rich K et al. Euro-American discussion document on entry-level and advance practice. Nucl Med Technol. 2011;39(3).

Tatsch K. Standardisation and harmonisation boost the credibility of nuclear medicine procedures. Eur J Nucl Med Mol Imaging. 2012;39:186–7.

DeSouza N, Hoekstra OS, Nestle U, et al. EORTC Imaging Group. Eur J Cancer Suppl. 2012;10(1):82–7.

Quality and Safety in Nuclear Medicine: The Vision of the Society of Nuclear Medicine and Molecular Imaging (SNMMI)

28

Bennett S. Greenspan, Frederic H. Fahey, and George M. Segall

Abstract

The Society of Nuclear Medicine and Molecular Imaging (SNMMI) is a non-profit, professional, and scientific organization that promotes the science, technology, and practical application of nuclear medicine and molecular imaging. The SNMMI is a leader in advancing, optimizing, and unifying nuclear medicine/molecular imaging, with the ultimate goal of improving human health. It has over 17,000 members worldwide, the majority of which are in the USA. The SNMMI is based in Reston, Virginia, USA.

The SNMMI has a comprehensive approach to quality and safety in NM. This approach can be divided into four main domains – education, clinical practice, training/certification, and advocacy and outreach. Quality crosses all four domains. Guidance, which includes technical procedure standards, appropriate use criteria, clinical practice guidelines, and radiation protection, includes activities in all four domains.

B.S. Greenspan, MD (✉)
Department of Radiology and Imaging, Medical College of Georgia at Augusta University, 1120 15th Street, Augusta, GA 30912, USA
e-mail: bgreenspan0708@gmail.com

F.H. Fahey, DSc
Division of Nuclear Medicine and Molecular Imaging, Dept. of Radiology, Children's Hospital Boston, Harvard Medical School, 300 Longwood Avenue, Boston, MA 02115, USA

G.M. Segall, MD
Stanford University, Stanford, CA, USA

Nuclear Medicine Service, VA Palo Alto Health Care System, 3801 Miranda Avenue, Palo Alto, CA 94304, USA

A.W.J.M. Glaudemans et al. (eds.), *Quality in Nuclear Medicine*,
DOI 10.1007/978-3-319-33531-5_28

Abbreviations

AAPM	American Association of Physicists in Medicine
ABNM	American Board of Nuclear Medicine
ABR	American Board of Radiology
ABSNM	American Board of Science in Nuclear Medicine
AC	Academic Council (of the Society of Nuclear Medicine and Molecular Imaging [SNMMI])
ACCME	Accreditation Council for Continuing Medical Education
ACGME	Accreditation Council for Graduate Medical Education
ACPE	Accreditation Council for Pharmacy Education
ACR	American College of Radiology
ARRT	American Registry of Radiologic Technologists
ASNC	American Society of Nuclear Cardiology
ASRT	American Society of Radiologic Technologists
AUC	Appropriate Use Criteria
CAMPEP	Commission on Accreditation of Medical Physics Educational Programs, Inc.
CER	Comparative Effectiveness Research
CME	Continuing Medical Education
CMS	Center for Medicare and Medicaid Services
CRCPD	Conference of Radiation Control Program Directors
CTN	Clinical Trials Network (of the SNMMI)
DICOM	Digital Imaging and Communications in Medicine
EANM	European Association of Nuclear Medicine
FDA	Food and Drug Administration
IAC	Intersocietal Accreditation Commission
IAEA	International Atomic Energy Agency
ICRP	International Commission on Radiological Protection
JNM	Journal of Nuclear Medicine
JNMT	Journal of Nuclear Medicine Technology
LLSAP	Lifelong Learning and Self-Assessment Program (of the SNMMI)
MI	Molecular Imaging
MIRD	Medical Internal Radiation Dose Committee
MOC	Maintenance of Certification
NCCN	National Comprehensive Cancer Network
NCRP	National Council on Radiation Protection and Measurements
NEMA	National Electrical Manufacturers Association
NM	Nuclear Medicine
NMPDA	Nuclear Medicine Program Directors Association (of the Academic Council of the SNMMI)
NMTCB	Nuclear Medicine Technology Certification Board
NR	Nuclear Radiology
NRC	Nuclear Regulatory Commission
PD	Program Director
PERCIST	PET Response Criteria in Solid Tumors

PQRS	Physician Quality Reporting System
QA	Quality Assurance
RADAR	RAdiation Dose Assessment Resource
RECIST	Response Evaluation Criteria in Solid Tumors
RRC	Residency Review Committee
SAMs	Self-Assessment Modules
SCCT	Society of Cardiovascular Computed Tomography
SNMMI	Society of Nuclear Medicine and Molecular Imaging
SNMMI-TS	Society of Nuclear Medicine and Molecular Imaging Technologist Section
SPECT	Single Photon Emission Computed Tomography
SPR	Society for Pediatric Radiology
TJC	The Joint Commission
VA	Veterans Administration
WMIS	World Molecular Imaging Society

28.1 Education of Members

The SNMMI holds two major educational and scientific meetings: the SNMMI Annual Meeting and the Midwinter Meeting. In addition, the SNMMI often holds additional workshops and smaller meetings, typically organized around a very focused topic. The educational sessions at these meetings cover a variety of topics ranging from the introduction of new technology to the appropriate use of established procedures. More recently, there has been more emphasis in these sessions on the maintenance of quality and safety, particularly radiation safety but also pharmaceutical safety.

The SNMMI Annual Meeting continues to be one of the largest international scientific and educational meetings dedicated to nuclear medicine and molecular imaging with over 6,000 attendees including physicians, scientists, technologists, and industry representatives. There are more than 80 scientific sessions, more than 900 scientific posters, and 100 continuing education sessions during the meeting. A number of the continuing education sessions are presented as self-assessment modules or "SAMs" that allow the participant to test their knowledge on the subject at hand and to compare their understanding to their peers. There are also full-day categorical seminars (about ten in all) prior to the meeting. In addition, there is a very large commercial technical exhibit as well as a variety of plenary, review, and highlight sessions. In the assembly of such a substantial program, much care is given to assure the quality of both the scientific and educational offerings.

The SNMMI Midwinter Meeting is a smaller, more topical meeting held in late January or early February in a city with a warm climate. In fact, it is a joint meeting between the SNMMI and the American College of Nuclear Medicine with between 300 and 400 attendees. At this meeting, there are only two or three parallel sessions that, again, focus on either advancements or the appropriate practice of the field.

The highlight of the year for the SNMMI is the annual meeting, usually held in June, which includes many educational sessions for nuclear medicine physicians, technologists, and scientists, including physicists, radiopharmacists, and radiochemists. The annual meeting provides attendees an in-depth review of nuclear medicine and molecular imaging clinical applications and imaging technologies, in addition to translational and advanced research topics (many of which will one day become part of routine clinical practice). The sessions are designed to evaluate and describe the most current indications and applications of NM and MI, and their impact on patient management, review advances in NM and MI, discuss new diagnostic and therapeutic agents that are impacting clinical practice, and review radiation dose and image quality. Many sessions during the annual meeting are recorded and can be viewed at a later date.

The SNMMI provides online lectures for physicians and technologists, presented with audio and PowerPoint presentations. These lectures include topics in basic science, breast cancer imaging and treatment, multimodality molecular imaging of prostate cancer, CT case reviews, basic principles of MRI, and therapy in NM. There is also a series of lectures on molecular imaging for residents. SNMMI also presents online lectures of review courses and also recorded sessions from annual meetings. Teaching cases are also available.

There are webinars given on various topics. These include the Clinical Trials Network, in which several sessions are offered to help facilitate the use of radiopharmaceuticals in clinical trials. There are webinars on quality and practice, designed to enhance the practice of NM by providing resources and tools to improve the quality of patient care. Some webinars are presented in collaboration with the IAEA, to provide timely information regarding the latest techniques in NM and molecular imaging. These webinars are currently presented in English and Spanish and will be presented also in French in 2014.

Online learning opportunities also include case studies. There are PET/CT case studies and diagnostic NM cases with DICOM images (DICOM is the international standard for distributing and viewing medical images). Teaching cases with slides are available. Amyloid brain imaging cases and cardiac cases will be available shortly.

A new self-assessment module (SAM) on nigrostriatal dopamine terminal imaging with dopamine transporter SPECT imaging is now available.

The above are all continuing education programs for physicians in practice. The SNMMI offers a review course for trainees (residents and fellows) at the annual meeting. The SNMMI also offers online lectures for NM residents in molecular imaging. Continuing education programs are also available for nuclear medicine technologists and for radiopharmacists.

Enduring materials are also available from SNMMI, which include books and journals. At this time (early 2014), at least two new textbooks on molecular imaging are in progress and are expected to be completed in 2016. A third book on molecular imaging is now available online. Journals include the *Journal of Nuclear Medicine*, the *Journal of Nuclear Medicine Technology*, and the *Molecular Imaging Journal*. Several newsletters are published at various intervals. Study guides are available for physicians on PET imaging and for technologists on PET and nuclear cardiology imaging.

The *Journal of Nuclear Medicine* has a section on continuing education. Some of these articles offer continuing education credits. The *Journal of Nuclear Medicine Technology* (JNMT) also offers continuing education articles.

The ABSNM produces a science syllabus as a study guide for the certification exam. It has a format appropriate for the ABSNM certification exam. Part I is a general nuclear medicine science section. This covers basic aspects of atomic and nuclear physics, instrumentation, radiopharmaceuticals, mathematics and statistics, radiobiology, radiation protection and (USA) regulations, basic anatomy, physiology and pathology, and clinical nuclear medicine. Part II has more detailed coverage of the subspecialty areas of nuclear medicine physics and instrumentation, nuclear pharmaceutical science and radiochemistry, radiation protection, and aspects of molecular imaging. While the purpose of the syllabus is to help prepare for the ABSNM certifying exam, it can also be used as a guide for others. The fourth edition is currently available, and a fifth edition is nearing completion. The syllabus is published by SNMMI.

Providers of continuing medical education (CME), which includes SNMMI, must comply with guidelines of the Accreditation Council for Continuing Medical Education (ACCME). The ACCME is committed to supporting the efforts of providers of CME to present high-quality CME programs, continuously improve those programs, and collaborate in quality and safety efforts.

Maintenance of certification (MOC) is a process mandated by the ABMS to promote continuous professional development. It has four parts: (1) Licensure and Professional Standing, (2) Lifelong Learning and Self-Assessment, (3) Cognitive Expertise, and (4) Practice Performance Assessment. Professional standing requires professional behavior in addition to a valid, unrestricted state medical license. Lifelong learning and self-assessment requires continuing education and comparison of knowledge to one's peers. Cognitive expertise is demonstrated by passing an initial certification examination and recertification examinations at regular intervals. Practice performance assessment requires use of best practices compared to peers and national benchmarks. SNMMI is committed to supporting this process and offers online courses, including self-assessment modules (SAMs), to assess competence as well as practice performance assessment projects, and journal continuing education articles.

28.2 Practice of Nuclear Medicine: Technical Procedure Standards

28.2.1 Technical Procedure Standards

One of the most important features of the overall quality and safety approach of the SNMMI is the formulation of technical procedure standards (formerly known as procedure guidelines), which provide guidance for best practice in nuclear medicine. They identify the key elements of the procedure and provide standardization with sufficient detail to enable performance of high-quality examinations. Cost containment is a side benefit. This standardization not only contributes to high quality in routine clinical studies, it also helps to improve the value of research studies in clinical trials. Some of these technical procedure standards were obtained in collaboration with other professional organizations, including EANM and ACR. The standards are updated every few years. The development process involves forming a committee for each standard within the Committee on Procedure Standards.

The following are current technical procedure standards (as of early 2014):

28.2.1.1 Cardiovascular

ASNC-SCCT-SNMMI Guideline for Cardiac SPECT/CT and PET/CT
ACR-SNMMI-SPR Practice Guideline for the Performance of Cardiac Scintigraphy
Myocardial Perfusion Imaging
Gated Equilibrium Radionuclide Ventriculography

28.2.1.2 Endocrine System

Parathyroid Scintigraphy
ACR-SNMMI-SPR Practice Guideline for the Performance of Parathyroid Scintigraphy
ACR-SNMMI-SPR Practice Guideline for the Performance of Thyroid Scintigraphy and Uptake Measurements
Scintigraphy for Differentiated Papillary and Follicular Thyroid Cancer
Thyroid Scintigraphy
Thyroid Uptake Measurements

28.2.1.3 Gastrointestinal System

EANM-SNMMI Practice Guideline for Small Bowel and Colon Transit
ACR-SNMMI-SPR Practice Guideline for the Performance of Gastrointestinal Scintigraphy
ACR-SNMMI-SPR Practice Guideline for the Performance of Liver and Spleen Scintigraphy
Hepatobiliary Scintigraphy
Gastric Emptying
Hepatic and Splenic Imaging

28.2.1.4 Genitourinary System

ACR-SNMMI-SPR Practice guideline for the Performance of Adult and Pediatric Radionuclide Cystography
Renovascular Hypertension

28.2.1.5 General

Guideline Development
ACR-SNMMI Technical Standard for Diagnostic Procedures Using Radiopharmaceuticals
General Imaging
Use of Radiopharmaceuticals
Procedure Guideline for SPECT/CT Imaging
Tele-nuclear Medicine

28.2.1.6 Infection and Inflammation

EANM-SNMMI Guideline for F-18-FDG Use in Inflammation and Infection
ACR-SNMMI-SPR Practice Guideline for the Performance of Scintigraphy for Inflammation or Infection

Gallium Scintigraphy in Inflammation

Tc-99 m Exametazime (HMPAO)-Labeled Leukocyte Scintigraphy for Suspected Infection/Inflammation

IN-111 Leukocyte Scintigraphy for Suspected Infection/Inflammation

28.2.1.7 Skeletal System

Sodium F-18 Fluoride with PET/CT Bone Scans (endorsed by EANM)

Bone Scintigraphy

28.2.1.8 Central Nervous System

Brain Death Scintigraphy

Dopamine Transporter Imaging with I-123-Ioflupane SPECT

F-18-FDG-PET Brain Imaging

Brain Perfusion SPECT Using Tc-99 m Radiopharmaceuticals

28.2.1.9 Oncology

EANM-SNMMI Practice Guideline for Lymphoscintigraphy and Sentinel Node Localization in Breast Cancer

Somatostatin Receptor Scintigraphy

Breast Scintigraphy with Breast-Specific Gamma Cameras (endorsed by EANM)

Procedure Guidelines for Tumor Imaging with F-18-FDG PET/CT

Breast Scintigraphy

Lymphoscintigraphy and the Use of Intraoperative Gamma Probe for Sentinel Lymph Node Localization in Melanoma of Intermediate Thickness

28.2.1.10 Pediatric

Pediatric Dose Consensus Guidelines

ACR-SNMM-SPR Practice Guideline for the Performance of Adult and Pediatric Radionuclide Cystography

ACR-SNMMI-SPR Practice Guideline for the Performance of Pulmonary Scintigraphy in Adults and Children

Diuretic Renography in Children

Renal Cortical Scintigraphy in Children

Pediatric Sedation in Nuclear Medicine

Radionuclide Cystography in Children

28.2.1.11 Pulmonary System

Lung Scintigraphy

ACR-SNMMI-SPR Practice Guideline for the Performance of Pulmonary Scintigraphy in Adults and Children

28.2.1.12 Therapy

Therapy of Thyroid Disease with Iodine-131 (Sodium Iodide)

Palliative Treatment for Painful Bone Metastases

The following are EANM Guidelines that have SNMMI endorsement:

I-131-Metaiodobenzylguanidine (I-131 MIBG) therapy
I-131/I-123-Metaiodobenzylguanidine (MIBG) Scintigraphy
Radioimmunotherapy for B-cell lymphoma with Y-90-radiolabeled ibritumomab tiuxetan (Zevalin)

The SNMMI also develops appropriate use criteria in collaboration with multidisciplinary groups. Appropriate use criteria (AUC) are statements that contain indications for when and how often an examination or therapeutic intervention should be used with consideration of the scientific evidence, clinical judgment, and patient values while avoiding unnecessary provisions of services. SNMMI uses a balanced multidisciplinary approach to guidance development by including various stakeholders in the development process. The first AUC to be established is for amyloid imaging in patients with suspected Alzheimer's disease.

28.2.1.13 Radiation Safety

SNMMI vigorously supports radiation protection and radiation safety in nuclear medicine. Elements of radiation protection and radiation safety can be found throughout SNMMI activities and initiatives. SNMMI collaborates with the NCRP, IAEA, ICRP, and the CRCPD in these activities. Optimization of radiation protection and radiation safety is found throughout the procedures guidelines. SNMMI established the MIRD Committee many years ago to develop standard methods, models, and mathematical schema for assessing internal radiation dose from administered radiopharmaceuticals. SNMMI uses guidance from the MIRD Committee for effective application of dosimetry techniques in clinical practice. SNMMI has also established the Radiation Dose Assessment Resource (RADAR) to develop information on dose assessment models and methods. In consideration of this guidance, SNMMI provides recommendations and guidance in providing the right test with the right dose at the right time for each patient. Included in this dose optimization process is the participation of the SNMMI in the Image Gently and Image Wisely campaigns.

28.2.1.14 QA Programs in Nuclear Medicine

SNMMI administers a quality assurance program to evaluate image acquisition, image quality, and image interpretation by the use of imaging phantoms. The SNMMI Quality Assurance Patient Simulator (Phantom) program designs, produces, and supplies phantoms for image evaluation. This program produces an unknown patient simulator "phantom" that demonstrates an actual clinical problem in technique and diagnosis. Participants image the phantom and submit images and answers to a questionnaire which are evaluated and graded. Results are tabulated and each participant receives a confidential, individualized report for each set of results submitted. This is a proficiency testing program in that it provides feedback on the participants' ability to acquire, process, and interpret the nuclear medicine images. This program assesses the proficiency of one or more technologists to acquire and process the images and of one or more physicians to interpret the images. It also evaluates performance of camera systems and other variables. The proficiency testing program compares the performance and analytical skills of each participant with others in the program and helps document participants' expertise and quality to regulatory agencies and third-party payers. Any nuclear medicine department can participate. Nuclear medicine departments in VA hospitals are required to participate under federal law that assures quality in VA nuclear medicine departments.

The SNMMI supports government initiatives to promote quality. One of these is the Physician Quality Reporting System (PQRS), which is a long-term quality initiative developed and implemented by CMS. The program is currently voluntary; however, there are payment incentives to promote participation, and there is the expectation in the community that participation will eventually become mandatory.

SNMMI participates in the Choosing Wisely campaign, which is led by the American Board of Internal Medicine Foundation. Each participating society develops recommendations on considering using certain tests or procedures less often or not at all if they are not necessary or effective.

The Clinical Trials Network (CTN) of the SNMMI seeks to improve the availability and quality of molecular imaging, typically FDG PET, acquired in the context of multicenter clinical trials. The CTN provides educational materials regarding the imaging within a clinical trial and provides a verification process for sites wanting to be included in the network. The verification process is, in some ways, similar to the accreditation of clinical sites in that the sites must demonstrate the ability to provide consistent, high-quality imaging data to the sponsors of the trial. As part of this process, the sites must provide image data of an anthropomorphic, quality control phantom and interpret the results.

28.2.1.15 Practice Resources

Accreditation of Departments of Nuclear Medicine

SNMMI is a strong proponent of accreditation of clinical nuclear medicine laboratories. The Intersocietal Accreditation Commission (IAC), American College of Radiology (ACR), and The Joint Commission (TJC) [formerly known as the Joint Commission for the Accreditation of Healthcare Organizations [JCAHO]] provide accreditation for departmental clinical programs to assure quality. These three organizations are approved by the Centers for Medicare and Medicaid Services (CMS, the federal agency that supervises Medicare) for Medicare reimbursement. Nuclear Medicine departments are accredited by IAC, ACR, or TJC, to assure quality of clinical studies. Hospitals are essentially required to have Joint Commission accreditation to receive Medicare funding.

IAC has several divisions. One of those is responsible for Nuclear Medicine and PET facility accreditation. SNMMI is a cosponsor of the IAC Nuclear Medicine/PET program. The American College of Radiology (ACR) also provides accreditation for nuclear medicine departments. The Joint Commission provides accreditation of hospitals and thereby all of the departments within a hospital.

In order to attain such accreditation, clinics must provide evidence that they have appropriate personnel, adequate imaging equipment, suitable quality assurance program, and standardized and appropriate protocols for each clinical procedure that the clinic performs. The accreditation process may also involve a site visit to the facility and the submission of images from clinical studies as well as quality control phantoms.

PET PROS

The PET Center of Excellence is one of the three Centers of Excellence within the SNMMI. The PET Utilization Task Force was charged with: identifying the factors responsible for the penetration and growth of PET/CT in oncology, cardiology, and neurology, identifying the opportunities and threats regarding PET/CT utilization, and developing short-term goals and long-range plans to increase appropriate PET/CT utilization. As a result of these efforts, PET PROS (abbreviated from PET PROfessionalS) was developed as a resource for referring and interpreting physicians to ensure easy access to important information and useful resources. The goal is to be a comprehensive resource for PET and PET/CT needs and questions.

PET PROS offers a tracer encyclopedia as a reference on new tracers in PET imaging. PET PROS offers a comprehensive guide on elements of PET/CT reporting, including sample reports. PET PROS offers practice guidelines summaries, which are intended to serve as an educational tool for referring physicians and for interpreting nuclear medicine physicians and radiologists. Practice guidelines are revised and updated periodically, and new guidelines are developed. PET PROS also offers an Oncology Practice Guidelines Summary from multiple organizations for major cancer types, especially the National Comprehensive Cancer Network (NCCN). There is also a Cardiac Practice Guidelines Summary. A Neurology Guidelines Summary is under development. PET PROS has educational brochures on various topics, including diagnosis of pulmonary nodules, non-small cell lung cancer, and radiation therapy treatment planning in lung cancer. There is also a collection of PET/CT PowerPoint presentations, which can be used for educational purposes. There are PET/CT NaF bone scan resources, which include a free webinar and the new SNMMI Guideline for Sodium F-18 Fluoride PET/CT Bone Scans. PET PROS offers samples of letters of medical necessity for educational use. There are multiple fact sheets for patients. The PET Center of Excellence has developed a PET e-library, an electronic library of key literature related to PET/CT. Topics include procedure guidelines, reporting, and cost-effectiveness. The PET Center of Excellence has also developed links to a dynamic imaging atlas. There is a response criteria page which includes response criteria articles, including RECIST, PERCIST, and Harmonization Projects I and II.

There are useful charts, tables, and diagrams for use by physicians as references in their PET/CT reading areas. These include Liver Segments, Neck Nodes, and Small Lung Nodules. Fleischner Society Recommendations and NCCN Clinical Oncology Guidelines can also be accessed.

Credentialing

SNMMI credentialing statements were developed in an effort to provide guidance for practitioners and institutions regarding the training required to perform, supervise, interpret, and report nuclear medicine studies and also relevant correlative imaging studies (such as the CT portion of PET/CT).

Image Gently

The Alliance for Radiation Safety in Pediatric Imaging was formed by the SPR, the ASRT, the ACR, and the AAPM. They launched the Image Gently campaign which is designed to maintain high-quality imaging studies while using the lowest doses and best radiation safety practices available on pediatric patients. The Image Gently campaign and the SNMMI created the "Go With the Guidelines" campaign to encourage the medical community to observe standardized guidelines on radiopharmaceutical dosage for pediatric patients. Physicians who perform nuclear medicine imaging exams on pediatric patients are urged to:

1. Follow the North American Guidelines for pediatric nuclear medicine
2. Create high-quality images with low radiation dose
3. Determine the appropriate radiopharmaceutical dosage by body weight

To increase awareness of this message, Image Gently and the SNMMI created and distributed thousands of posters reminding medical practitioners to use these new guidelines for 11 frequently performed nuclear medicine imaging studies in children. A companion Image Gently/SNMMI publication "What You Should Know About Pediatric Nuclear Medicine and Radiation Safety" can help families and also referring physicians better understand the complex factors involved in providing safe and effective nuclear medicine exams in children.

Image Wisely

Image Wisely is a collaborative initiative of the ACR, the RSNA, the ASRT, and the AAPM. Following the success of Image Gently, this campaign was launched to address similar issues for adult patients. SNMMI, SNMMI-TS, and ASNC collaborated with the Image Wisely campaign to develop educational materials to help practitioners use the lowest radiopharmaceutical dosage necessary to perform nuclear medicine exams on adults. The Image Wisely nuclear medicine initiative urges nuclear medicine physicians to:

1. Perform nuclear medicine procedures only when clinically indicated
2. Individualize doses based on the specific clinical task
3. Employ maneuvers to minimize radiation dose
4. Familiarize themselves with recommended administered activities

Scope of Practice

An SNMMI-TS Task Force developed a scope of practice for nuclear medicine technologists. The scope of practice in nuclear medicine includes, but is not limited to, the following areas and responsibilities: patient care, quality control, diagnostic procedures, radiopharmaceuticals, in vivo diagnostic testing, in vitro diagnostic testing, transmission imaging, and radionuclide therapy and radiation safety. This scope of practice is intended to serve as a concise outline of nuclear medicine technology skills and responsibilities.

Webinars, White Papers, and Journal Articles

Webinars are offered on a variety of topics including the effective use of nuclear medicine procedures, dealing with new guidelines, compliance with regulations, and effective use of molecular imaging radiopharmaceuticals in clinical trials. White papers are authoritative reports that help readers understand issues, solve problems, and make decisions. Journal articles in the peer-reviewed publications help provide SNMMI members with information, reports, and updates on issues related to quality and practice.

28.3 Training, Certification, and Recertification

Generally, people are certified and institutions/programs are accredited. Certification of an individual indicates that the diplomate has acquired, demonstrated, and maintained a required standard of knowledge, understanding, skill, performance, and experience essential for safe and competent practice. SNMMI does not technically engage in training and certification; however, it is strongly supportive.

Residents in nuclear medicine are trained in nuclear medicine residency programs. The residency is 3 years for those students who have completed an internship, 2 years for those students trained in other fields, such as internal medicine, who are eligible for board certification in those fields, or 1 year if trained and eligible for board certification in radiology. These nuclear medicine residency programs are accredited by the Nuclear Medicine Residency Review Committee (RRC) of the ACGME.

There are also nuclear radiology fellowships. Trainees in these programs have completed a residency in diagnostic radiology, which includes 4 months of nuclear radiology, and take one additional year of training in nuclear radiology. These fellowship programs are accredited by the diagnostic radiology RRC of the ACGME (see below).

Currently (early 2014), there are 47 NM programs and 20 NR programs.

The SNMMI also supports the training of other professionals in the field of nuclear medicine, including technologists, radiopharmacists (or nuclear pharmacists), and medical physicists.

Students in nuclear medicine technology complete an accredited training program and earn an Associate degree or a Bachelor's degree. Most of these programs are in universities or community colleges. The students are then eligible to sit for a certification exam. There are two options. One is the Nuclear Medicine Technology Certification Board (NMTCB) which provides the CNMT credential (Certified Nuclear Medicine Technologist). They are also eligible to sit for the registry exam of the American Registry of Radiologic Technologists (ARRT) and obtain the NMT credential (Nuclear Medicine Technology). The SNMMI has a closer alliance with the NMTCB. The majority of nuclear medicine technologists are certified by NMTCB, probably approximately 75 %. A substantial number are dual certified by NMTCB and ARRT, probably approximately one-third.

Radiopharmacists are required to have an active pharmacist license and have either received didactic instruction of 200 h in the practice of nuclear pharmacy or have had supervised professional experience of 500 h in the practice of nuclear pharmacy. Nuclear pharmacy programs are accredited by the Accreditation Council for Pharmacy Education (ACPE).

The training of nuclear medicine physicists has historically been quite varied. Some individuals are trained specifically in medial physics graduate programs. Others received their graduate degrees in traditional fields of physics such as atomic/nuclear physics or in related fields of study including mathematics and engineering augmenting this training with a postdoctoral fellowship in medical physics that included the clinical aspect of nuclear medicine. More recently, there has been a push toward more formal training in medical physics including nuclear medicine physics. In the near future, individuals will have to have attended an accredited medical physics program in order to be considered "qualified medical physicists." The American Association of Physicists in Medicine (AAPM) and the SNMMI have recently formed a task force to look at the current state of training and certification in nuclear medicine physics and the steps that should be taken to assure an appropriate number of qualified nuclear medicine physicists in the future.

28.3.1 Certification in Nuclear Medicine

Shortly after finishing the nuclear medicine training programs, the graduates sit for the certification exam by the American Board of Nuclear Medicine (ABNM). The exam is generally given in September/October each year.

ABNM The ABNM is an independent nonprofit organization and is one of the 24 medical specialty boards that form the American Board of Medical Specialties (ABMS). The ABNM was formed as a conjoint board in 1971 with sponsorship by the American Board of Internal Medicine, the American Board of Pathology, the American Board of Radiology (ABR), and the Society of Nuclear Medicine. ABNM became a primary board in 1985 and an independent board in 1990. Further information on the ABNM can be found at www.abnm.org.

ABR The ABR is an independent not for profit organization and is also one of the 24 medical specialty boards of the ABMS. The ABR was founded in 1934. Fellows in nuclear radiology are eligible to sit for the ABR certification exam if they are already certified in diagnostic radiology by the ABR and have completed the Nuclear Radiology Fellowship. The ABR provides study guides for candidates.

Of the approximately 3,000 physician members of the SNMMI, roughly half are dual board-certified by the ABNM and the ABR. The SNMMI recognizes and supports the efforts of the ABNM and the ABR.

There are two certification boards that certify individuals in nuclear medicine physics: the American Board of Radiology (ABR) and the American Board of Science in Nuclear Medicine (ABSNM). Currently, the ABR requires individuals to have attended a medical physics residency in addition to proper educational credentials in order for them to sit for the certification exam. The ABSNM bases its eligibility criteria on academic and professional experience.

Within the SNMMI are ten councils. One of these is the Academic Council (AC). The mission of the AC includes support for education and training in NM. The AC is an advocate for NM education and training to organized radiology and NM. It also provides an avenue of communication for program directors and NM coordinators to the ABNM, ACGME, other societies, and government agencies. The AC meets twice per year, at the SNMMI annual meeting and the SNMMI Midwinter meeting (MWM). These meetings are intended to inform program directors and other interested faculty of new regulations and requirements and to discuss issues and problems of mutual interest and concern.

A subgroup within the AC is the NM Program Directors Association (NMPDA). This group meets twice per year, at the SNMMI annual meeting and MWM, in addition to the AC meetings, to discuss issues regarding training programs, requirements, regulations, etc., and other issues and concerns.

The SNMMI provides substantial resources for support for the AC and the PDs of NM programs. This support includes a new molecular imaging resident training series (particularly useful for those programs that do not have the resources to present this information to their trainees), an NM residency curriculum resource compendium, an advanced curriculum for residents interested in expanding their knowledge of molecular imaging, references for MI, links to imaging science programs, and online lectures and workshops offered by various academic institutions.

28.3.2 Accreditation of Training Programs

The Accreditation Council on Graduate Medical Education (ACGME) is the agency responsible for accreditation of medical residency programs in the USA. This is done through the residency review committees (RRCs). Each specialty has its own RRC. The RRCs review information submitted by the residency or fellowship programs and also provide a site visit to obtain information on the program. The RRCs meet several times a year (twice for the NM RRC and three times for the diagnostic radiology RRC) to determine if the program meets the criteria for accreditation. The RRCs assure quality by confirming that the programs meet all required criteria, including an appropriate curriculum and evaluation of resident progress. The nuclear medicine RRC has six members, two of whom are from the SNMMI. The Radiology RRC has ten members and a resident member. One of the members represents nuclear radiology.

The Commission on Accreditation of Medical Physics Education Programs (CAMPEP) accredits graduate programs and residencies in medical physics including nuclear medicine physics. CAMPEP also approves continuing medical physics education. In this way, CAMPEP is similar to both the ACGME and ACCME but within the field of medical physics.

The ACGME, through the RRCs, reviews the training programs of residents in all medical fields. CAMPEP reviews graduate programs and residencies for medical physics graduate students.

28.4 Advocacy and Outreach to Promote Quality and Safety

In addition to its efforts regarding the education of its members and others in the fields of nuclear medicine and molecular imaging, the SNMMI considers it essential to provide outreach to other medical professionals who rely on nuclear medicine in their clinical practice and to patients and their families so that they can best appreciate the benefits of the procedures as well as any potential risks. The SNMMI also strives to provide the most useful and up-to-date information to our public servants so that they can make informed decisions regarding our profession.

The SNMMI partners with a variety of other medical, professional, and educational organizations including the American Society of Clinical Oncology, the American Association of Physicists in Medicine, the World Molecular Imaging Society, the American College of Radiology, the Alzheimer's Association, and the American Society of Nuclear Cardiology with regard to education, quality, and safety. The SNMMI often collaborates on education offerings at the annual meetings of these other organizations in order to inform their members as to the state of the art in our field. Likewise, the SNMMI often invites specialists in other medical fields to present at its annual meeting as to how nuclear medicine is utilized for the betterment of their patients.

The SNMMI recently partnered with the Alzheimer's Association to develop appropriateness criteria for the imaging beta amyloid radiopharmaceuticals. In this partnership, the SNMMI brought its expertise regarding molecular imaging while the Alzheimer's Association offered insight with respect to the patients who may best benefit from this new technology. Such cross-specialty collaborations are very useful in yielding high quality in the practice in our field.

The SNMMI has also participated in the Choosing Wisely project to assist physicians and patients regarding the proper use of nuclear medicine. The Society underwent a thorough review to arrive at a list of five things that physicians and patients should question regarding nuclear medicine.

With regard to radiation safety, the SNMMI has partnered with both the Image Gently and Image Wisely campaign with respect to keeping the radiation dose to our patients as low as possible while still providing excellent clinical information to our referring physicians. The SNMMI worked with the Image Gently group to develop the North American consensus guidelines for children and adolescents that were published in 2011. More recently these guidelines and those of the European

Association of Nuclear Medicine have been harmonized. The SNMMI also worked with the Radiological Society of North America, the American College of Radiology, the American Association of Physicists in Medicine, the American Society of Radiological Technologists, and the American Society of Nuclear Cardiology on the development of the Image Wisely nuclear medicine site which was launched in 2012.

In 2011, the SNMMI established a patient advocacy advisory board to help in direct outreach to patients. This board which consists of representatives from a number of patient advocacy groups initially assisted the Society in the development of a patient-centered website. In addition, the group organized a very successful patient-centered program at the SNMMI Annual Meeting and patient oriented visits to Capitol Hill.

The SNMMI has constant interaction with a variety of government agencies, especially the NRC and FDA regarding regulations and CMS regarding reimbursement, with the goal of promoting and protecting quality and safety in NM. The SNMMI has also partnered with the NIH on a variety of workshops ranging from molecular imaging as applied to cardiology and targeted radionuclide therapy.

Lastly, the SNMMI provides organized visits to Capitol Hill for its members allowing them the opportunity to provide their congressional representatives information on a number of topics that affect the practice of nuclear medicine and molecular imaging.

References

The SNMMI website www.snmmi.org. Most of the material presented in this chapter comes from the SNMMI website.

The ACR website www.acr.org.

The ABNM website www.abnm.org.

The ABR website www.theabr.org.

29 Nuclear Medicine Training: Imagine the Future

Imene Zerizer and Arman Parsai

29.1 Introduction

Nuclear medicine established itself as an independent specialty in several European Union (EU) countries since the 1970s and was endorsed by the European directive of 1988 (Cuocolo et al. 2007). Despite this, the practice of nuclear medicine (NM) remains as variable as the cultural diversity across Europe, and many countries were slow to embrace it as a recognised monospeciality. In fact, in several EU countries nuclear medicine did not become a separate entity until the 1990s and 2000, for example, in Austria it became a recognised speciality in 1994 and in France this came into force in 2000 (Leith 2013; Gremillet et al. 2013). This variability in the practice of nuclear medicine, local infrastructure and national regulations resulted in huge variability in training provision. With the introduction of the free movement of workers in the European economic area (EU directive 2004/38/EC), it is becoming ever so important to ensure harmonisation in training and experience (Directive 2004). This will ensure that new nuclear medicine graduates are well prepared to take on the responsibilities of a nuclear medicine specialist in any EU country they choose to practise in.

The first attempt to harmonise nuclear medicine training was proposed following the EU directive of 1988. A curriculum for training in NM was defined with a minimum period of 4 years of postgraduate training (Cuocolo et al. 2007). Despite this, the training of NM continues to be hugely variable across the EU countries with differences in the entry requirements into the speciality, rotations undertaken and time spent in each subspeciality. Moreover in the past decade, NM has undergone

I. Zerizer (✉)
The Royal Marsden Hospital, Fulham Road, London SW3 6JJ, UK
e-mail: imene@doctors.org.uk

A. Parsai
Barts and the Royal London NHS Trust, Whitechapel road, London E1 1BB, UK

A.W.J.M. Glaudemans et al. (eds.), *Quality in Nuclear Medicine*,
DOI 10.1007/978-3-319-33531-5_29

major changes mainly the introduction of hybrid imaging which is both exciting and challenging particularly in terms of raining requirements and clinical practice. Our speciality also continues to face new challenges with a recent emphasis on multidisciplinary care. Nowadays nuclear medicine imaging is an integral part of the patient pathway, and NM specialists are required not only to have comprehensive knowledge of NM but also to have a thorough understanding of their affiliated specialities.

Therefore, there is an even greater need to harmonise NM training across Europe and tailor the curriculum to face the future challenges of our speciality.

29.2 Conventional Nuclear Medicine Training

Nuclear medicine training has evolved in the past decade to meet the demands of a growing speciality; however, great variation in the provision of training within Europe remains. A document published by the European Association of Nuclear Medicine (EANM) in 2007 has attempted to address this variation and define a common syllabus (Cuocolo et al. 2007). Although this paper gave a framework of the requirements of training and achieving competencies, it remains underutilised in many EU countries as training is regulated by national bodies. An important shortfall of this document is the lack of insight into the challenges facing nuclear medicine as a speciality, particularly greater involvement in clinical practice with multidisciplinary meetings (MDTs) and hybrid imaging.

First of all, the entry criteria into nuclear medicine are extremely variable across Europe. This ranges from no prior experience as a resident to enter NM training in countries such as France and Italy to the need for completion of core medical training in the UK and Germany with completion of specialist exams such as membership of the Royal College of Physicians (Leith 2013; Gremillet et al. 2013; Vieira and Costa 2013; General medical council 2010).

The 2007 EANM syllabus acknowledges the need for acquiring a good background in internal medicine and developing more detailed knowledge of conditions that are commonly treated and investigated by nuclear medicine physicians such as thyroid disease. However, it did not specify the length of the training required in internal medicine or the competencies to be achieved. This is left to the national training bodies to decide, and often this is based on historical facts rather than the needs of NM trainees. For example, in France, the residents are required to rotate for one semester in internal medicine, whilst in Italy there is no such requirement but it is preferable (Gremillet et al. 2013).

In our opinion, this requires better definition by national regulatory bodies and harmonisation across the EU states particularly in view of the rapid changes in our speciality. NM physicians are now required to work within a multidisciplinary team in a subspeciality-based framework, and therefore a good understanding of the clinical questions and patient management plan is becoming mandatory. Hence, prior experience in the medical and surgical specialities is essential to fulfil this role. This can provide the trainees with the basis of becoming a core member of the multidisciplinary team with a strong and valuable clinical opinion well-respected by clinical colleagues.

The syllabus of core nuclear medicine training is less controversial as most countries across Europe agree that trainees need to develop an understanding of basic science, radiochemistry, instrumentation, NM physics, radiation protection and the clinical applications of NM. The clinical training often includes theoretical foundations and general principles of NM including in vitro studies and practice in protocoling, understanding image acquisition and interpretation of NM procedures.

The EANM syllabus also gives a good outline of how each year of training should be spent, the objectives to be achieved and the number of studies required to acquire competency.

Several EU countries have adopted the EANM syllabus or have similar national curricula such as in France, Portugal and Austria (Leith 2013; Gremillet et al. 2013; Vieira and Costa 2013). In addition, a log book of cases is kept by the trainees in several EU nations such as the UK, Switzerland and France (Gremillet et al. 2013; General medical council 2010; http://www.bag.admin.ch/themen/strahlung/10219/10312/10347/index.html?lang=fr).

Overall, the conventional nuclear medicine training detailed in the EANM syllabus does give the necessary knowledge and skills for trainees to become independent NM physicians. However, due to the variation on the application of the syllabus and the challenges facing our speciality, further harmonisation work is required.

29.3 Assessment of Competencies

Although it is well recognised that trainees must pass a qualifying test covering both theoretical and practical knowledge to become independent practitioners, again this is hugely variable across Europe. Some countries such as Italy rely on work-based assessments to evaluate the abilities of trainees to perform and interpret procedures without the need for a national formal assessment. The disadvantage of such method is that it often does not cover the theoretical knowledge and is subjective depending on the institution where training is undertaken. Other countries have more robust methods of assessment which consist of work-based evaluations, end of year tests and final examination covering the theory and practice of NM. National examination takes place in several EU nations, for example, in Portugal the trainees are required to pass an oral examination each year before proceeding to the next stage of their training and also take a final national test which consists of three parts: a curricular discussion, a practical test and a theoretical knowledge exam (Vieira and Costa 2013). In France, the trainees are required to pass an examination of fundamental training which includes short answer questions on physics, radioprotection, dosimetry, instrumentation, radiopharmaceuticals and a clinical examination assessed with 100 multiple choice questions on both the diagnostic and therapeutic applications of NM (Gremillet et al. 2013).

The European Union of Medical Specialists (UEMS) and European Board of Nuclear Medicine (EBNM), which are the representatives of nuclear medicine specialists in the European Union and associated countries, have introduced a fellowship examination with the aim of promoting free movement in the EU and harmonisation of training (http://uems.eanm.org/index.php?id=87). This fellowship assesses the candidates' clinical ability and knowledge in nuclear medicine. This consists of an multiple choice question (MCQ) paper covering all aspects of nuclear medicine including basic sciences, instrumentation, physics and radiochemistry as well as an oral exam assessing the candidate's ability to interpret a variety of NM studies. Perhaps this is the most comprehensive method of assessment that should be adopted by all EU and non-EU member states. Regrettably it is not compulsory for obtaining a certificate of completion of training, and throughout the years the number of candidates taking this board examination remains low. For example, in France nine residents passed the fellowship, whilst in Austria no resident has undertaken this examination (Leith 2013; Gremillet et al. 2013). Moreover, this fellowship has not yet been acknowledged for an automatic agreement of movement across EU states.

29.4 Hybrid Imaging Training

The introduction of hybrid imaging modalities (PET/CT and SPECT/CT) into clinical practice had a major impact on the expansion of nuclear medicine especially in oncology and musculoskeletal. These new imaging modalities are providing more accurate diagnoses by combining anatomical and molecular information. With the introduction of more novel PET tracers, advances in CT and increased availability, it is likely that the use of these imaging modalities will further increase in the future to encompass wider clinical applications. In addition, PET/MRI has recently been introduced into clinical practice in neurology and oncology. As these imaging modalities are becoming disseminated, there is a need for defining appropriate training to prepare future NM specialists to become competent in reporting and performing research in hybrid imaging.

Since hybrid imaging modalities cross both specialities radiology and nuclear medicine, it is becoming an increasingly controversial topic in terms of ownership and competencies. It is therefore highly important that NM trainees achieve competencies to face this challenge and that they do not lag behind resulting in these modalities being lost to radiology.

This need has been recognised by the EANM and the European Society of Radiology (ESR) who published a joint position white paper (Bischof Delaloye et al. 2007). In this paper the authors acknowledged that reporting hybrid imaging requires competencies in both radiology and nuclear medicine and have provided an overview of the training requirements to be achieved (European Association of Nuclear Medicine (EANM) and European Society of Radiology (ESR) 2011). The authors have recognised that there are several pathways, but the final choice remains with the countries where training is undertaken depending on their national legislation.

The training options proposed in the white paper include:

1. Undertaking training in both specialities in countries where nuclear medicine and radiology can be practised either simultaneously or in a single speciality. This means the trainee will undertake the entire curriculum of both specialities making the duration of the speciality very lengthy. Economically this will represent a burden on many European countries.
2. Training in a primary speciality such as radiology or nuclear medicine and undertaking a further period of training in a designated programme to acquire the skills of the second speciality. Economically this will be the most effective approach to achieving the required competencies to practise both specialities. The additional years of training will be dedicated to hybrid imaging rather than radionuclide therapy or interventional radiology. Nuclear medicine trainees will undertake years 4 and 5 in radiology whilst maintaining their nuclear medicine skills. Radiology trainees will undertake nuclear medicine training also during years 4 and 5. Both will spend an additional year 6 dedicated to the second speciality to be accredited to practise both specialities. The length of training will be determined by the local societies and regulatory bodies in each individual EU state.
3. A complete merger of the two specialities with a new training pathway designated to produce individuals who can competently practise both radiology and nuclear medicine. This will be achieved with core training in radiology and nuclear medicine followed by 2 years of nuclear medicine training. Such programme is being introduced in the Netherlands this year and will be implemented in the UK in 2015 (General medical council 2010). This new training model has gained approval from the countries' regulatory bodies. In the UK, the training programme will consist of 6 years, three of which will be spent in general radiology gaining core knowledge of anatomy and diagnostic conventional imaging. This is followed by training in nuclear medicine whilst maintaining the acquired radiology skills. The trainees will be expected to complete the fellowship of The Royal College of Radiologists and the diploma in nuclear medicine or the fellowship of European Association of Nuclear Medicine (UEMS/EBNM) to be accredited with a licence to practise both specialities.

The introduction of hybrid imaging and its rapid expansion as well as the job market in Europe are most probably the single most important factors driving the reshaping of the nuclear medicine training to incorporate all imaging in a single speciality. A survey conducted in the UK amongst newly qualified NM specialists has demonstrated that most participants felt they lacked confidence in reporting hybrid imaging and faced great difficulties in finding specialist positions after completion of postgraduate training in nuclear medicine (General medical council 2010). In fact, a good number of these trainees decided to undertake further radiology specialist training. This was the main factor that had resulted in introducing the new combined training curriculum in the UK.

The future of nuclear medicine trainees in Europe following completion of training in many European countries is also less optimistic. Trainees are facing a tough competitive job market with many nuclear medicine departments having no vacancies and closures. In Austria, two departments of nuclear medicine have recently closed and three departments have been merged with radiology (Leith 2013). Job prospects in radiology are however more optimistic with many European countries having a shortage of radiologists such as in France and the UK.

Despite this situation and the need for reconfiguring NM training to include competencies of hybrid imaging, the vast majority of European nations remain resistant to the merger of radiology and nuclear medicine (European Society of Radiology (ESR) and European Association of Nuclear Medicine (EANM) 2010). This is understandable as this will lead to the extinction of nuclear medicine as a speciality; however status quo is not sustainable and an approach that would allow nuclear medicine to maintain its identity whilst providing the highest quality of service and research in hybrid imaging is much needed.

29.5 Future of Nuclear Medicine

Nuclear medicine has undergone major changes in the last 50 years from being embedded into the clinical specialities to becoming a recognised speciality on its own rights. Although this resulted in rapid expansion of imaging techniques, treatments, clinical applications and available number of specialists, nuclear medicine somehow dissociated itself from many of the medical specialities in several countries. However, in the recent years, there has been a refocus on personalised medicine and multidisciplinary care to deliver the best treatment to patients. This has resulted in a team of specialists each one providing unique skills that follows the entire patients' journey, from diagnosis to treatment to determine the most appropriate management plan for each patient. This is the era of "individualised medicine"! As a result, nuclear medicine specialists are required to adapt to this model and ensure they become a core member of this team. For trainees, this will mean that more time should be spent acquiring sound knowledge of the affiliated medical specialities such as endocrinology, oncology, cardiology and neurology. This will ensure that they comprehend the needs of referrers and will be able to deliver patient-specific imaging to answer the important clinical questions. Moreover, nuclear medicine nowadays offers a comprehensive range of radionuclide treatment options from cancer to benign conditions which are likely to further increase in the future. This makes nuclear medicine specialities at the hub of the future of personalised medical care.

As previously mentioned, hybrid imaging and its rapid expansion are likely to be the major challenge facing nuclear medicine. A number of new imaging techniques such as PET/MRI are also becoming disseminated and are finding an increased number of clinical applications. NM has to rise to this challenge and embrace it to ensure it does not lose ownership of hybrid imaging and PET/MRI. As such nuclear medicine training will inevitably have to change to ensure competencies in this field and increase the confidence of NM specialists in cross-sectional imaging reporting in particular MRI. Despite the publication of the white paper on hybrid imaging, the right path to follow is still unclear in many European nations, and perhaps the UEMS/EBNM will need to play a bigger role in providing better definitions of training requirements and regulations across European nations.

The job market in Europe in nuclear medicine and the economic situation are also an important driving force, likely to influence training. As currently there is an imbalance between NM specialist and radiology posts, many countries will have to reconsider their position on filling vacancies and avoiding unemployment of highly skilled professionals.

To summarise, NM is an exciting and thriving speciality attractive to many trainees across Europe. Although the core competencies in NM are well covered in most countries, further harmonisation work is required to ensure consistency. The future of NM is both exciting and challenging. NM and training will need to be adapted to individualised medicine, hybrid imaging and the job market.

References

Cuocolo A, Milcinski M, Bischof Delaloye A. Syllabus for postgraduate specialisation in Nuclear medicine 2006/2007 update. Eur J Nucl Med Mol Imaging. 2007;34:433–6.

Leith T. Nuclear medicine training and practice in Austria. Eur J Nucl Med Mol Imaging. 2013;40:817–8.

Gremillet E, Lemaire B, Prigent A, Vuillez JP. Nuclear medicine training and practice in France. Eur J Nucl Med Mol Imaging. 2013;40:976–8.

Directive 2004/38/EC of the European Parliament and of the Council of 29 April 2004 on the right of citizens of the Union and their family members to move and reside freely within the territory of the Member States"(in English). 2004-04-29. Retrieved 17 Dec 2008.

Vieira R, Costa G. Nuclear medicine training and practice in Portugal. Eur J Nucl Med Mol Imaging. 2013;40:1135–8.

General medical council: approved curriculum and Associated Assessment system. 2010. http://www.gmc-uk.org/education/nuclear_medicine.asp.

Office federal de la santé publique: formation medicine nucleaire. http://www.bag.admin.ch/themen/strahlung/10219/10312/10347/index.html?lang=fr.

Certificate of Fellowship of the European Board of Nuclear Medicine. http://uems.eanm.org/index.php?id=87.

Bischof Delaloye A, Carrió I, Cuocolo A, Knapp W, Gourtsoyiannis N, McCall I, et al. White paper of the European Association of nuclear medicine and Medicine (EANM) and the European Society of Radiology (ESR) on multimodality imaging. Eur J Nucl Med Mol Imaging. 2007;34(8):1147–51.

European Association of Nuclear Medicine (EANM), European Society of Radiology (ESR). Multimodality imaging training curriculum- general recommendations. Eur J Nucl Med Mol Imaging. 2011;38:976–8.

European Society of Radiology (ESR), European Association of Nuclear Medicine (EANM). Multimodality imaging in Europe: a survey by the European Society of Radiology (ESR) and the European Association of Nuclear Medicine (EANM). Insights Imaging. 2010;1:30–4.

Index

A.W.J.M. Glaudemans et al. (eds.), *Quality in Nuclear Medicine*,
DOI 10.1007/978-3-319-33531-5

Made in United States
Orlando, FL
06 June 2022

18558588R00268